CLEAN UP YOUR ACT

From Sickness to Vitality without Medication

Revised & Expanded

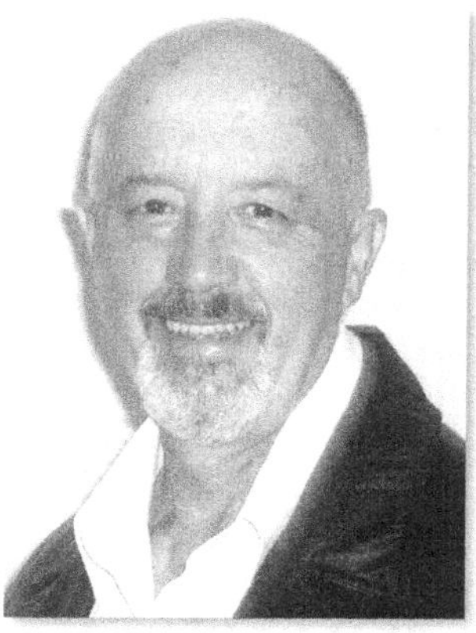

2012 (56 years)

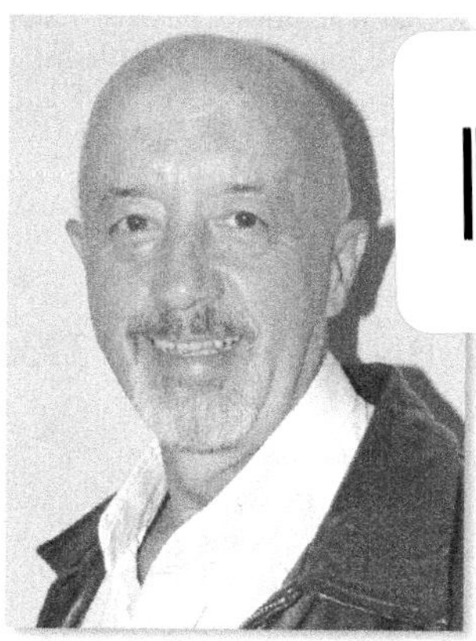

2016 (60 years)

2020 (64 years)

By ***Ramiah J Selwood***

(Pronounced 'Rama' or 'Rami')

With selected illustrations by Ramiah J Selwood

v.200930 (Revised & Expanded)

Disclaimer

The author is not a qualified doctor, nutritionist or healthcare practitioner. He does not claim to diagnose, advise, heal or cure diseases but simply wishes to guide you towards improvements in lifestyle to give your body the best chance of allowing its natural healing resources to come forth. The publisher and author do not accept responsibility for the use or any misuse of any information in this book.

You are totally responsible for any choices you make (or don't make) from the information presented. The author is legally obliged to recommend that you always seek advice from your healthcare practitioner before using any product or therapy recommended in this book and note that results from testimonials may not be typical and results may vary from person to person.

If you don't resonate or align with the information in this book, then please feel free to treat the information as opinion only and move on with your life. It is not the author's intention to convince you of anything; this book is simply a reflection of his journey towards better health and what he has found that worked for him. The author encourages you to check and question all information presented.

The information in this book and other platforms, are not intended to replace advice from qualified healthcare professional and is not intended as medical advice. The guidance within is intended as a sharing-of-knowledge and information from the research and experience of the author, Ramiah J Selwood and Quantum Knowledge Pty Ltd.

Copyright

Queensland State Library ~ J 615.5 Sel

National Library of Australia:

Selwood Ramiah, 1956, Clean Up Your Act, From Sickness to Vitality without Medication

ISBN 978-0-646-91323-0

ISBN 978-0-646-91323-0

9 780646 913230 >

Published by

Quantum Knowledge Pty Ltd

www.cleanup-your-act.com

Ph: 0427 443 302 ~ quantumk88@gmail.com

Dedication

This book is dedicated to my parents, my grandparents...
and my parents-in-law

Through their journeys of illnesses and passing, they have inspired me to choose an alternative path by becoming informed, allowing me to take control of my health using
natural products, diet and moderate exercise.

I won't need the pills and surgery that my parents chose to have!

I loved them dearly, but I love my wife and my two children even more. I love them so much in fact; I don't want to put them through what I experienced with my parents...

I want to be a grandfather for my children.

Hopefully you will find your truth amongst these pages.

I invite you to conduct your own research, question everything and prove the information mentioned for yourself.

Has your doctor ever proposed such an invitation?

Enjoy your journey...

It costs money to stay healthy...
But, it's even more expensive to get sick!

Good Health Costs Less

Written by the Actual Author

Only about 30% of non-fiction books are written by the actual author. Most non-fiction books are written by a ghost writer who interviews and writes on the author's behalf. In fact, I have ghost-written for others too.

There is also a plethora of books on the internet that have the same content, but given a new title, format, cover, author and ISBN number then marketed by anyone for a quick buck.

As a reader, you don't fully receive the author's knowledge. Instead you read limited information filtered through the interpretation, experiences, prejudices and emotions of the ghost writer, who is not the expert.

THIS IS <u>NOT</u> ONE OF THOSE BOOKS!

Over three years, I have personally written over 98,600 words and drawn numerous diagrams so that I can personally relate my learning from my personal experiences and research. Trust one who has been there!

WHY SELF-PUBLISH?

When distributing through a **publishing company**, the author only receives around 3-10% of the sale price of the book - maybe. The remaining 90% or more goes to the merchant and publisher for printing, promotion and distribution. Most bookshops will only sell books from publishing companies.

I've chosen to **self-publish** so I am not limited in what I can say and so that I, the person who invested time, effort, risk and money, am rewarded for my years of investment — it's called free enterprise, i.e. taking a risk based on passion and belief in receiving a return.

This does however limit my ability to distribute and promote my book. You can help by telling family, friends and outlets about this book. Word of mouth is **the most powerful** form of marketing. Thank you for your trust and support, I am most grateful☺

SELF PUBLISHED BEST SELLER

Finally; to claim best seller status in Australia, you need to sell 5,000 or more copies. Registered publishers and retail outlets keep track of sales and are then listed on the 'New York Times Best Seller List' (for example). Because this book is self-published and therefore outside the 'official system,' the best I can do is show my printing invoices to demonstrate over 5,000 copies printed, distributed and sold.

Acknowledgements

I would like to recognise and appreciate the input from special people...

Ela Gold (colon hydrotherapist and natural therapist) of Vitalis Health in Murwillumbah, NSW Australia

Rosemary Greer (colon hydrotherapist - retired) formerly of Oasis Colon Hydrotherapy Clinic, Nerang, Gold Coast Australia

Stacey Roberts (physiotherapist, herbalist, author, speaker and natural fertility expert) of Milwaukie, Wisconsin USA

Peter Edwards (naturopath, professor, author and speaker of Pan Harmony) Mudgeeraba, Gold Coast Australia

"Diseases are not really diseases, they are symptoms of the body's adaptation to a toxic, deficient environment"

Dr John Bergman

One Paragraph Summary...

"Disease derives from early experiences that give rise to negative emotions, creating feelings that seek relief (creating beliefs). Feelings lead to actions (food, behaviour, etc) that become habitual and ultimately make up your body and your life. Your subconscious mind is actually your body – built through habits derived from your original emotions and reactions repeatedly revisited. Over several years you begin to feel unwell as your body morphs to reflect your choices (karma) and you develop negative thoughts and a victim attitude, so you seek more relief – and the cycle continues. Over decades your body becomes toxic, deficient and blocked – beginning in your bowel, then liver, kidneys and circulatory system. Toxins spread to other organs and impacts your brain, eyes and feet especially. Then you pass our inherited beliefs, habits and 'diseases' onto your children. Why be normal? Why be average? It doesn't have to be this way..."

Ramiah J Selwood

Contents

Introduction

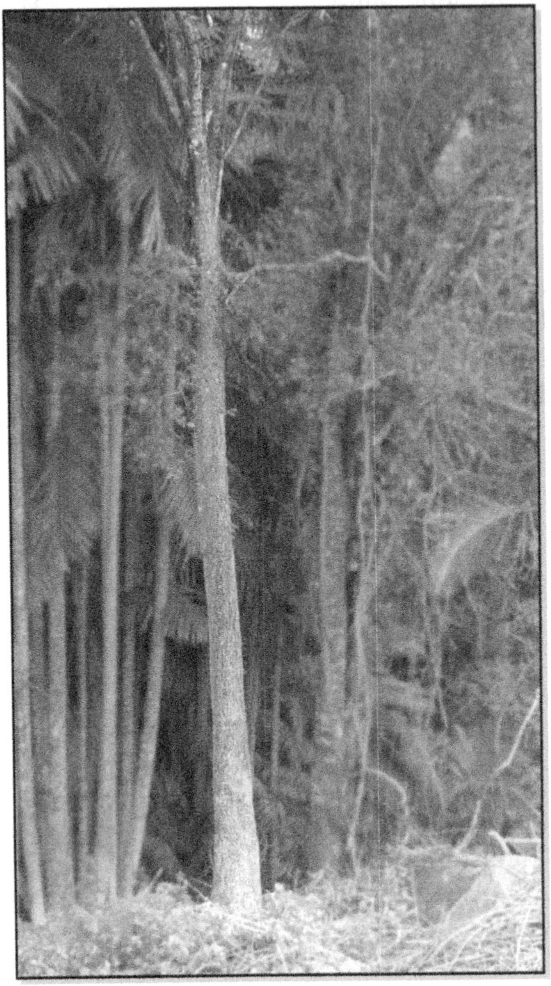

Take a look at this tree. It stands about 8 metres (26') tall.

It stands tall and, straight doesn't it?

After all, you can see with your own eyes — from your point of view — this is a tall, straight tree. No one could argue otherwise!

Now keep an open mind and turn the page...

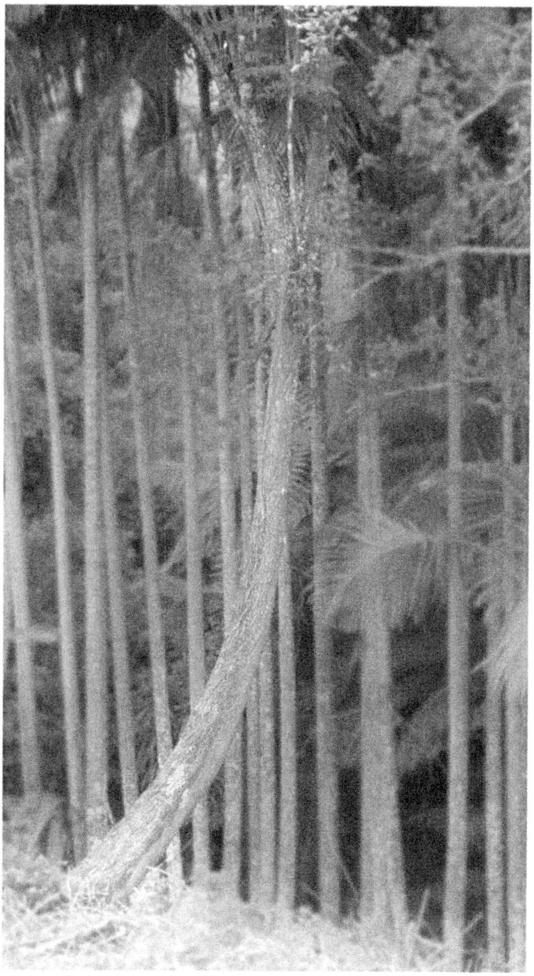

Photos of trees — Contour Rd, Eagle Heights, Tamborine Mtn, Queensland Australia (near where I live)

This photo is of the same tree, taken from a different angle.

A person viewing the tree from this angle would argue that this tree is curved, and it would be totally unacceptable that it could be anything else to anyone else.

It's only when you allow yourself to **move your point of view** that you allow the full range of evidence to be presented and absorbed, and you can make a better, more educated choice. You are closer to the truth.

If you hold firm, rigid and never shift from your old viewpoint, never open yourself to other possibilities, then you will never know the whole truth or understand why someone else may have a different view. Being rigid, dogmatic and interested in your point of view only is often referred to as being a 'Redneck'.

Continually looking down at one point on the ground gives you a sunburnt neck – a redneck.

When you look from one point of view to the other, the evidence can be different, and you can begin to understand alternate possibilities. But it's during the journey itself of moving your perspective that the full evidence of the situation reveals itself bit by bit, so you can digest the new information as you go, adding to your overall knowledge and personal growth.

Incidentally, the above tree (which I passed every day on my walks where I live on Tambo) has since fallen during a storm ☹. Thankfully we now have these photos to preserve its memory.

Chapter 1

My Journey Towards Better Health

Why My Family History is Important

I want to give you an understanding of my linage; my heritage and how it gave me the genes, habits and thoughts that ultimately grew my body and therefore my ailments. If my family has a history of heart disease, diabetes, rheumatoid arthritis and cancer, then medical research indicates that I will be more susceptible to contracting the same diseases. I'll also show you what I did to release myself from my family's seemingly inevitable path of terminal illness and early passing.

In telling my story, I want to emphasise the **impact ill-health and early passing has on the surviving, supporting family members.** In our case, our children grew up (essentially) without grandparents, and we as a family unit, spent a large amount of money and several years supporting the low quality of life passing of our parents, instead of creating a future for our children, though (of course) we did this with unconditional love.

My Grandparents

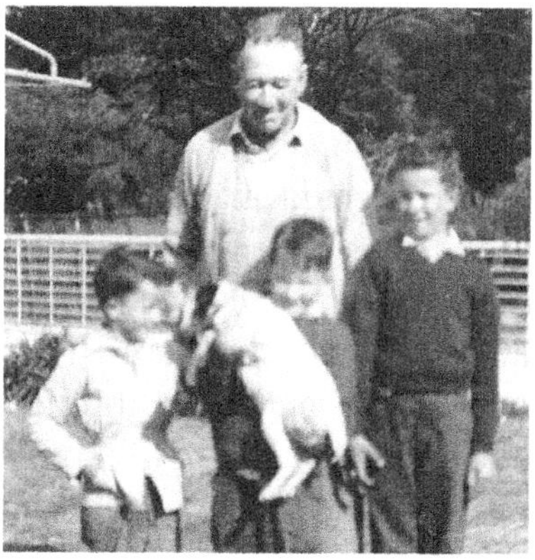

Pop with me (centre) and my brothers

Both my grandfathers were orchardists, so during my childhood I grew up around sprays and pesticides. Each weekend and school holidays, you would find me in the packing shed making boxes, grading and packing, or out on the tractor pruning and picking cherries, apples, pears, peaches and grapes. Most of these activities involved touching spray residue on the fruit or tree with my hands. The skin is very absorbent.

From the age of five, I enjoyed trips with Pop into the cool-stores and shops where he dropped off fruit to friends who owned shops in Orange, NSW Australia.

I didn't know it at the time, but Pop was a respected and influential man around Orange, owning three properties in the district and was once chairman of the local growers' association. Before my time he owned a sheep station and citrus orchard in Bourke, NSW where Mum was born. I remember him covering up in his yellow raincoat, hat and breathing apparatus to spray the trees on his tractor and returning hours later soaked in white spray residue.

In 1971, when I was just fifteen, the world fell from under my feet when my cousin arrived late in the evening (on my brother's birthday, just after Christmas) to inform us that Pop had suddenly dropped dead from a heart attack. This was devastating to me and my family, as it was my first experience of death. Only four days earlier we had celebrated Christmas with Gran and Pop; we didn't know it would be our last Christmas with him.

Pop was always happy, generous, and joyful and gave us horsey rides on his knee, 'sour lollies' (Fruit Tingles) and 'hot lollies' (Steam Rollers) from the jar on the sideboard cabinet. Now this jolly-old kingpin of our family was gone forever, overnight at just 66 years old.

Because my grandmother (Gran) depended greatly on Pop, she slowly passed away over the next four years, finally ending up in a nursing home with dementia. When I was sixteen, Mum asked me to spend my summer holidays 'granny-sitting' instead of picking fruit, which enabled mum to pack fruit and earn money. That was the most boring school holiday of my life, but precious time was spent alone with Gran watching cricket on TV. In Gran's younger days, she was the typical farmer's wife — often found at the sink or stove, always cooking a Sunday lunch with lots of baked meat, potatoes, dairy, pastry and sugar. She used to boil the life out of the few green vegetables she served. I vaguely remember seeing one of her gallstones in a jar after numerous bouts of surgery.

My other grandfather (Grandad) was a war veteran who served as a medic in New Guinea during World War Two and was foreman on an orchard in Orange for around forty years. He was also well respected in Orange and could tell you anything you wanted to know about trees and fruit. Grandad had a depth of knowledge about the world and was easy to chat with about anything. He worked until he was over 70 and died at 86 years, but sadly lived his final ten years with fading eyesight (macular degeneration) through diabetes. I recall him sitting on his lounge with the TV only a metre (3') from his chair so he could see. My brother and his wife (who lived around the corner) would visit daily to support and comfort him in his passing years.

His wife, my Grandma, passed away ten years before Grandad, just after their 50th wedding anniversary, with diabetes, though she wasn't overweight.

Every night they would have supper which consisted of hot chocolate in milk and biscuits or cake before bed; unknowingly creating havoc with their digestive system and slowly creating their diabetes.

My Mum

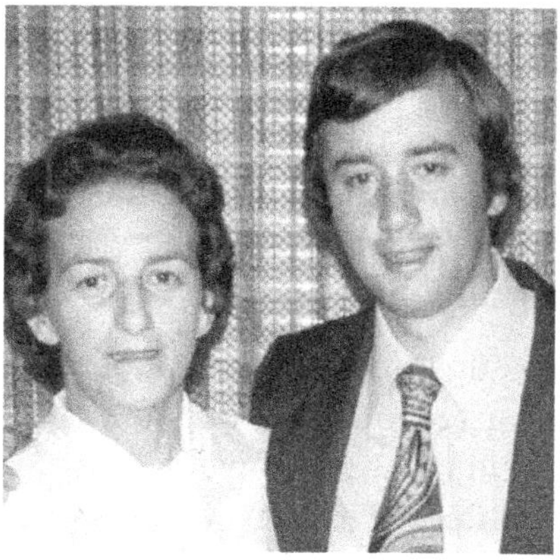

Mum was diagnosed with rheumatoid arthritis in her early 30s. Pop's sister (Mum's aunt) also suffered from arthritis, with swollen knuckles and had repeated surgery, including archaic removal of joints and even a leg amputation. Mum believed she inherited the affliction, so expected she'd live a similar fate as her Aunt, and therefore did.

I remember Mum having archaic surgery when the surgeon broke all her toes and inserted pins along them in a vain attempt to reset them straight. Mum went through months of agony, but the joints continued on their crooked way. Often, we had to lift Mum out of bed and rub her joints so she could get started for the day and I learnt how to NOT complain or whinge about anything. She took copious amounts of prescription drugs to ease the pain in a vain attempt to regain mobility. Every drug added to her body's toxicity and provided side-effects. My older brother has also been diagnosed with this inflammatory disorder and has been taking drugs and had surgery to combat the disease for several years with limited success.

Being single, Mum was the number one woman in my life at the time. My brothers married and left home in their early twenties and having a great relationship with my parents, I stayed at home with Mum and Dad until the age of twenty-six. Dad and I anguished internally to see Mum suffer daily and in a strange way, it was a relief to see her taken in a car accident, so she didn't suffer the pain any longer.

I have since learned that rheumatoid arthritis is not inherited as such, rather your genes might be predisposed to developing this autoimmune disease where the body attacks itself. Rheumatoid arthritis is mainly triggered by the acidic food we eat, especially dairy, grains, sugar and excessive omega-6.

According to the book *The China Study*, foreign invaders that enter the body are protein molecules called antigens, which can be bacterium, viruses or molecules of food. One of these antigens (or foods) commonly consumed is cow's milk, which contains a protein called casein (87% of milk), that mimics the body's own healthy proteins. Some antigens can leak through the bowel wall without going through the proper digestion process, which results in the production of amino acids. The immune system makes 'moulds' to identify and remember unsupportive antigens, but under some conditions (like overconsumption of dairy and sugar, and a dysfunctional bowel) the mould can be seen to fit the body's own similar proteins and the white blood cells start attacking the body in error.

Overconsumption of excessive dairy, grains and sugar creates an over-acidic system and an excess production of uric acid from the kidneys. Seed oils (commonly known as vegetable oils) in general are acidic to the body and sugar produces uric acid in the kidneys; the excess uric acid gathers in the joints causing inflammation — swelling and painful movement.

Mum loved her dairy, sugar and cakes, adding sugar to watermelon, bananas and cucumbers. Homemade mayonnaise consisted of a tin of sweetened, canned condensed milk, extra sugar, vinegar and mustard — we had this on every salad. She was a great believer in dessert after the evening meal (served at exactly 6pm, "or you'll miss out") which usually included ice cream, custard and preserved fruit from Pop's orchard.

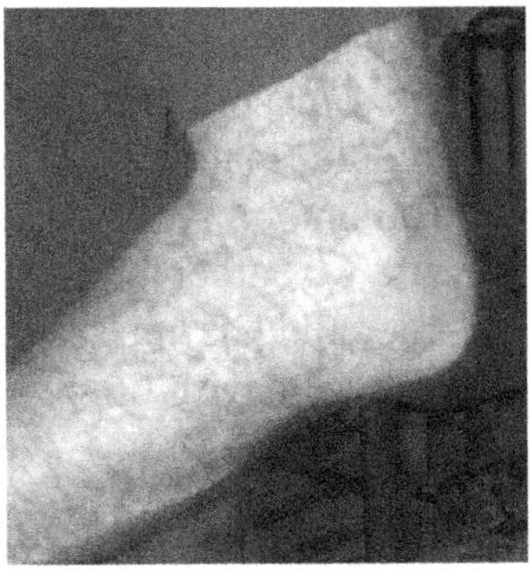
Early signs of arthritis in my elbow

I inherited Mum's patterns of sugar, cake and dairy consumption, and in January 2010 (at the age of 53) I started developing signs of arthritis in the elbow *(see photo)*. It was amazingly painful, and I literally couldn't bring my left hand to my mouth.

Instead of succumbing to this hideous autoimmune disease and going to the doctor for drugs and surgery, I started supplementing with a combination of herbs and fibre called AIM Herbal FiberBlend® to clean out my colon and started detoxing my liver. I also took AIM BarleyLife® and AIM LeafGreens® — which are excellent at detoxing and providing nutrients. Along with this I took omega-3 supplements, I reduced my dairy, grain and sugar consumption and increased regular exercise, when pain allowed. Over the course of a year, the swelling in my elbow has reduced and the pain gone. I am now, 10 years on, easily lifting heavy weights with my left arm.

I don't believe you necessarily inherit diseases; I believe you inherit the habits that trigger disease, including lifestyle, attitude and diet.

Mum used to take vast quantities of legally prescribed drugs. After the car accident in which she died at just 52 years old, my brothers and I drove to Bellingen in northern NSW to bring Dad home from the hospital, along with their luggage (they were heading from Orange to Tweed Heads to retire). Upon arriving back in Orange, we found one of Mum's suitcases absolutely crammed with prescription drugs — nothing else. Mum was able to work around the pharmacy system's safeguards against over-prescribing and convert all her prescriptions and repeats into a suitcase full of chemicals to meet her addiction and perceived needs for the near future.

My Dad

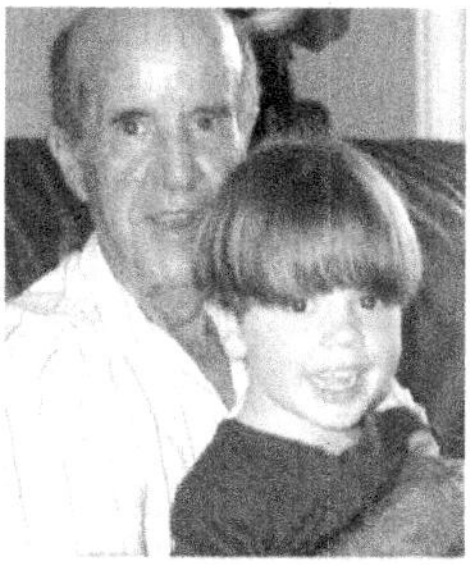

Dad (the bald one)

As a result of a lifetime of smoking and eating Mum's cooking for 32 years, Dad had double bypass heart surgery and retired from driving trains at just 48 years of age. Even after his heart surgery, Dad continued to have angina attacks, which limited the effort he could put into any project. It's worth noting that Dad had his heart surgery and retired 15 years younger than I am now, as I update this book.

I didn't want to leave Dad alone in his new house in Tweed Heads after Mum's death, so I sold my house in Orange and lived with Dad for two years. Dad outlived Mum by 19 years.

In 2004, at the age of 71, Dad was diagnosed with liver and bowel cancer (with a spot of lung cancer). After diagnosis, Dad was referred to an oncologist who recommended chemotherapy and radiation treatment (as the cancer industry recommends). Dad and I went for a quiet lunch at the Dolphins Hotel in Tweed Heads and chatted; he asked my opinion and I suggested there was very little chance of a cure and the drugs would make him feel ill and he would be unable to enjoy his last days with family. The only bonus was that losing his hair was not going to be a problem☺. I said I would support him in whatever choice he made — after all it was his body and his life.

Dad trusted the (false) up-beat information of the doctors and he chose orthodox treatments and I busily drove him between hospitals on the Gold Coast and Tweed Heads. Our family purchased a second car to handle the extra attention Dad required during this period, allowing my wife to drive our children to and from school and to complete other errands like shopping.

I remember one occasion at the Tweed Heads Hospital where a dozen cancer patients were lined up, side by side, each receiving their prescribed dose of chemicals (known as 'FU5' — read what you want into that). The energy was morbid, and I knew in my heart this was a futile attempt at extending Dad's life. But the doctor insisted that there was a reasonable chance of success, though I've since found that his chance of survival was only improved by 2% by taking the chemotherapy and radiation option. The chemo made dad very ill, very quickly and after fitting a colostomy bag (which didn't work as promised), Dad passed just six weeks after diagnosis.

Dad's cancer must have been growing in his liver for many years. Dad often complained of the discomfort he felt when bending over and tying his shoelaces and yet he was a very slim man. When diagnosed, the scan showed his liver was twice the size of a normal liver because of the cancer growth.

Dad also had difficulty hearing and both my parents had their teeth extracted in their mid-30s. I believe if there is something going astray internally, it may manifest firstly in places where the inside meets the outside — the orifices: namely the mouth, ears, eyes, hair, skin, nails, anus or genital areas.

My Brothers

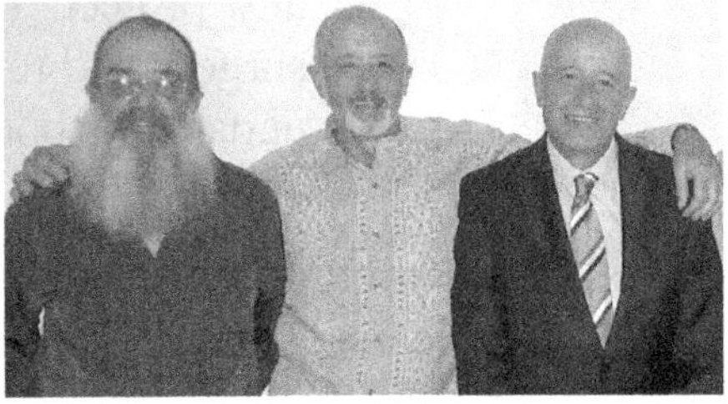

I have two brothers living in Orange, one older and one younger, about 18 months apart.

I won't go into too much detail to respect their privacy, but I thought I'd include a photo from a recent family gathering.

We all support our family's notorious hairline.☺

My Inheritance

So, if you believe the statistics, because of my genealogy I was a **prime candidate for diabetes, heart disease, bowel cancer, liver cancer and arthritis.** If I had followed my parents' (and grandparents') lifestyle choices and pursued their orthodox treatments and diets, there is a strong chance that I would now be retired, incapacitated in movement to some degree and on prescription drugs for my arthritis, heart disease and/or diabetes after numerous bouts of surgery.

I'm so pleased I stopped the cycle and chose an alternative way.

My In-Laws

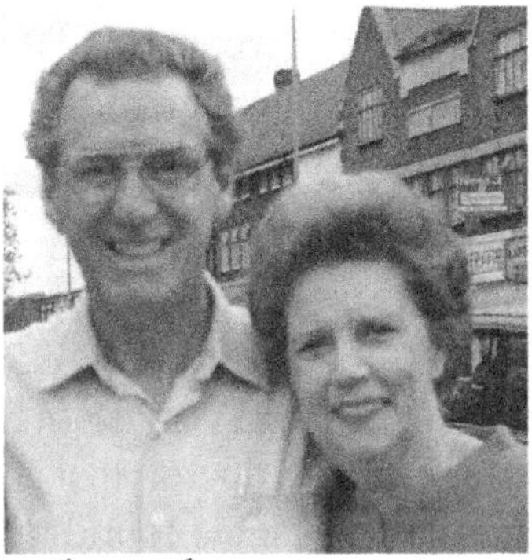

Though not related by blood, my mother-in- law and her husband's experience on their journey towards ill health and passing had a significant impact on our family and was the main encouragement we chose to seek alternative ways to prevent illness and disease.

Rex was my wife's stepfather and he loved his sweets and cream. He would seem to tempt fate by ordering two or three chocolate thick shakes at a time when we went out.

In 1998, just after our son was born, we received a late-night phone call from my mother-in-law (Shirley) to inform us that Rex had been admitted to hospital (again) with severe pain in the abdomen and this time it was really serious. As my wife was breastfeeding at the time, I went to Redcliffe Hospital in Brisbane to sit with Shirley all night, as Rex had been sedated to relieve the pain and to get some rest.

I remember the doctor telling Shirley that there was a good chance of recovery for Rex, and recommended surgery and procedures that I felt were dubious. Numerous previous scans and ultrasounds never showed any gall bladder issues until Rex was opened surgically. I remember Shirley replying to a doctor, "I'll be guided by your advice".

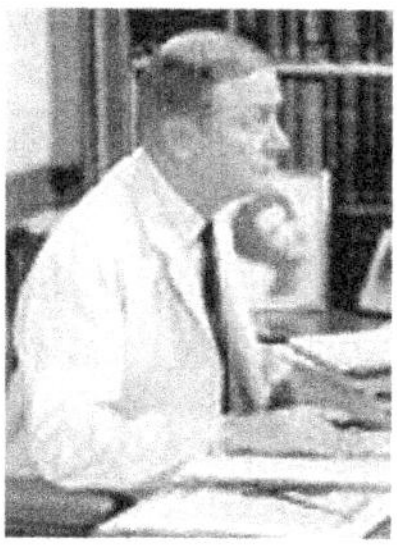

Marcus Welby MD from the 1960s

Shirley's generation trusted doctors implicitly, encouraged by images from her favourite shows about the caring doctor in a white coat who had their patients' best interests at heart, as portrayed in Marcus Welby MD and Dr Kildare on TV. They also genuinely respected bankers, lawyers and priests for some reason — haven't times changed!

The doctor gave Shirley hope where I believed there was little, and for the next eight weeks we made countless trips to Redcliffe Hospital with two babes in tow. Rex's gall bladder had turned gangrenous, which had contaminated the pancreas and killed other tissue around that area (liver and colon). This probably explained Rex's strong breath — we thought was mouth related halitosis.

I remember thinking there was little hope as, after the final surgery, the doctor left the wound open with a plastic sheath over the opening so they could access the area more easily next time without cutting through stitches again.

After eight weeks of extreme pain in intensive care, Rex passed away leaving Shirley alone and our children with one less grandfather. This was the first passing of our children's surviving grandparents.

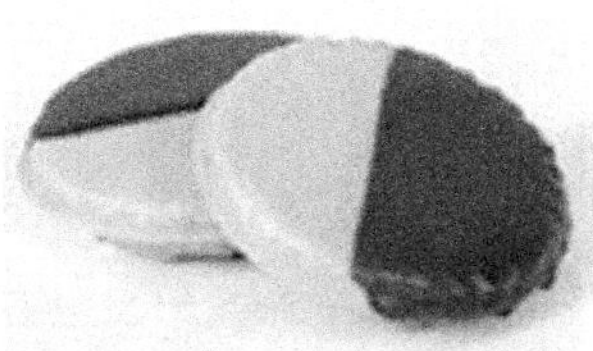

Neenish Tarts

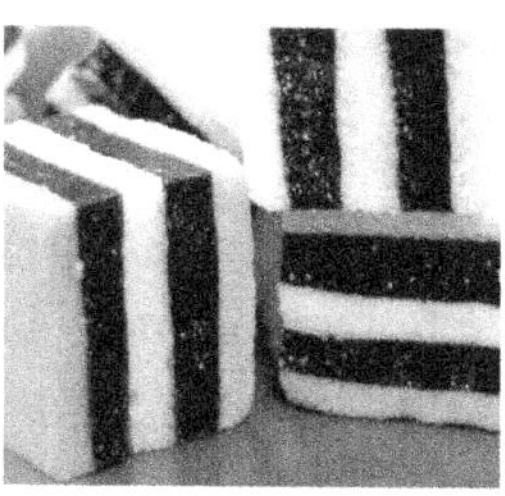

Liquorice Allsorts

Shirley continued to the best of her ability creating a life around playing indoor bowls and her new grandchildren. Unfortunately, within fifteen months (in the year 2000), Shirley was diagnosed with liver cancer. Shirley loved her sweets and dairy too. When we visited, we were often served neenish tarts (sweet cream and icing on pastry) or bright pink-iced cupcakes fresh from the supermarket.

She once explained, "A lady at the health food shop recommended we eat more liquorice," as she served us liquorice allsorts covered in brightly coloured sugar icing. She also used artificial sweeteners under the guise of losing weight. *(I will explain more about sugar and find out why this doesn't work, later in this book)*

Shirley was offered chemotherapy and radiation treatments for her liver cancer (of course). After going through two treatments, her hair started falling out and reality hit — she wasn't going to get better. We read in her diary later, "I had the colours of the rainbow go into me today and I feel awful".

At this time, we recommended Shirley take kelp to help boost her immune system; however, her doctor advised her against taking kelp as he didn't know enough about it, to which we replied, "for goodness sake, it's only food!"

My wife advised her mother not to have the third treatment and enjoy whatever time she had left with our family, including my wife's sisters, who had flown from England to be with her. But Shirley opted for the third and final treatment which lowered her immune system, and introduced a blood infection, which put her into palliative care. Just five months after diagnosis, Shirley passed away — again leaving our children with one less grandparent.

There was another woman in palliative care at the same time as Shirley. She was the same age and had the same diagnosis and prognosis; however, she chose not to have chemotherapy. Rather, the nurses managed her pain and she was allowed to pass her time with dignity. She had a full head of hair, walked around, played cards with her grandchildren and chatted with her daughter.

Meanwhile on the opposite side of the room, we were standing around, holding Shirley's hand while we chatted amongst ourselves. She was bald, a dark shade of yellow, with black circles around her eyes, incapacitated and totally bed ridden.

My Father-In-Law

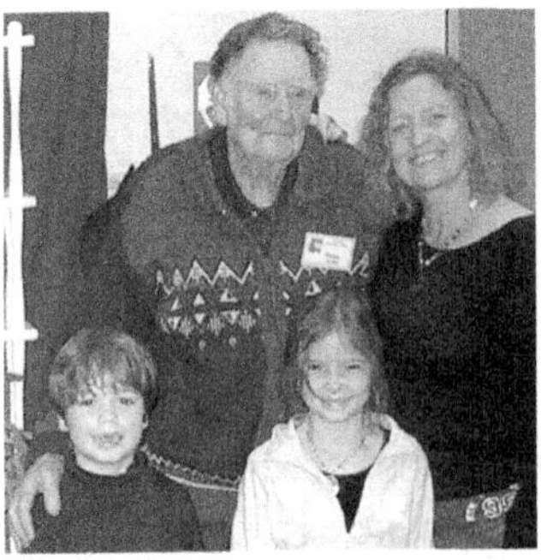

In 2011, my wife's father Doug, who lived in New Zealand, was diagnosed with an enlarged heart (inflammation) along with bowel and liver cancer, just short of his 85th birthday.

Most healthcare professionals have told me that the majority of cancers start in the bowel and the cancer contagion is spread to other organs via the blood filtered by the liver. The liver is the first organ to receive blood from the bowel and acts as a filter for the body's blood. The liver can seem to function normally, even when up to 90% diseased. The kidneys operate in a similar manner. Usually by the time we receive pain feedback, it's too late.

It was just three weeks from the time of diagnosis to Doug's passing. This doesn't mean that disease suddenly appeared overnight; it's more an indication of how insensitive we can be to feedback from our digestion and elimination systems. Like my father, Doug's cancer would have been brewing for many years, with his body giving little feedback until it was too late.

I've concluded that there is a definite need to continually nurture, clean and maintain the bowel and liver, even if you think everything is alright, you're having regular motions and you feel well. Personally, I do this through daily servings of fibre, water and exercise to keep my bowel and liver squeaky clean. I also supplement my diet with stem cell enhancement, wholefood nutrition powders and nutraceuticals that detoxes and supports my liver. Nutraceuticals are natural, nutrition-based products that have pharmaceutical benefits without the side-effects of chemical-based pharmaceuticals. Along with the above, I take regular coffee enemas and gall bladder flushes.

I haven't bothered having a colonoscopy (like my brothers did) as recommended by the government and doctors following our father's bowel cancer, because I feel this procedure is very invasive, uncomfortable, inconclusive and doesn't always recognise constipation, irritations, strictures, diverticulitis, mucoid plaque, early cancers or parasites which can cause the underlying conditions for future disease.

Doug was offered chemotherapy and radiation treatment by the medical industry (of course), but declined, as he did not consider the addition of toxic chemicals and deadly radiation as beneficial in his situation.

We visited New Zealand in 2004 and observed Doug eating plenty of deep-fried food, dairy and wheat products, like most New Zealanders. He scoffed at the supplements we brought with us.

Doug related over the phone to my wife, shortly before passing, that he was standing on tiles in hospital and, "got the fright of his life" to find a puddle of liquid at his feet. Initially he thought he'd unknowingly urinated, but was surprised to find that sores and abscesses on his ankles and calves had burst and leaked. The sores were from toxic build-up, which gravitated to the lowest point, and due to poor circulation, sat stagnant in the feet and putrefied. The only way the body could release these toxins was through ankle sores.

Doug went through an uncomfortable passing in constant pain, which the hospital tried in vain to relieve using morphine.

I have a theory...

Doctors may tell you chemotherapy and radiation have a good chance of working, because that's what they've been told at medical college by the suppliers of the chemicals — Big Pharma. But as with me and my father, if you do your research you will find that chemotherapy treatment may only improve your chances of living beyond five years by about 2%.

An article published in the *Clinical Oncology Journal*, December 2004 quotes the Department of Radiation Oncology, North Sydney Cancer Centre:

"Results of Study: *The overall contribution of curative and adjuvant cytotoxic chemotherapy to 5-year survival in adults was estimated to be 2.3% in Australia and 2.1% in the USA.*

Conclusion: *As the 5-year relative survival rate for cancer in Australia is now over 60%, it is clear that cytotoxic chemotherapy only makes a minor contribution to cancer survival. To justify the continued funding and availability of drugs used in cytotoxic chemotherapy, a rigorous evaluation of the cost-effectiveness and impact on quality of life is urgently required."*

To clarify this, statistics show that the chance of living beyond five years, following a diagnosis of cancer, has improved over the last few decades to around 60%. However, this can be explained with improved imaging, regular screening and so on. Cancer is being discovered earlier; therefore, patients are living longer than five years from diagnosis.

A few decades ago, patients might have been diagnosed at say, three to four years into their cancer's progression, after they eventually felt a lump, they would die soon after diagnosis and treatment. Nowadays with CT scans and imaging, the smallest cancer can be spotted within its first year of growth, and therefore survival beyond five years is far more likely. The survival rate beyond five years has really only improved due to new and earlier detection processes and statistics, not necessarily from improved treatments. Many patients who receive treatment and survive also change their lifestyles significantly and it's difficult (via cognitive dissonance) for the sickness fraternity to credit such changes as contributing to life extensions.

The following statement may seem a little callous; but I'll stick my head on the block (along with several friends who have had similar experiences): I believe doctors prescribe chemotherapy to move elderly, terminal patients who have little chance of recovery towards passing sooner, to free up hospital beds while Big Pharma continues to milk profits from government-subsidised chemotherapy and hospitals — a type of euthanasia. My theory evolved through my own experiences and those of many friends. I am a great believer in studying statistics and watching what the sickness industry does, rather than believing what they say.

And the figures back this up... There was a recent study by the UK-based

National Confidential Enquiry into Patient Outcome and Death (NCEPOD) which found that: *"40% of patients who received chemotherapy treatment towards the end of their life died from the treatment, not cancer. The NCEPOD also reviewed over 600 cancer patients who died within a month of receiving chemotherapy treatments and they found chemotherapy to have accelerated or caused the death of 27% of patients."*

Quoting a 1994 patent application (#5 605 930) from the US government Department of Health, *"Current approaches to combat cancer rely primarily on the use of chemicals and radiation, which are themselves carcinogenic and may promote recurrences and the development of metastatic disease."*

Caught early enough, it has been proven that cancer can be prevented, stopped and reversed through diet, supplementation and lifestyle changes. If you don't provide a sugar-based (carbs), acidic environment in which cancer can flourish, cancer can't sustain its own growth — alkalise and oxygenate the body, the less-favourable the environment for cancer growth.

Diabetes and heart disease can also be prevented and reversed through diet, supplementation, lifestyle changes too. There are over 700 scientific, peer-reviewed references with evidence to back this up. Do your research!

Our Family's History Summarised

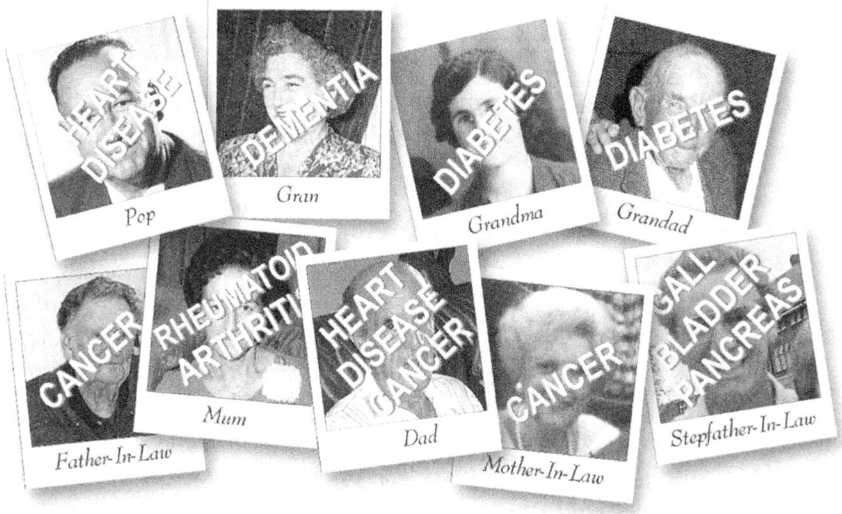
HEART DISEASE
Pop
DEMENTIA
Gran
DIABETES
Grandma
DIABETES
Grandad
CANCER
Father-In-Law
RHEUMATOID ARTHRITIS
Mum
HEART DISEASE CANCER
Dad
CANCER
Mother-In-Law
GALL BLADDER PANCREAS
Stepfather-In-Law

I watched our families' parents die from bowel and liver cancer, heart disease, diabetes and dementia.

I was determined not to go the same way!

But my prognosis was not looking good — please read on...

My Wife

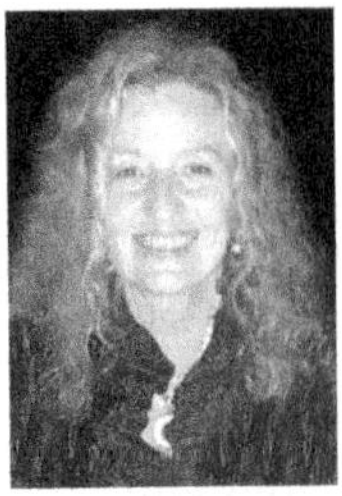

A few years before I met my wife Shakti, she had seen several doctors trying to find reasons for her constant aches and pains, moods, lack of energy and chronic digestive and bowel complaints. Doctor after doctor offered ideas, but no answers and prescribed numerous pills and treatments. Finally, Shakti was referred to a psychiatrist — the doctors' conclusion was that her problems were all in her head. I recall her relating to me, "Is this the best modern medicine can do for me?"

Tapeworm

After we married, we arranged an appointment with a kinesiologist who diagnosed parasites in Shakti's bowel and recommended AIM Herbal FiberBlend®. After using the supplement for three months, Shakti passed a two-metre tapeworm (along with hundreds of intestinal fluke) that had been present in her bowel for years. Her chronic constipation had provided a perfect nest-bed for parasites and caused most of her ailments. AIM Herbal FiberBlend® relieved her chronic constipation and cleaned out her bowel, making it no longer comfortable for parasites to reside or breed.

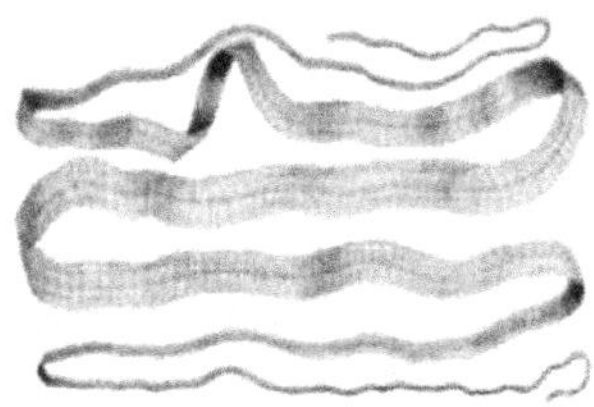

Tapeworm

Constipation... I got to the Bottom of it!

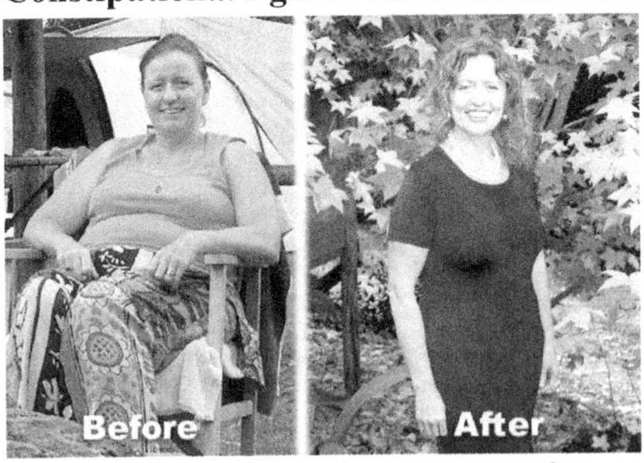

"Working in country Victoria, single and 30, I had visited doctors, chiropractors and osteopaths seeking relief for abdominal and back pain, headaches, mood swings, lethargy, flatulence, belching, overweight, cravings, itchy anus and ears, haemorrhoids, lack of sleep, anxiety and chronic constipation that had plagued me for many years. The visit to my sixth doctor left me with a referral to a psychiatrist. "Am I going mad?" I asked myself. The psychiatrist charged $150 an hour and left me grossly despondent.

After ten years, I moved to Queensland, married and gave birth to two children. My bowel problems intensified. Following the death of my mother from bowel and liver cancer, I had a colonoscopy. The specialist diagnosed irritable bowel, leaky gut and diverticulitis and told me to increase my intake of psyllium husk. It didn't really help, and I still felt bloated.

In 2003 a kinesiologist assessed parasites in my bowel and recommended AIM Herbal FiberBlend®, which I was to take for at least three months.

Within days I noticed about 100 white lumps in the toilet bowl after each motion, rather like I had eaten loads of blanched almonds. These were intestinal fluke.

I started to feel lighter, happier, and experienced less belching, gas and bloating. I also had noticeably more energy and vitality. Within a few weeks, I had lost three kilos, my appetite had decreased, and I seemed to want to drink more water. The pain in my joints had gone completely, though my lower back still had pain. By this time, my husband and our children, who were five- and six-years-old at the time, had joined me in my daily servings of Herbal FiberBlend®.

That Tapeworm!

Then something happened that changed my health, wealth and quality of life. Upon my second visit to the loo for the day, I felt a large lump moving under my rib cage. Then I felt a huge release. I looked into the bowl and immersed in white mucus was a two-to-three-metre tapeworm.

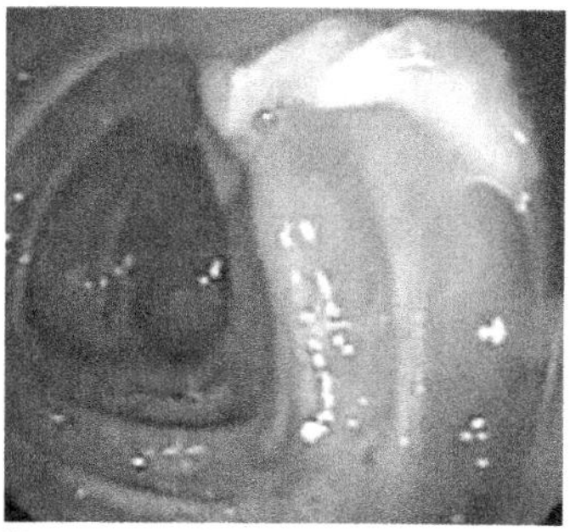

Tapeworm shown inside the colon top right (white)

Instantly I felt a completely different person and have never looked back. I still take Herbal FiberBlend® daily, because health practitioners recommend a minimum of 30–70 grams of fibre a day. I feel that Herbal FiberBlend® also strengthens the lining of my bowel. After many years of constipation, my bowel lining was very thin and weak, and besides, I did not want parasites to reinfest.

Now I am 12 kg lighter and my back and joint pain, headaches and my many other ailments have all gone.

Sometimes we must hit the wall before we take responsibility for our own health, or we can learn from what has happened to others and take action."

Shakti — Gold Coast, Qld

Testimonials should not be construed as representing results everybody can achieve. Results may not be typical and may vary from person to person.

Tumour and Hysterectomy

After giving birth to our two beautiful children and feeling run-down, Shakti visited her doctor and had a full-body check. The doctor found a small cyst on her ovaries about 25mm (1") in diameter and she was advised that this was a common occurrence and it would "go away" or "dissolve itself" in time. A few years went by and despite removing her tapeworm; Shakti began to feel unwell again. New scans revealed that the cyst on her ovaries had grown to a potentially life-threatening tumour (cancer) about the size of a grapefruit *(see document inset)*.

Shakti was scheduled for surgery six weeks later, but in the meantime, she ate a pristine diet, meditated and exercised daily and took copious amounts wholefood supplements. She also conducted daily coffee enemas. Though she didn't know it at the time, Shakti shrank her tumour *(see second document below)*, which wasn't revealed to her until after surgery.

During surgery, the surgeons decided to perform a full hysterectomy as the tumour appeared to be benign and could have burst during removal, causing an even greater risk.

SOUTH COAST RADIOLOGY

Exam Date: 11th December 2006
Report date: 11th December 2006

NERANG 4211
RE: Ms SELWOOD
BEECHMONT 4211
Birthdate: /59

UPPER ABDOMINAL & PELVIC ULTRASOUND

There is enlargement of the right ovary which measures approximately 10.5 x 4.2 x 3.5cm. There are multiple cystic spaces within the right ovary, the largest single cystic space superiorly measures approximately 4.2cm in diameter. There is a further similar sized cyst

OPERATION:
Date: 24.01.07
Operative diagnosis: Frozen section of right paraovarian cyst benign: haemorrhagic +/- torsion, possible endometriosis.
Operation: TAH/BSO, pelvic washing
Surgeon: DR N
Operator: DRS N
Assist: DR H
PROCEDURE: IDC inserted. Midline laparotomy. Exploration of upper abdomen normal pelvic washing, fluid sent for cytology. Right parovarian cyst 5x6cm adhered to right ovary. Cyst removed sent for

Shakti was already shrinking her tumour through serious lifestyle changes and supplementation and may have even dissolved it completely. However, as she was not aware that her lifestyle changes were having such a momentous impact, she opted to go ahead with the surgical procedure, which involved removal of organs that were not vital to sustain her life.

In the same hospital ward were three other women who had undergone the same surgery (hysterectomy) on the same day. Shakti was released just four days after surgery, as her bowel was functioning correctly, and her blood count and vital signs were impressive. Meanwhile, the other three women stayed on in hospital because they were yet to walk, pass a motion or eat and drink without vomiting.

Shakti put this down to daily supplementation she had lined up on her bedside table. We were surprised that after such an obviously positive effect, none of the other patients, doctors or nursing staff enquired further about the products she was taking.

Hernias

Since she had lost weight, Shakti could feel a hernia at the end of the stitches from her hysterectomy and was referred to a specialist surgeon. Just 12 months after her original surgery; she was scheduled for surgery again. While waiting for her results in the waiting room after her appointment, Shakti read a book which showed common hernias and realised she possibly had another hernia in her groin area which the specialist had not checked for or noticed.

Against the specialist's advice, Shakti insisted on another scan, which revealed a second hernia. Shakti believes this hernia possibly happened when trying to save her mother from a fall in the months prior to her passing. The surgeon charged us many thousands of dollars for this "quality of service".

My Own Health

Work History

Before I discuss the health issues I had, I want to briefly mention my work history so you gain a perception of the chemicals and toxins I may have absorbed into my body. Beyond my childhood working on my grandfathers' orchards and being in regular contact with pesticides and fungicides, I started an apprenticeship as a fitter and turner/toolmaker in 1974. During my employment, I worked around paint, glue, acetone, turpentine, mentholated spirits, kerosene, soluble oil, fibreglass, vinyl, plastics, petrochemicals, petrol, diesel and degreasers. In the tool-room there was an area for casehardening which utilised cyanide and arsenic. I breathed in fumes from welding galvanised pipe and flux from braising metal.

In the late 1970s I ignorantly believed I would inherit Mum's rheumatoid arthritis and so upon completing my apprenticeship I embarked on a thirty-year journey in drafting and engineering in the whitegoods, boat manufacturing and food processing industries. I was also a licensed building designer (draftsman) with the Queensland Building Services Authority. At the time, I thought that a sedentary, less physical lifestyle would support my arthritis in old age, but this wasn't to be — I was extremely misguided by the expectations of the medical mind-programming machine – *see chapter 10.*

I'm currently director of our company and I write and speak. I live a meaningful, fulfilled life through my work by personally growing as a human-spirit, inspiriting people to take responsibility and providing knowledge and opportunities. If they are attracted to my energy, they will find their passion and purpose too and live a more meaningful, fulfilled life – inspiring others.

Tonsillitis

Like most children of the 1950s and 60s, I had a tonsillectomy at five years with the promise of as much ice cream as I could eat after surgery. The tonsils are external lymph glands at the back of the throat that eliminate external threats from the mouth and are one of the first organs of the body to repel germs and bacteria that the body can't utilise. Occasionally, while performing these functions, they become inflamed and very often in those days, the solution was to 'rip them out' surgically, leaving the patient vulnerable to bacteria and phlegm for the rest of their life.

Tonsils are the storehouse for sulphur, so if you had yours ripped out like I did, you should eat plenty of eggs and cruciferous vegetables containing sulphur which will help support the liver and balance estrogen levels in men (especially). Foods such as broccoli, cauliflower, brussels sprouts, kale, rocket (arugula), cabbage, onion, garlic, turnips, watercress, horseradish, etc.

School Lunches and other meals

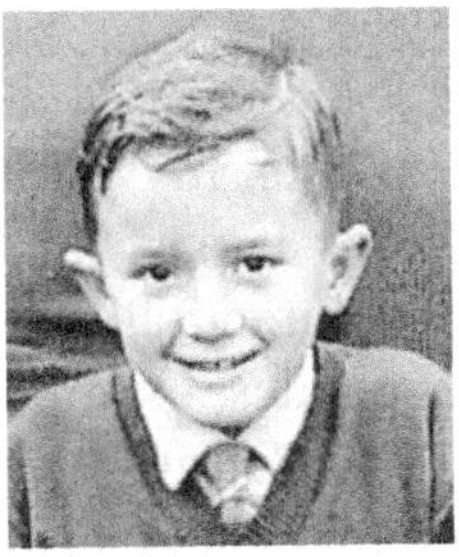

Back in the 1960s, the standard school lunch consisted of white bread with jam (jelly), cheese, Vegemite, peanut butter or honey. This wasn't really food; it was more like a filler, containing very little nutrition or fibre. Just something to fill me up, which tasted sweet and kept me happy; mum didn't know any better.

Today with a plethora of knowledge at everyone's fingertips, I still observe many parents unconsciously pursuing the same habit (introduced by their parents) for their own children, because they haven't considered the impact the lack of nutrition and fibre has on young, growing bodies and brains. With today's access to information, ignorance is no longer an excuse, but is often a reason.

Mum would make an iced chocolate cake on Sunday that would see our morning tea through all week. In primary school, we were provided with free milk and hot chocolate in winter. Occasionally I was 'spoiled' and enjoyed a ham sandwich with a can of Coke or was allowed to buy lunch from the school 'Tuck Shop' — usually a meat pie, sausage roll or hotdog with flavoured milk. After school, my brothers and I would race home and demolish a packet of biscuits and a pint of flavoured milk. Nothing green so far...

For breakfast, I would have cereal with honey or sugar, or toast, honey and jam (carbs). For dinner, we would eat meat and three veg (boiled excessively), followed by dessert, then we'd snack until bedtime. I ate as little veg as possible, except potato. Although my grandparents were orchardists, we ate little fruit. We took fruit for granted so never ate it regularly, though I do remember opening my lunchbox once whilst apple picking and found an apple inside☺ - Mum was like that.

Today, as I reflect on this diet, I see nothing supportive for my health. I don't blame Mum; she was only doing what her parents (Pop and Gran) taught her. Yet this ignorant diet laid the foundations for my future health issues.

Ignorant or not, with love or not, with trust or not; this level of knowledge and belief, and the relative actions still had a karmic impact on my health.

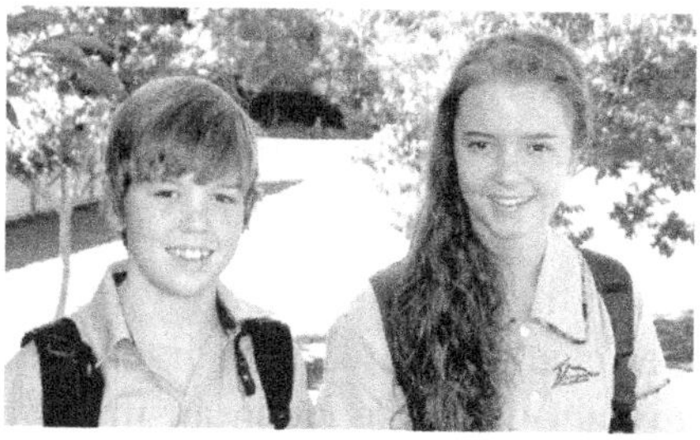

As parents, when our children attended school, my wife rose early and prepared a healthy lunch containing lots of quality meat and vegies with low carbs for school meals every day. We broke the cycle and have given them a better start for their health span.

Haemorrhoids

At the age of just seventeen I had haemorrhoid surgery because of my poor diet. I condescendingly referred to salad as "rabbit food!" I have since found out that haemorrhoids mostly happen due of a lack of bile from the liver and fibre and water in the diet. Fibre is not present in animal products and can only be found in plants. Stimulating bile production and a simple increase in both fibre and water would have helped resolve these issues and remove the need for surgery. I've spared you from viewing any images.☺

Blocked Sinuses

Not long after my haemorrhoid surgery, I felt a significant blockage in my throat, just above the larynx on the left side, that restricted swallowing and was quite painful. After searching for fish bones and prescribing antibiotics, my doctor gave me two massive shots of penicillin, which reduced the pain and blockage; however, the blockage remains (to a lesser extent) today.

Coupled with my throat, I had always experienced sinus problems and a blocked nose. I continually produced phlegm and needed to clear my throat constantly. Immediately after I had my throat and sinuses checked by a specialist doctor, I was booked in for sinus surgery. Fortunately, following advice from a friend who had similar surgery (which didn't improve his situation), I cancelled my surgery. Perhaps my throat and sinus problems were caused from my tonsillectomy? I have since found that acidic refined carbohydrates (like grain products, sugar) and dairy create mucus and block the sinuses. My ear, nose and throat specialist didn't tell me this, he just wanted to 'commit' surgery on me.

Hernia

At eighteen years, I had surgery for a hernia I'd had for as long as I can remember. I had only realised the lump in my groin area was a hernia after viewing a safety film during my apprenticeship.

Pilonidal Cyst

At the same time as the hernia, I discovered a lump on my intergluteal cleft (the crease between the buttocks colloquially known as a 'bum crack') — a repeating pilonidal cyst that I had surgically removed three different times over four years. This lump resembled a large, permanent boil or pimple with a large whitehead and was extremely painful at times. After my three bouts of surgery, I still had similar problems, and found that a basic pimple cream worked best to restrain its symptoms.

I see the cyst as my body attempting to eliminate toxins through my skin, because my bowel and liver were dysfunctional. Since I started cleaning up my act there has been an improvement, but I still had a painful pimple/boil rise a couple of times a year. Finally, after taking stem cell nutrition for 18 months, the pimple recently rose again to a painful head for a few weeks, then it hardened to a head about 2mm in diameter and popped out for good.

Doctors

At around this age I suffered my first significant injury, when I injured my knee playing first-grade hockey. My family paradigm at the time was to visit my doctor to get better, so I did. I was surprised at how little knowledge the doctor had about my injury and how to treat it. He prescribed anti-inflammatories and antibiotics and told me to go home and rest.

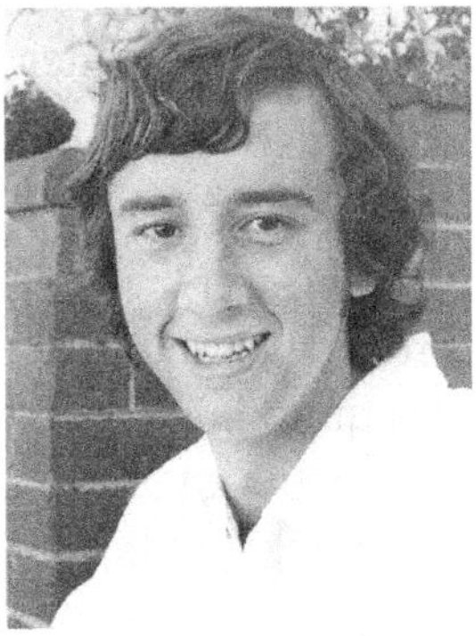

Though at 17 years I looked rather 'handsome' and healthy on the outside, internally I was wearing the health effects of my ignorant choices — which were to unfold in the years to come

After speaking with the club 'strapper' (a 50-year-old sports veteran), I found out that doctors have little training or knowledge about sports injuries. The strapper gave me advice about ice, Hirudoid cream, peroxide and stretching, which I implemented. I fixed my injury within days – thanks 'Patto'.

Tap on My Shoulder

At just 17, my perceived need for surgery was the first 'tap on my shoulder', warning me that I had to make changes, but I wasn't ready to listen — yet.

At this stage in my life, surgery as a solution to my problems was okay, as my life-experience had involved my mother going through regular surgery, as did my grandparents. It was part of normal life back then.

From 18 years to about 26, I tended to drink too much alcohol and ate poorly, although I was fit from playing representative hockey. Though I was fit and slim, my body was being built from my poor food choices, alcohol and toxins from my work environment. I didn't know it at the time, but I was building a toxic overload for my body to deal with at some time in the future (30 years later) and was setting myself up for future ailments.

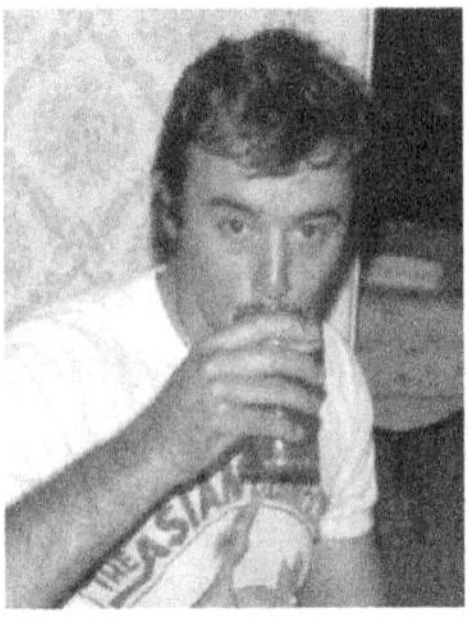

At the age of 21, fresh out of my apprenticeship, I borrowed $1000 and did the 'Asian Fling', as many young Aussie males do. I still hold the world record for the greatest number of Sakes (Japanese rice wine) on a rice barge cruise in Bangkok – 21 Sakes in three hours. As far as I know, the record still stands, which is a good thing — I think?☺

At this early age, I thought I was bullet proof. I really couldn't physically feel any of the abuse I was heaping onto my body; instead my body simply absorbed it for later distribution through seizures (30+ years later) when finally, my organs had enough and were overloaded.

I see a similar attitude in the same age group of the current generation of millennials and Gen Ys, however, the current generation can add to the mix concentrated high-caffeine and sugar energy drinks, recreational drugs, extra sugar, artificial sweeteners, cheap takeaways, trans-fats, electro-magnetic fields, GMOs and heavy reliance on the convenience of processed foods. In modern society, many people are too busy (or lazy) to cook. The tradition of preparing wholesome, healthy meals seems to have somewhat been replaced with regularly eating out and microwaving 'healthy choice' frozen meals. There's a big problem waiting to unfold over the next few decades. This probably explains why supermarkets are investing heavily into selling spectacles, to take advantage of the ensuing diabetes epidemic.

Mouth Injury

In 1985 I was hit in the mouth with a hockey stick. My lower front-four teeth were bent backwards from a horizontal fracture line about a centimetre (half inch) below the base of my teeth. Over the next year, I visited the dentist repeatedly and wore a fibreglass brace, culminating with one tooth being capped with a root canal.

At the time root canals were a new procedure and there was little evidence of negative side-effects. It seemed better than wearing a plate with a false tooth.

Over the next 30 years, research and studies have shown root canals and teeth implants are major contributors to long-term, chronic health issues as you will read in the *'mouth' section* later.

I believe this root canal was the major contributor to my seizures in the decades to come.

Bell's Palsy

At 29 years, I was diagnosed with Bell's palsy, which temporarily, partially paralysed one side of my face. The doctor prescribed steroids, which made me rather anxious and uptight — the opposite of what I needed.

Bell's palsy is a nervous complaint. At around that time, Mum died, I sold my house in Orange and had problems with payment. I had just relocated to South East Queensland and started a new job, all the while supporting Dad through his grief, not to mention my own grief I had to deal with. No wonder I was stressed, but we do what we must do to cope, don't we?

These days I would have consumed more electrolytes, applied transdermal magnesium and increased my stem cell levels *(more on this later)* which relaxes and repairs nerves. The side-effects of steroids made me short-tempered, agitated, angry and aggressive at a time when I needed to relax. I remember on one occasion angrily ripping into one of the guys I was car-pooling with — sorry John.

My Liver

I had given blood for two decades, then in the early 1990s I received a letter from the blood bank saying they couldn't use my blood as the gamma glutamyl tanspeptidase (Gamma GT) reading was more than double the recommended reading. They suggested I visit my doctor.

High gamma GT readings indicate a stressed liver, usually associated with excessive alcohol. At that time, I was not drinking much; but perhaps my earlier years of excessive drinking had taken a toll on my liver. The doctor and I did a series of tests over a few months and the readings didn't change significantly. This was my 'second tap on my shoulder' and now I was a little older, wiser and more willing to listen. I decided to get on with life and start detoxing my liver.

After four decades of bachelorhood and an advert in a 'lonely hearts' newsletter, in 1996 at the age of 40, I met my wife and we married just four later. We gave birth to two children and over 10 years moved house four times. Over the course of our relocations, three of our parents passed away, one after the other (over six years). After observing how our parent's lack of basic health-knowledge and 'handing themselves over' to the sickness industrial complex had let them down, we started looking at alternative ways of improving our health. Though at times the changes were stressful, my health seemed alright over this decade until I neared my fifties...

Seizures

Just after Easter 2003 (at 47 years) at around midnight, I became conscious lying on the floor beside my bed, with my wife and our friend Helmut — a male nurse who lived nearby — leaning over me. I had blood running out my mouth from biting my tongue and felt incredibly sore all over. My brain was thumping with an incredible headache. Helmut explained that I had just had a seizure.

I really feel for people with epilepsy, as it literally takes many months to recover from just one seizure. Every muscle, tendon and ligament in the body aches, and there is always a certain group of muscles where the seizure was most intense that is particularly painful for many more months. Headaches occur for months afterwards, triggered by the simplest effort or stress.

I tried to find the reason for the seizure but came up with no answers at the time. Later I realised that a liver flush I had performed had released a mass of toxins (stored in my liver) into my body, effectively poisoning my system internally, though at the time of doing the flush, I didn't know it could cause such a situation.

I believe toxins are the cause of epilepsy and repeated seizures? We may never find this out, as there is little money to be made in simply detoxing the liver, therefore research may never happen.

I took life a little easier after my first seizure and I went for four years with no complaints, until November 2007 when I had two seizures in one night, again for no apparent reason. At the time I assumed it was stress.

Earlier that year, my wife had a tumour surgically removed, necessitating a hysterectomy *(see 'My Wife' previously)* and I was carrying the load of maintaining our property, running our business, caring for my wife and children, including driving our children to school (up and down our mountain, 30 minutes each way, twice daily). We assumed this was too stressful for me, so we sold our semi-rural property and moved into the suburbs where we were closer to school and life would be easier – or so we thought.

We moved to our new suburban house on the Gold Coast in March 2008, but with the move, the stress continued. The Global Financial Crisis (GFC) hit just as we doubled our mortgage and our income halved overnight.

I had several (what I called) 'stress attacks' where I had episodes of heart palpitations, high blood pressure, extreme headaches, I was dizzy, my temperature was very high and all I could do was lie down in front of a fan with a bucket nearby.

Aussie blokes are notorious for avoiding doctors but, I finally succumbed and had every test possible. I had a full blood count, blood folate levels checked, haemoglobin test for diabetes, cholesterol test, blood tests for lead, arsenic and other heavy metals, gamma GT test (which was still double what is considered normal, although it had reduced), a PSA prostate test, thyroid function test, tumour markers, an ECG test to measure my brain patterns for possible epilepsy, ultrasound scans on my liver, CT scans to check for aneurisms in the brain, and finally a stress test during which I had another 'stress attack' with all the probes attached.

The end result — the doctors couldn't find anything wrong with me. Everything they measured was within the 'normal' range, for a man my age and I was apparently healthy. In fact, I measured healthier than most men my age. So, what was wrong?

I rested even more, avoiding stress and continued to detox my liver — again, a little too hard unfortunately. At the time, I didn't know that severely detoxing the liver too quickly was going to cause a crisis. I somehow knew however, that my dysfunctional bowel and toxic liver were at the centre of all my problems and if I didn't clean them up, they were going to affect my future health, including causing possible heart disease, plus bowel and liver cancer like my father.

I nearly didn't make it. I believe if I had a weak heart, thin blood vessels or clogged arteries I could have easily passed away through this intense period. Oh, and my death would have been recorded as a heart attack (for example), rather than the real cause, a clogged bowel and toxic liver caused by decades of poor choices and continual contamination caused by a root canal.

In July 2008 I conducted a major detox over a couple of days, which alkalises the blood and shifts toxins quickly. My thinking was that if I could clean the toxins out of my liver quickly, the rest of my body would have a better chance of recovery. However, this may have been too much at once, throwing my body into a 'healing crisis' (which sometimes happens during the curative or healing stage of a treatment, when the body detoxes too quickly and displays temporary symptoms that appear to be worsening the situation. If the symptoms go too far, they can have a temporary, negative impact on the healing process or person) and possibly triggering another two seizures which I had in one night. This time the seizures were focused around my diaphragm and I stopped breathing for a long time.

My wife said I didn't inhale for several minutes during my seizure and **if I hadn't come out of my unconscious state within the next minute or so, I would have certainly suffocated and died or been left with brain damage.** Even today, sometimes my communication and cognitive abilities can be a little slow, but I am so lucky to have survived 95% intact.

Working with a naturopath, we concluded that over the years my liver had accumulated a concoction of waste and toxins that couldn't really be measured or categorised by medical laboratories. The toxins were no specific heavy metal, just a compound of everything I had accumulated from my childhood working around pesticides on my Grandfather's orchards, my apprenticeship, too much alcohol in my younger years, poor nutrition for four decades, toxins from my root canal and consequently a clogged, constipated bowel and possibly leaky gut.

I had moved incredible amounts of toxins too suddenly and the noxious concoction had moved from my liver into my blood, poisoning my body, causing the seizures and 'stress attacks'. I learned that it is important to change your diet before doing a food fast or other radical detoxes.

Armed with this information, and knowing I had to continue detoxing my liver, I started detoxing again, but this time more slowly and steadily. I corrected my diet by eating less dairy, more meat, fat and vegetables and avoiding fruits, sugar and refined grains (carbs). I began exercising regularly, alternating walking, and time in our home gym.

As mentioned earlier, our business was hit by the GFC, so we sold our suburban house at a significant loss (yet more stress) and decided to rent on Tamborine Mountain in the hinterland of the Gold Coast.

Since then, enjoying a happier life, slowly cleaning out my colon and liver, eating better, increasing my stem cells, taking high-nutrient wholefood supplements and exercising regularly (I walk 4km *(2½ miles)* daily), my health has improved significantly and 2008 was my last seizure. I believe that at 64 years old, I am healthier than I have been for over two decades.

I've reversed my declining health without medication or surgery.

If I didn't make changes, I was certainly heading for the same future as my parents – early retirement, limited movement from arthritis, surgery, heart disease, cancer, general low quality of life and an early passing, leaving my children prematurely fatherless.

In early 2012, I repeated the above blood tests, and everything again showed within normal range. The normal range for the gamma GT reading is between 10–70u/l — my 2008 reading was more than twice the high mark at 146u/l. After focusing on detoxing my liver for several years, my liver gamma GT reading was back to normal at 41u/l for the first time in 20 years, showing the value of steady, consistent bowel cleansing and liver detoxification through lifestyle improvements, supplementing and regular coffee enemas.

Parasites

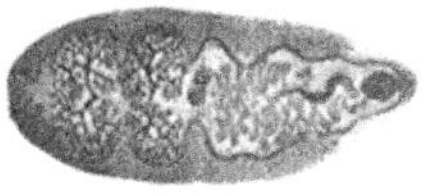

Intestinal fluke

As part of my colonic detox program and following my wife's success with removing her tapeworm, I took AIM Herbal FiberBlend®. After a few weeks, I too noticed hundreds of white almond-shaped intestinal fluke parasites in my motions. I had no idea I was infested with parasites. Experts claim that some type of worm exists in the intestines of over 75% of the world's population.

Plaque (Mucoid) Lining my Colon and Strictures

Upon continued use of AIM Herbal FiberBlend®, one morning I noticed a black ribbon (like thick, black twine) running through my stool. This I believe was part of the mucoid lining off my colon wall, a plastic-like material which is a build-up of chemicals, mucus, stale faeces and toxins accumulated over the decades and which blocks the uptake of nutrients and hinders the removal of toxins through the colon wall. It is often called 'mucoid plaque'.

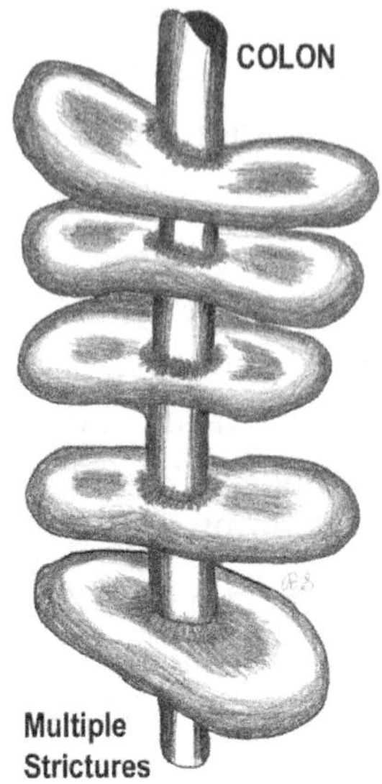

A few months later I released one amazing motion, which at the time made me feel quite ill. It was in the shape of multiple segments and strictures from my sigmoid/descending colon *(see sketch, right)*.

The photos *(below)* show further plaque removal. The stool released in 2007 was rubbery, elastic, shiny, smooth and dark maroon in colour, looking similar to the outside of a liver, but emulating the contours of my bowel — it was probably from my sigmoid or cecum section of my colon.

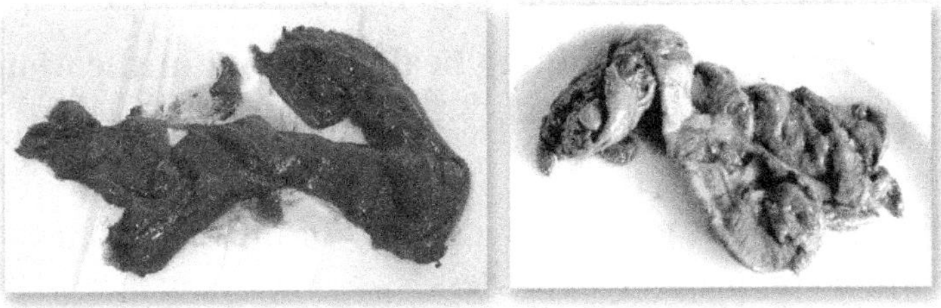

Mucoid plaque removed from my colon wall in 2007 (left) and 2011 (right)

The photo on the far right is a stool I removed in 2011 and again shows an elastic, rubbery covering containing most of the faeces. This stool was much lighter, almost a dark yellow in colour and was flattened in some areas, possibly from my sigmoid area.

I believe if I had not relieved my constipation, this plaque would still be residing inside my colon today, hindering my body's ability to uptake nutrients and release toxins. Removing this plaque has allowed my body to begin to heal itself.

Eyesight Improvement

In the year 2000, at 44 years, I began to develop headaches when reading or using the computer. So, I had my eyes tested and purchased reading glasses costing $210. I wore them for about five years until I started to develop headaches again whilst

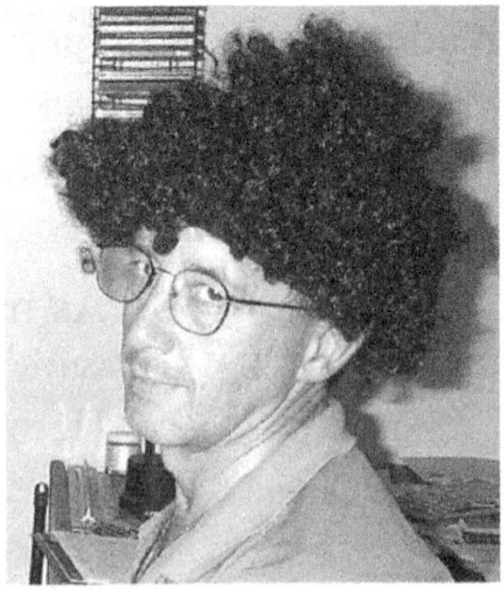

2002 when I wore glasses (and hair — yes it's a wig)

reading. As a result, I took my glasses off and very rarely use them now at the age of 64.

My eyesight has improved following my detoxing, exercise, nutrition and wholefood supplementation. I also started taking quality omega-3 regularly. I found that when you eat poorly and therefore store toxins, fat and sugar float in the bloodstream as small toxic particles of fat and tend to clog the finest capillaries first. This is generally known as circulation or fluid retention problems.

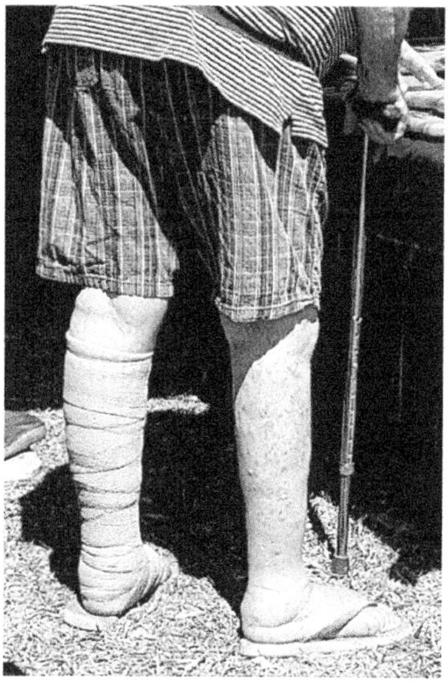

Many of the finest capillaries are in the feet and hands and when circulation slows, we can end up with cold feet and hands. Many years of toxins in the blood, which blocks capillaries, leads to purple-coloured feet and ankles with abscesses that won't heal — often resulting in amputations as diabetes or cancer sets in, as with my father-in-law.

However, some of the finest capillaries are also in the retina of the eyes and when blocked by fat in the blood (especially from fructose and carbs), excess omega-6 and toxins, eyesight declines. This is commonly known as macular degeneration, again a symptom of diabetes, which can ultimately lead to blindness.

The sickness industrial complex may tell you that from the age of around 45, it's common to find it difficult to read small print, requiring glasses. Because of my experience, I feel this is more a result of clogged capillaries built up from decades of consuming carbs, sugar and omega-6 (i.e. not enough omega-3), which can be reversed through a change in lifestyle — as I did. Smoking significantly accelerates eye problems through the same blocked-capillary process.

I did notice that during periods of significant detoxing, my eyesight temporarily diminished, and my eyes were sore and watering, but there was an overall improvement afterwards.

Sometimes during a detox, I find that for about one hour, the centre of my vision becomes blurred or missing, and I can't read the words I try to focus upon. Over the course of an hour, the central spot turns into a whitish-transparent ring around the centre of my vision, and then moves to the outside peripheral vision before disappearing. I've had this happen occasionally during detoxes, so I know what is happening and relax into the situation.

Afterwards I may have a headache and feel a little lethargic (a sign that toxins had been shifted into my blood for release), but my eyesight was crisp, clear and improved. I conduct a coffee enema afterwards and over the ensuing hours, the lethargy goes away, and I usually feel better than ever.

Skin Cancer

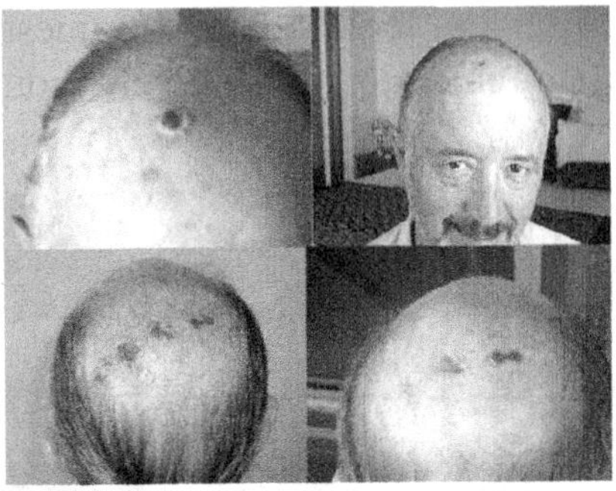

With a hairline like mine, it was probably inevitable that sunspots (skin cancers) developed, especially with my toxic system, which had been trying to eliminate through my skin as explained previously. I had one spot removed by the orthodox freezing method in 1998, but it is still irritated today when exposed to sunlight.

I had several spots across the top of my head, along my former part line — as I often failed to wear a hat as a child — which became very irritated when exposed to direct sunlight. I removed them using what is commonly called 'black salve'.

(refer to video One Answer to Cancer *at* ***www.oneanswertocancermovie.com*** *where you can find the recipe).*

I removed around ten irritations using this natural paste and have had no recurrence. I simply applied a little on each spot and covered with a Band-Aid, repeating this process three times. If the cancer is active, the natural products in the paste may trace all tentacles of the cancer and raise them to the surface forming a scab, which eventually falls out and leaves a small 'hole in the skin' which usually closes in without scarring (in my case).

Using the salve can be very painful (like having a drawing pin stuck in the skin) and can make you feel irritable and unwell during treatment, which can take three to four weeks. But I have found it beneficial over the long term.

Others have used this technique for breast and bowel cancer with success.

Again, if you have skin cancers you should seek advice from your healthcare professional. Because of issues outlined in Chapter 10, black salve is not approved for human use by government administrations in Australia but can be found overseas on the internet. If faced with a similar situation, I strongly suggest watching the video *One Answer to Cancer*, so you are more informed before visiting your healthcare provider. Ultimately it is your choice.

Through my experience I believe melanoma develop due to a dysfunctional elimination system that uses the skin (as a last resort) to expel toxins. Upon reaching the skin surface, toxins are triggered by excessive sunlight and air allowing the melanoma to activate. Again, this is my theory; perhaps soon science will catch up with my view and prove me correct? But this will only happen if Big Pharma can make money from it.

Chapter 2

Sickness and Wellness Cycles

It's not what happens to you, it's how you handle what happens that matters

You Create Your Own Reality — in Sickness or in Wellness
Since writing my first book, 'The Inside Scoop on Bowel Health', I've come to understand that a dysfunctional bowel is a consequence (symptom or result) of your choices which depend on your ongoing attitude that ultimately create your habits that build your body.

Over my years of experience and research I have found that stress is the original cause of illness, but here's the tricky bit — you cause most of your own stress through your thought patterns and resultant actions which develop into habits that construct your life.

If you aren't pleased with your current situation, take responsibility and know that where you are today is an end result of how you have chosen to handle events in your life. Your choices have created your current level of health, wealth and happiness — your life. If you don't like it; change it.

If you get anything out of this book, my subtext is: take responsibility for your life and stop relying on or blaming others for your situation.

You have a choice of how you handle every event in your life...

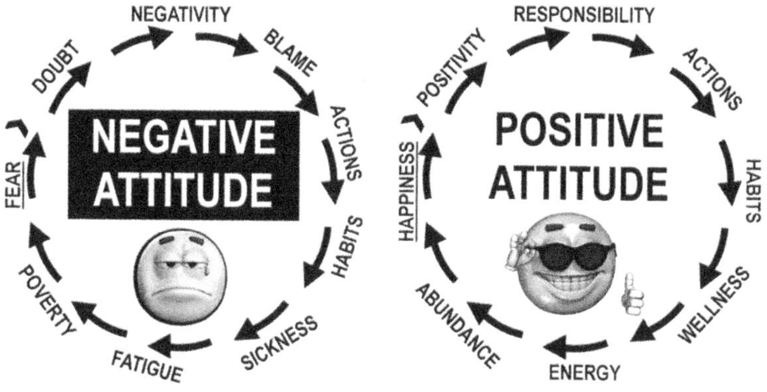

The diagrams on the following pages demonstrate this clearly. Take your time to study my diagrams. It took me many weeks of 'sage-like-thinking' to compile a complicated idea into simple diagrams to help you understand.

Understand that we are all born relatively equal and can grow into what we want to be, but through our response to what life throws at us, we progressively create our reality; positive or negative.

Go through each individual point and ask yourself where you stand firstly in the **Sickness Cycle,** then secondly, what **three things** you could do to begin your **Wellness Cycle**. Just three things to start with — that's all.

If you don't make plans and drift from day-to-day being a typical Aussie 'battler', you are more likely to end up broke and create lifestyle-related diseases like heart disease, diabetes and cancer. Your 'health span' or quality of life will be low, and your happiness will be reliant on escape addictions like alcohol, drugs, gambling, sex, sport or the internet.

On the other hand, if you **take responsibility** for your thinking, make better lifestyle choices, detox and supplement to rebuild your body cell-by-cell; you will improve your thought processes and become happier, leading to better choices and less stress, therefore will have an improved chance of creating an abundant, happy, healthy, fulfilled life.

Your body totally replaces almost all its 100 trillion cells every 120 days (4 months). Every day, around 40 billion cells die and are replaced through natural attrition. Your body will always utilise a higher quality nutrient to replace dead cells over a lower, toxic or waste nutrient or chemical – if there are enough stem cells present. Stem cells will trigger the replacement of dead cells and they will be replaced with whatever you are eating, drinking, breathing or thinking at the time. *See Acid/Alkaline section later.*

If you consistently change your thought patterns to being higher, happier and more positive for long enough, eventually you create more supportive habits, allowing the ultimate possibility of **habitual, hypnotic, positive drifting** (positive subconscious) where everything you eat is exactly what you want (because you only want health), feel fulfilled and create an amazing life that is in the flow with natural laws. **Your subconscious IS your body!**

Procrastinating?

Things will stay about the same, on the same trajectory and will continue to cost you in dollars and health, unless you make changes. You must do something different to achieve more or improve your wealth and health span.

Two Identical Cars

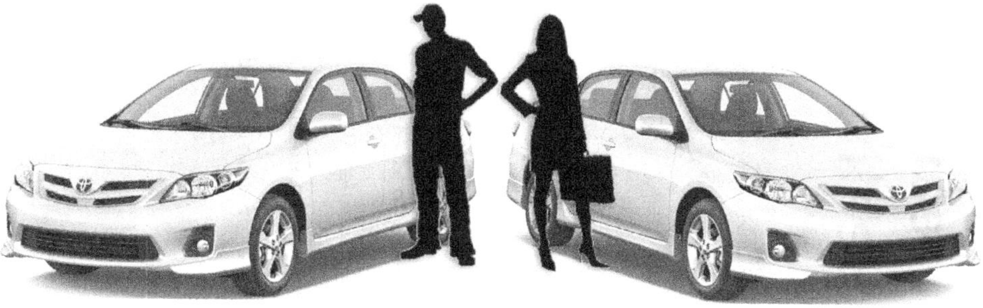

Picture two identical cars, both produced in the same factory on the same day.

One is purchased by the parents of a 17-year-old teenage 'lad' (Frankie) as a gift for finishing high school. The other is purchased by a 25-year-old woman (Trish) who has worked hard and saved for a few years to pay for her car.

Frankie, taking little responsibility for his car (because he didn't pay for it), immediately spends what little money he has on altering the wheels, suspension, exhaust and sound system. He uses the cheapest fuel and he can't afford servicing. He places stress on his car by driving it hard into corners, speeding away from lights and breaking hard at the next set. Most nights he takes his mates on joyrides around the streets, eating fast-food and leaving litter on the floor and seats and empty Coke cups in the cupholders.

Trish drives her car to and from work daily and parks it in a garage. On weekends she catches up with friends in cafés and visits family. She takes responsibility for her new car by using premium fuel, has the car serviced twice yearly. She never eats in her car and drives carefully because she knows how much it costs for repairs.

Which car will last the longest, be cheaper to run and need least repairs?

Our bodies are similar. Run them on chronic stress and fatigue, fill them with junk-food, alcohol, drugs and medication, drink little water and avoid exercise… you will pay the price in dollars, happiness and health.

You have a choice to take responsibility, be at peace, exercise regularly and eat and drink good quality food and water, with just a few social drinks occasionally. You are rewarded or pay a price for everything you do, positive and negative and your body, life and finances will distort to reflect your choices – karma.

Your health is not a debt you can cancel; your body eventually collects.

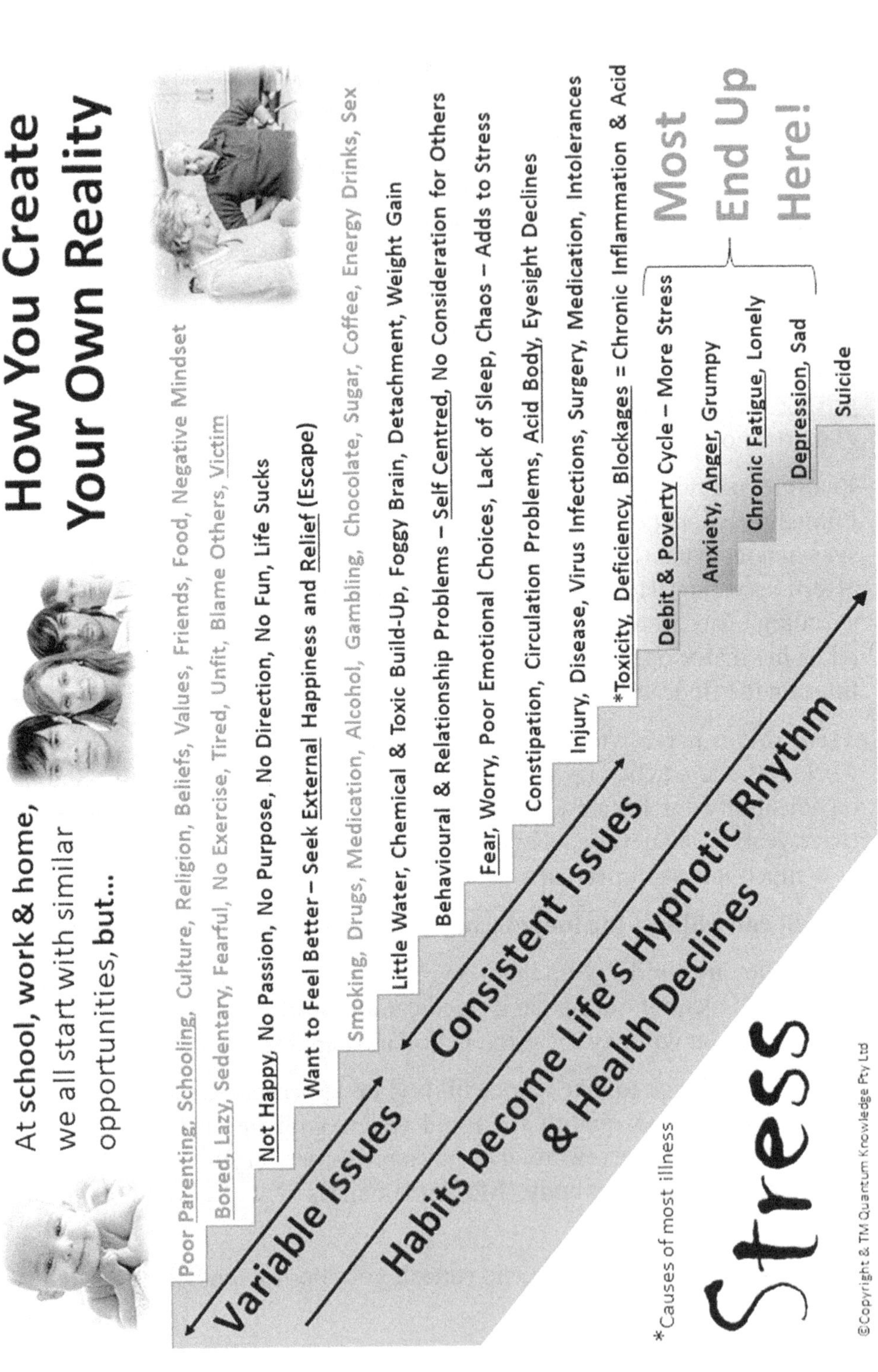
How You Create Your Own Reality
At school, work & home, we all start with similar opportunities, but...
Poor Parenting, Schooling, Culture, Religion, Beliefs, Values, Friends, Food, Negative Mindset
Bored, Lazy, Sedentary, Fearful, No Exercise, Tired, Unfit, Blame Others, Victim
Not Happy, No Passion, No Purpose, No Direction, No Fun, Life Sucks
Want to Feel Better – Seek External Happiness and Relief (Escape)
Smoking, Drugs, Medication, Alcohol, Gambling, Chocolate, Sugar, Coffee, Energy Drinks, Sex
Little Water, Chemical & Toxic Build-Up, Foggy Brain, Detachment, Weight Gain
Behavioural & Relationship Problems – Self Centred, No Consideration for Others
Fear, Worry, Poor Emotional Choices, Lack of Sleep, Chaos – Adds to Stress
Constipation, Circulation Problems, Acid Body, Eyesight Declines
Injury, Disease, Virus Infections, Surgery, Medication, Intolerances
*Toxicity, Deficiency, Blockages = Chronic Inflammation & Acid
Debit & Poverty Cycle – More Stress
Anxiety, Anger, Grumpy
Chronic Fatigue, Lonely
Depression, Sad
Suicide
Most End Up Here!
Variable Issues
Consistent Issues
Habits become Life's Hypnotic Rhythm & Health Declines
*Causes of most illness
Stress
©Copyright & TM Quantum Knowledge Pty Ltd

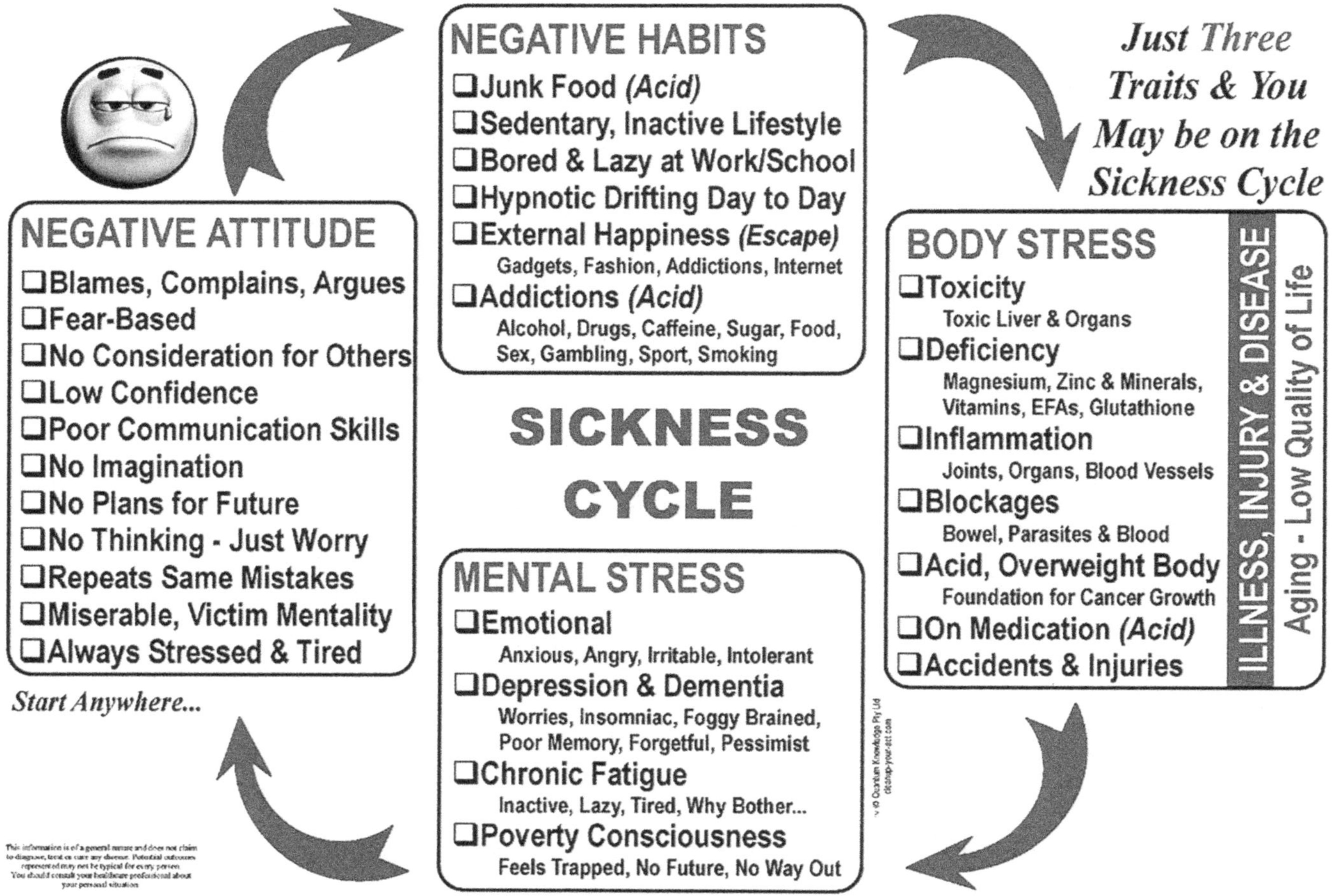
NEGATIVE ATTITUDE
❑Blames, Complains, Argues
❑Fear-Based
❑No Consideration for Others
❑Low Confidence
❑Poor Communication Skills
❑No Imagination
❑No Plans for Future
❑No Thinking - Just Worry
❑Repeats Same Mistakes
❑Miserable, Victim Mentality
❑Always Stressed & Tired
Start Anywhere...
NEGATIVE HABITS
❑Junk Food (Acid)
❑Sedentary, Inactive Lifestyle
❑Bored & Lazy at Work/School
❑Hypnotic Drifting Day to Day
❑External Happiness (Escape)
Gadgets, Fashion, Addictions, Internet
❑Addictions (Acid)
Alcohol, Drugs, Caffeine, Sugar, Food, Sex, Gambling, Sport, Smoking
SICKNESS CYCLE
Just Three Traits & You May be on the Sickness Cycle
BODY STRESS
❑Toxicity
Toxic Liver & Organs
❑Deficiency
Magnesium, Zinc & Minerals, Vitamins, EFAs, Glutathione
❑Inflammation
Joints, Organs, Blood Vessels
❑Blockages
Bowel, Parasites & Blood
❑Acid, Overweight Body
Foundation for Cancer Growth
❑On Medication (Acid)
❑Accidents & Injuries
ILLNESS, INJURY & DISEASE
Aging - Low Quality of Life
MENTAL STRESS
❑Emotional
Anxious, Angry, Irritable, Intolerant
❑Depression & Dementia
Worries, Insomniac, Foggy Brained, Poor Memory, Forgetful, Pessimist
❑Chronic Fatigue
Inactive, Lazy, Tired, Why Bother...
❑Poverty Consciousness
Feels Trapped, No Future, No Way Out
This information is of a general nature and does not claim to diagnose, treat or cure any disease. Potential outcomes represented may not be typical for every person. You should consult your healthcare professional about your personal situation.

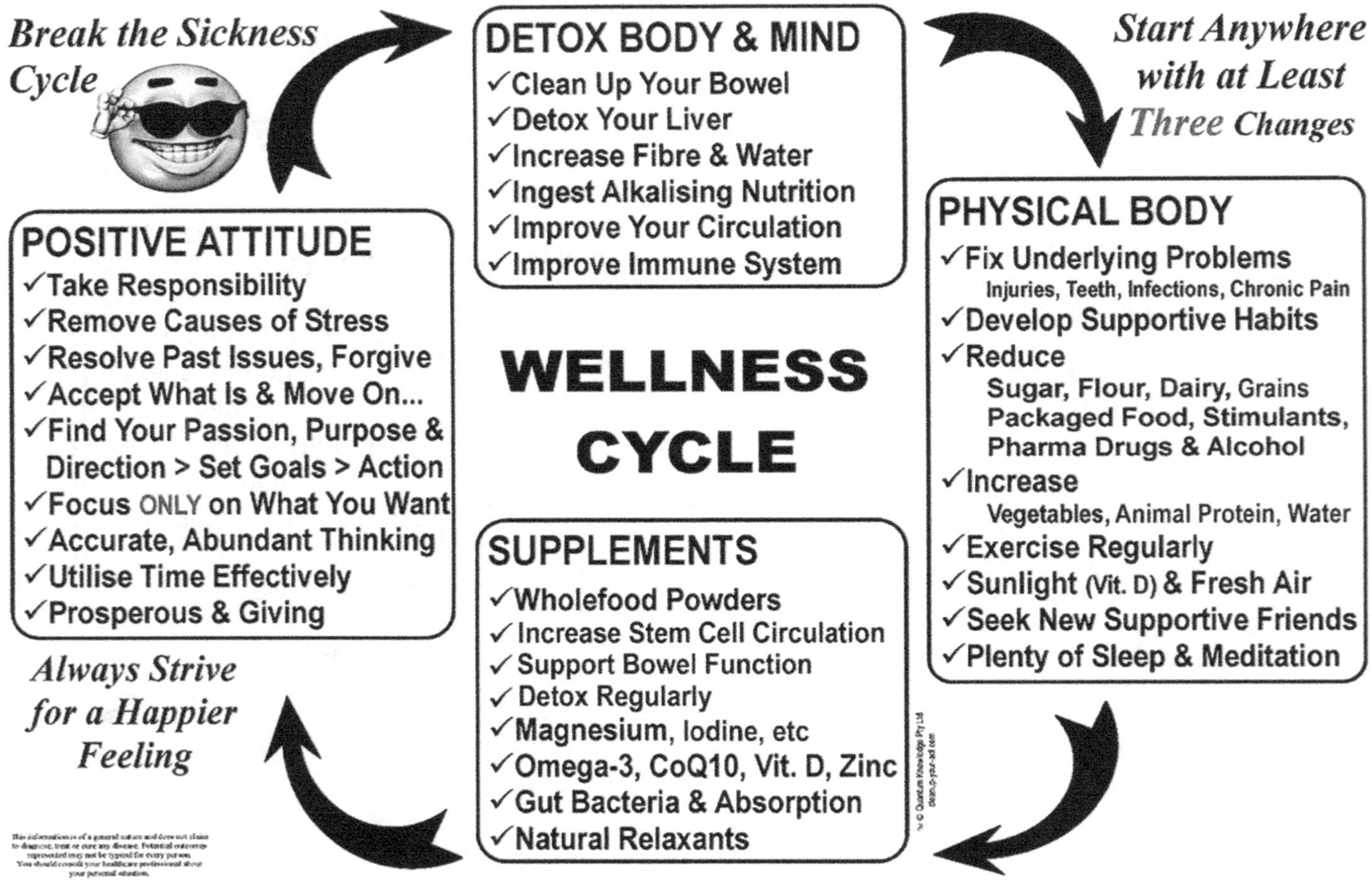
Break the Sickness Cycle
DETOX BODY & MIND
✓Clean Up Your Bowel
✓Detox Your Liver
✓Increase Fibre & Water
✓Ingest Alkalising Nutrition
✓Improve Your Circulation
✓Improve Immune System
Start Anywhere with at Least Three Changes
POSITIVE ATTITUDE
✓Take Responsibility
✓Remove Causes of Stress
✓Resolve Past Issues, Forgive
✓Accept What Is & Move On...
✓Find Your Passion, Purpose & Direction > Set Goals > Action
✓Focus ONLY on What You Want
✓Accurate, Abundant Thinking
✓Utilise Time Effectively
✓Prosperous & Giving
WELLNESS CYCLE
PHYSICAL BODY
✓Fix Underlying Problems
Injuries, Teeth, Infections, Chronic Pain
✓Develop Supportive Habits
✓Reduce
Sugar, Flour, Dairy, Grains
Packaged Food, Stimulants,
Pharma Drugs & Alcohol
✓Increase
Vegetables, Animal Protein, Water
✓Exercise Regularly
✓Sunlight (Vit. D) & Fresh Air
✓Seek New Supportive Friends
✓Plenty of Sleep & Meditation
SUPPLEMENTS
✓Wholefood Powders
✓Increase Stem Cell Circulation
✓Support Bowel Function
✓Detox Regularly
✓Magnesium, Iodine, etc
✓Omega-3, CoQ10, Vit. D, Zinc
✓Gut Bacteria & Absorption
✓Natural Relaxants
Always Strive for a Happier Feeling

Attitude — the Only Thing You have Absolute Control Over

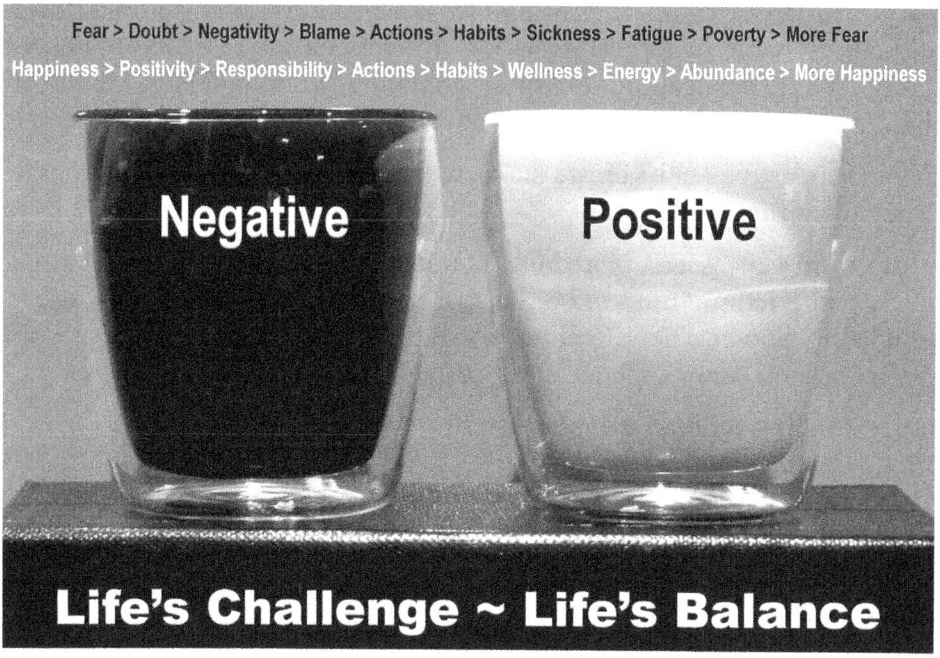
Fear > Doubt > Negativity > Blame > Actions > Habits > Sickness > Fatigue > Poverty > More Fear
Happiness > Positivity > Responsibility > Actions > Habits > Wellness > Energy > Abundance > More Happiness
Negative
Positive
Life's Challenge ~ Life's Balance

We are conditioned to believe a positive or negative attitude depends on our perception of a glass being half full or half empty.

This has blinded us to the possibility that there may be a much more abundant view of two glasses, one full of black negativity and the other full of white positivity — when in balance.

Nature's laws require opposing forces for resistance to build strength for learning and growth, therefore the negative glass has a purpose. Negative aspects and thoughts should alert us to possible danger, instigating thought, triggering us to do something different — avoid injury; learn something.

When out of balance, we begin to work against nature's laws and become sick, worry, develop debt, argue, blame others and create stress, rather than take responsibility for the void we created in our positive glass.

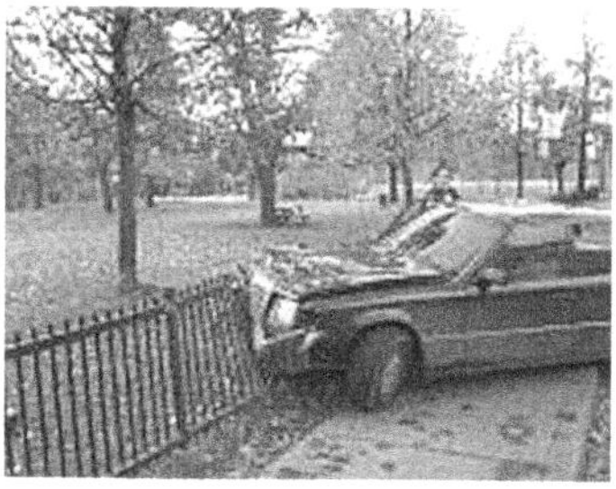

We allow ourselves to drift along in a hypnotic, negative (grey) trance chocked full of unsupportive habits (undisciplined subconscious body); causing us to run off-track, crashing into fences, repairing the damage and starting over again. Every such incident is a waste of **three times** your resources; your first effort, the repair effort and what you could have been doing to positively build your life instead of repairing.

This grey hypnotic drift leaves us unfulfilled, creating cravings in an effort to feel better (escape or forget), resulting in overindulgence of food, alcohol, tobacco, drugs, medication, sex, sport, gambling, work, holidays, fanatically religious, obsessive, the next Guru — anything to escape our inner emptiness.

Such unsupportive habits create sickness and diseased, unhealthy bodies — we begin our **Sickness Cycle**.

Negative influences are incredibly dominant, from our overly emotional friends with victim attitudes, politicians, institutions, religions, lamestream media entertainment, news and advertising. 98% of external influences are negative, which compound our inner, negative thoughts and feelings.

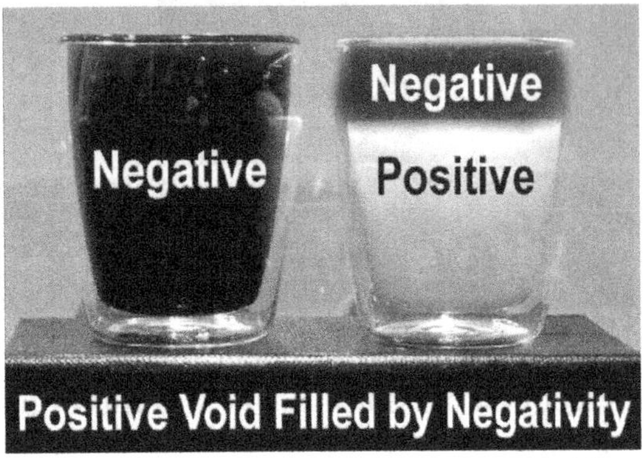

Positive Void Filled by Negativity

To negate this continual external barrage of negativity, we need to keep our **positive glass totally full — all the time**. Make it a habit to **catch yourself** upon any negative thought creeping in and instantly turn it around to a positive. Even having a neutral thought will leave a positive void that **WILL be filled** by something, most likely negativity.

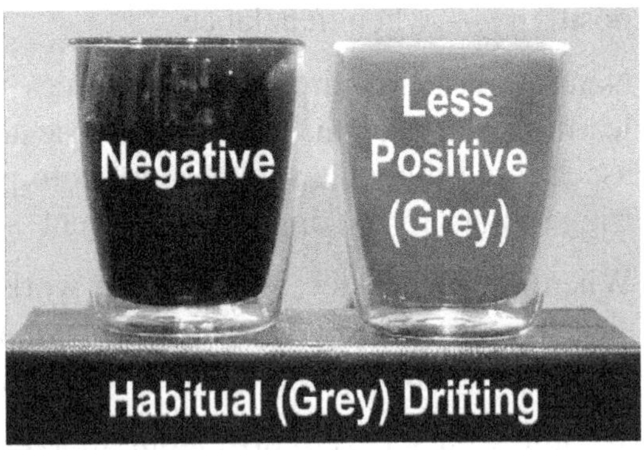

Habitual (Grey) Drifting

Lack of positivity (i.e. any negative thought) will create a void in the positive glass, allowing some negativity to creep in and fill the void. Eventually black negativity combines with white positivity, greying (clouding) our thinking, supporting negative emotional responses, making it difficult to purify your thoughts and understand our values.

Fear is the vehicle used by negativity to contaminate your positive glass, and **doubt** fuels fear. **FEAR of ANYTHING,** - relationships, heights, darkness, death, the unknown, spiders, etc. Any fear will allow doubt in, which will attract black, negative thinking (worry). When you're thinking negatively, you cannot be positive; therefore, you create a greater void in the positive glass which will be filled by more negativity, displacing some of the white positive (love) energy. Like a blackhole, nature will always fill a void and that's why you might feel empty, unfulfilled — in real terms.

Do this for days, weeks and months, then you progressively become confused and negative; off colour - feeling blue. Doctors may diagnose depression, anxiety, etc. and refer you to a psychiatrist or prescribe antidepressants, sedatives or sleeping pills to relieve symptoms, but won't fix the cause.

The secret to keeping your white positive glass full is having fulfillment and meaningfulness in your life, which leads to purpose and direction. Working backwards, finding your passion, having a definite purpose (seeking meaningfulness and fulfillment) and therefore reasons to be positive and proactive is a good place to start.

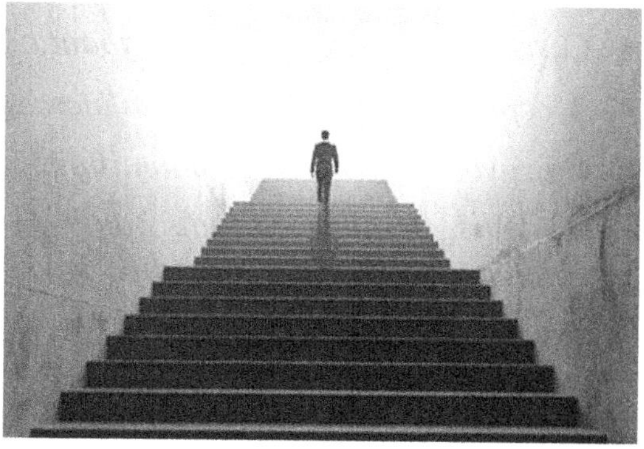

Always make your next step a higher step, **upstairs to the penthouse** (happiness), rather than downstairs to the basement where there is nothing to see or do (depression). It takes more effort to climb stairs, but that's called exercise and will eventually make you stronger.

Emotional Memory

Fear is born from initial events that spark **emotions**. A single event at (say) three-years-old (that you may not even remember), can be the trigger of the majority of your fears for the rest of your life. Stress issues facing your parents or grandparents at the time of conception, can also reflect in your DNA and energy too as shown in survivors of prison camps in WW2. The good news is that you can release your fears and emotions within 30 minutes…

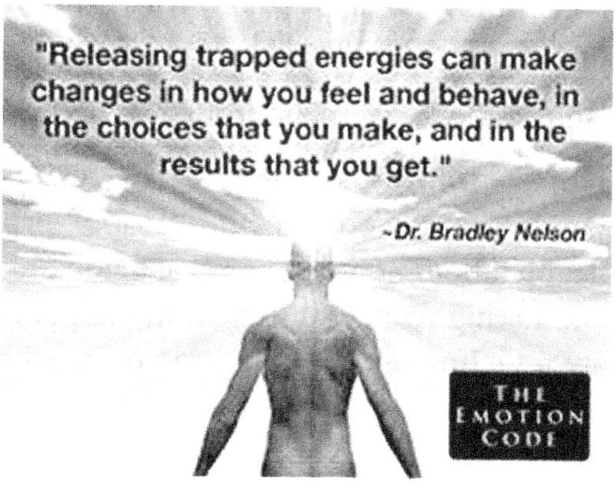

This area of research is amazing and <u>almost magical</u>☺; I was sceptical until I experienced a session. When a negative event happens, emotions are trapped in a specific organ or area of the body via the nervous system and through the release of these trapped emotions, you can clear up numerous health issues and release triggers for cravings, unhappiness, anger, etc. **Dr Bradley Nelson** has conducted some amazing work on **The**

Emotion Code and **The Body Code** at www.drbradleynelson.com *(see resources section in the back of this book for practitioners)*

Fear – the Master Disabler

How do you relinquish fear? Isaac Lidsky has some other suggestions…

- *Hold yourself accountable for every moment, thought, emotion and action*
- *See beyond your fears*
- *Recognise your assumptions*
- *Harness your internal strength*
- *Silence your internal critic*
- *Correct your misconceptions about luck and success*
- *Accept your strengths and weaknesses and understand the difference*
- *Open your heart to your bountiful blessings*

Your fears, critics, villains and heroes – they are your excuses, rationalisation, shortcuts, justifications and surrender. They are fictions you perceive as reality.

Choose to see through them. Choose to let them go. You are the creator of your reality. With that empowerment, comes complete responsibility.

- *What do you fear?*
- *What lies do you tell yourself?*
- *How do you embellish your truth and write your own fictions?*
- *What reality are you creating for yourself in your career, personal life, relationships and in your heart and soul.*

Fear exacts a momentous toll *in missed opportunities and unrealised potential. Fear engenders insecurity and mistrust where you seek fulfilment and connection through the prism of insecurity and disconnection.*

Bottom line; be true to yourself, be kind, giving and take responsibility.

Hope – Don't Get Sucked In!

Don't get sucked into the "Hope" propaganda and paradigm. If you think deeply about hope, hope means you aren't truly accepting your current reality and taking responsibility to make plans and create change. Hope means you are a victim of your past and you must continue on your path and hope things will change. But things can't change, as your victim thought forms create your reality, therefore you have no hope.

Politicians, finance, media, entertainment and the sickness industrial complex have used the 'hope tactic' for decades and have been very effective in creating a society of victims – some might call them consumers.

Depression is NOT a disease, but is created by progressive negative steps downstairs, and it ALWAYS starts with your first step down, followed by your next. Gossip, judgment, selfish thinking (me, me, me) and a subservient, victim attitude is the starting point as often portrayed on 'reality' TV shows.

The original thought for depression is, "I'm not worthy, I'm not enough" often cemented emotionally during childhood. That encourages you to want to be something or someone because you feel like you're nothing and no one. If you have this thought pattern, you can never achieve what you want because you know you don't deserve it, so you struggle and get depressed.

On top of thought aspects, I believe many depressive mental states like dementia, bi-polar, Alzheimer's and Parkinson's are born of a toxic body which begins in the bowel with our lifestyle choices.

Meanwhile, progressively making better lifestyle choices and supplementing to detox and fix nutrient imbalances will assist on a physical level. As you will read later, the clarity and happiness of your mind originates through proper levels of magnesium chloride absorbed through the skin and from the bowel, where 95% of your body's serotonin (used in the brain) is produced.

Very few people independently think before acting. Generally, we blindly follow old habits (our subconscious mind which becomes our body) and go with the comfortable norm. Governments, bureaucracies, corporations, institutions and lamestream media all welcome us to be part of their system, so (as a population) we are easier to control and sell things to, even if their things are not good for us.

Systems have their positive aspects, like utilising credit cards to make purchases, however, when used without accurate thinking, can leak negativity into the positive glass, allowing you to increase debt and live beyond your means. The negative side of debt is that you relinquish control and begin to mindlessly drift further away from being in control. You become subservient.

You can relate your need to take action as being similar to arriving at a T-intersection on the road. You have choices, which, if not accurately thought through, you will go the same old comfortable, habitual way.

Thinking brings in the realisation that you actually have a **minimum of three choices; turn left, turn right or do nothing.** Habitually doing nothing is often your first choice which has ongoing consequences. Just a little accurate (unemotional) thinking will reveal other opportunities hitherto unconsidered.

Whenever you are feeling a little down, simply change your focus to something that makes you feel a little happier. Perhaps some comedy, positive music, a hobby, walking, a supportive friend, etc. Be careful not to confuse striving to feel happier with old, comfortable, unsupportive habits.

Studies have shown that synthesising happiness (introducing or visualising happiness) changes neuro-patterns in the frontal lobe of the brain and creates positive chemicals that actually change your attitude and habits in a positive direction over time. Simply sitting with positive, open body-language for two minutes, changes neuro-patterns in the brain too.

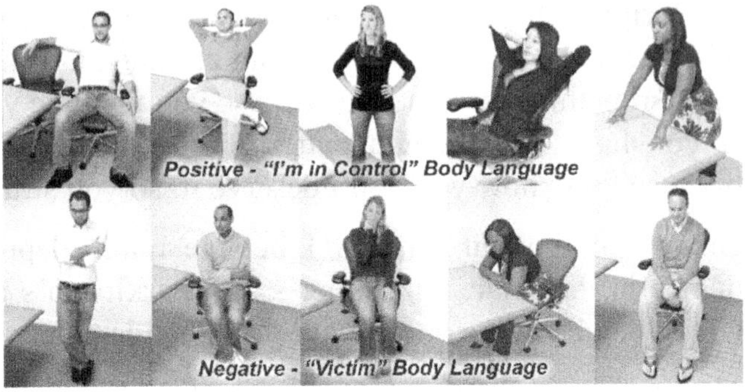
Positive - "I'm in Control" Body Language
Negative - "Victim" Body Language

By doing this every time you are feeling down, your actions will keep your white positive glass full, so there is no chance of encouraging the grey mix.

Choices made in a happier mood are always better choices. This will lead to less repairs, more supportive action, more control, healthier thoughts and you begin your **Wellness Cycle.**

Do whatever you are passionate about for your income and you will never have to work another day in your life. Become happy and your problems will go away.

Dung Beetles and Tall Poppies

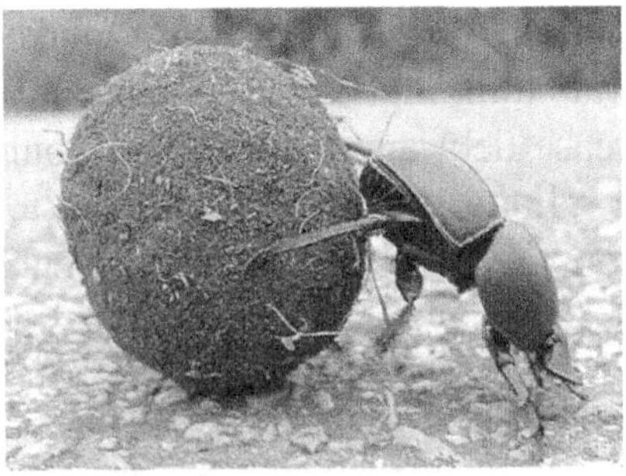

You are where you find yourself at this moment, because of one overriding truth... Every choice you have made to this point, has created where you are today. You are totally responsible; no one else is to blame.

Sure, we're all dealt a hand to play from the card-deck of life, but it's your attitude and how you play those cards that creates either an exciting life or a miserable existence. Even not making a choice is a choice to submit to mediocrity.

The **Dung Beetle Principle** is where a person continually returns to roll the same old ball of crap throughout life because it's familiar, safe, comfortable and, *"that's what I do"*.

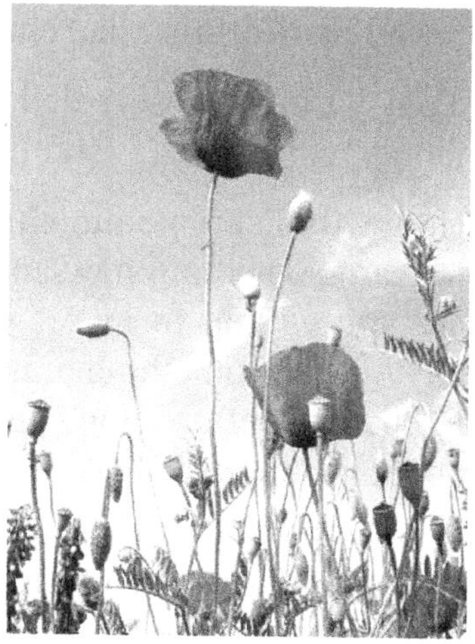

Change frightens many of us as there are risks involved and, in Australia especially, you should not stick your head above the rest and shine, exhibiting your best! If you do so, your mates might cut you down and bring you back to their level, commonly known as the **Tall Poppy Syndrome**.

To escape and justify our submission to mediocrity, we occasionally indulge in distractions and addictions like alcohol, gambling, blame, footy and shopping in an effort to have a perception of enjoyment/escape.

If you want things to change in your life, **you must change**. Events, opportunities and people surrounding your life will not change unless you move out of your comfort zone and make a move towards a better future.

It's not what you do, and it's not even what you give away that matters. It's what you eventually become as a result of your choices that matters. So, ensure your choices and actions match what you want to become.

First thing you can do is to ask yourself, **'what really makes me happy?'** Find your passion, set goals and make plans to pursue your livelihood through your passion.

Your **passion** may be a specific skill; it might be an overall feeling of wellbeing when doing something or when certain events happen. Identify such feelings and link them to your work. Passion is when you are doing something, and your sense of time disappears.

Keep focused on your goals, write them down and experience them in your mind regularly. Don't focus on today's boring mess, instead focus on where you 'will be' in the future and live those emotions now. Accept where you are for the moment, be as happy as you can and focus on your higher goals.

Secondly consider the people with whom you **associate** and from whom you receive **advice**. Are they successful? Have they achieved something similar to what you want out of life? Would you ask a bricklayer financial advice or ask an accountant to lay bricks?

You should especially trust advice from someone who has actually experienced what you might be about to launch yourself into. Watch out for armchair experts or university graduates who have only learnt from professors who are told what to say and are teaching from a book rather than experience. Check out the agenda of the people who wrote the professor's book. This goes for **all institutions**, like churches, support groups, etc.; not just universities.

Your future is closely tied to the people with whom you associate - friends, family, colleagues, work, education, groups, clubs, churches, etc.

How willing are you to **change and learn**? What are you willing to give up to learn something new and do something different? What time and money are you willing to invest into your change? If you are not willing to give anything up something or invest any time, money or effort, you are not willing to change (yet), so don't complain and go back to rolling dung, but be happy about it – and STOP WHINGING!

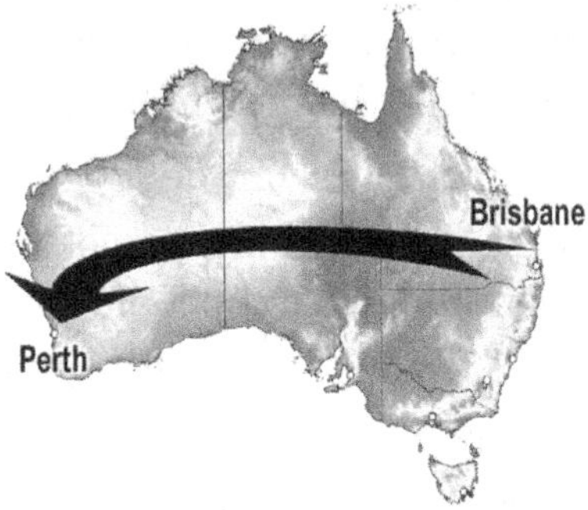

Your **attitude and thinking** are 99% of your future. **Thinking precedes every action**. Good thinking (and advice from someone experienced) can save a lot of time, effort and money. For example, if your goal is to travel from Brisbane to Perth (or New York to LA) and without thinking, you hopped in your car and started driving west. Your action would be immediate, purposeful, positive and heading in the right direction, but would take you five days, four nights' accommodation, plus $1000 in fuel.

However, just an hour's thought, research and planning would reveal that you could fly direct from Brisbane to Perth in just five hours from just $260.

Massive planning followed by massive action is the key.

As you make changes and learn new things, understand that there are four stages to learning:

1. **Ignorance** (you don't know that you don't know)
2. **Information** (you now know something about it)
3. **Knowledge** (you put what you know into practice)
4. **Wisdom** (you habitually do it without thinking)

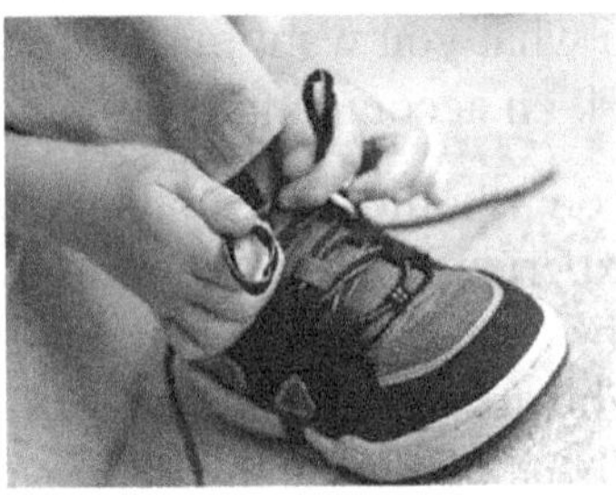

You can easily relate this to learning to tie your shoelaces as a child. You started not knowing there was any issues with laces at all. Then you found that tied shoelaces were more comfortable and safer. Your parents showed you how to tie your laces and repeatedly stayed with you until you could consciously do it yourself. Now you can tie your laces whilst talking to someone else and not even thinking about it.

Understanding the current stage of your learning process relieves most frustration and fear, giving you more confidence.

And lastly, above all, as much as possible, be **happy and grateful** for your current situation. Know that change is in the winds. Things will be different soon. Be at peace with current events and accept what is.

If you find yourself a little depressed, listen to music, go for a walk, think of happy events from the past or watching something funny will often help lift your mood. I know this is repeated, but it gets in, it gets in, it gets in.

Through the above techniques, nature's **law of attraction** will bring situations towards you that match your attitude.

If in the past, your thoughts have been negative, negative outcomes have often resulted. Now that you have happy, positive thoughts, more positive people and outcomes are likely because that is your new focus. A truly happy, positive person with purpose and direction doesn't look for a drug dealer.

The thing that will differentiate you from your current friends in five years is that you made small changes and practiced those changes every day. **This is the secret to changing your life** and making your dreams come true.

For example, if you eat a piece of cake today, will it make a difference to your life tomorrow? Probably not. If you ate a piece of cake every day, would it make a difference at the end of the week? Maybe a little. If you continued eating a piece of cake every day for a month, you would begin to notice weight gain and lower energy. By the end of the year, you will be several kilograms fatter and unhealthier.

This works in reverse too. If you don't eat your piece of cake today, you won't notice a difference tomorrow, etc., etc. By the end of the year, you will be several kilograms thinner. Sort of a sustained, long-term instant karma – consequences for actions.

Focus on the above foundations every day, and the scoreboard of life (health, wealth and happiness) will look after itself. ☺

Why Aren't We Thinking?

Reflecting back to my high school days in the early 1970s, I recall cherry picking all summer and receiving a $200 cheque for my efforts (about $1,000 today). I set my goals on buying a writing desk and trundled into Walton's department store, handing over my cheque as payment and expecting change. However, the salesman politely informed me that he could not accept my cheque and I would need to go to my bank and make a deposit, wait five days for it to clear, then withdraw the cash and pay for my desk that way.

I remember exclaiming with frustration, "Why wasn't I taught this at school?" I spent months learning logarithms which I have never used since but wasn't taught basic life-skills like banking!

Recently I had the opportunity to chat with several teachers and students from a large public school on the Gold Coast in Queensland, Australia and they lamented their frustration at the education system too.

The word "educate" originates from Latin where 'educe' means to bring out and develop a latent condition from within. Our current education system operates in reverse and was developed from the top down to suit industry and management systems, moulding students into industry's needs.

Students are rewarded for learning how to memorise and recite information in order to pass exams, upon which the school and teachers are also rewarded with more funding and wage rises. The present assessment-based system is subjective and fragmented leaving large gaps in students' knowledge. What is required is a holistic, inquiry-based system which allows students to become critical **THINKERS** not just copy and paste robots - future rednecks.

Students are not taught via the passage of learning from **ignorance > information > knowledge > wisdom.** Knowledge and wisdom develop through practical utilisation (practice and benefits) of information and are often left out of the process.

The students I spoke with stated they spent many weeks recently rehearsing for their NAPLAN (National Assessment Program – Literacy and Numeracy) exams and thus, their school scored well and should receive improved funding.

One student quoted a teacher saying, "You will probably never use this, however it's in the curriculum and I've got to teach you, so let's all just get through it so we can get to the interesting stuff."

The teachers are frustrated too, being forced to teach a curriculum they know is mostly meaningless to the majority of students. This means students are bored, misbehaving, distracted, disillusioned and depressed about their future.

This extends into university and college where young adults weighed down with HECs debits of $100,000 or so and family expectations, struggle to find enthusiasm in their chosen vocation. Then they experience difficulty finding employment in their chosen field because they don't have the experience, just a diploma or degree like everyone else.

The quality of teachers coming out of our universities has also declined. Forty years ago, you had to be in the top 10% of the state and have a literacy course as part of your degree. Today they can have an OP (Overall Position) score of around 13-19 (depending on the university). Low wages provide poor quality teachers, provide poor quality education and dull citizens who just follow the system because that's all they know - the dung beetle principle. Also, most teachers go from school, to school (university), then go back to school to teach. They have little real-world experience other than academia.

Of course, there is always going to be the need for basics of reading, writing, maths and science. Beyond that, students should be directed towards fulfilling their passion through developing skills to suit their passion through vocation. Lessons should be directed **by the student's interests,** rather than **at them**.

If a student has a fascination with insects, they should be steered towards the biology grouping, numbers towards calculus, artistic towards creative, puzzles toward physics, plants toward environmental/agriculture, ethical/righteous toward law, etc. I'm not the expert here, but there can only be (say) 20 or so groupings that would suit 95% of students' fascination areas. Within this system there needs to be curriculum settings and criteria that should be taught and checked along the way via self-managed inspection system that can't be corrupted.

Along with this, students need to understand our economic and political systems too, so they can ask questions of leaders and know their rights.

Imaginative ideas are going to come from independently thinking, confident individuals who can sell their ideas. At the moment, we are producing a lot of children who are only able to ask, "Would you like fries with that?"☹

Beyond education, but relevant, is **parenting**. We can't blame the education system for a lack of **'tough love, routine, security and consequences for actions'** parenting. There is a myriad of books available on this topic to help guide parents. We especially like Steve Biddulph's guidance and Rudolph Steiner's education principles which we utilised with our children.

If Australia wants to be a world-leader over the next century, we need to have genuine reform of the whole education system, not just the funding, facilities and resources. Currently, Australia is ranked below the OECD average for education assessment, where we used to be ranked second.

For two years, we once interacted with a high-profile university professor who was on the board that set the curriculum for Queensland schools (the state that is falling behind most in Australia). This guy was so dry, detached, inconsiderate, had high expectations and few social skills. His own children were drug addicts and suicidal – and he was helping direct the future of five million people, but he was 'qualified'.

Following are a few suggestions on how we could better serve our students from the bottom up, where the child learns to find his/her passion and is fed the necessary tools to pursue their direction in life...

Suggestions for a better curriculum:

- How to think critically, accurately and solve problems
- Ideas are an evolution, teach them to think logically, discuss and expand concepts
- The difference between failure and defeat
- How to make decisions promptly and take responsibility for their choices
- Question everything they don't understand and rely on their own judgement
- How to build relationships and communicate needs and feelings in a positive manner
- Channelling emotions for positive outcomes
- How to sell and meet your customer's needs
- Utilise activity-based methods making lessons interesting and interactive
- How to budget and organise money & time
- How the banking system works and how to avoid debt
- How to find their passion, set goals, plan strategies, act and review
- The real consequences of their lifestyle choices: health, wealth and happiness
- The value of self-control and how habits evolve - positive or negative
- Teach them the dangers and consequences of mindless drifting without thinking
- Intelligence without morals is extremely dangerous

14 Principles for Health, Wealth and Happiness

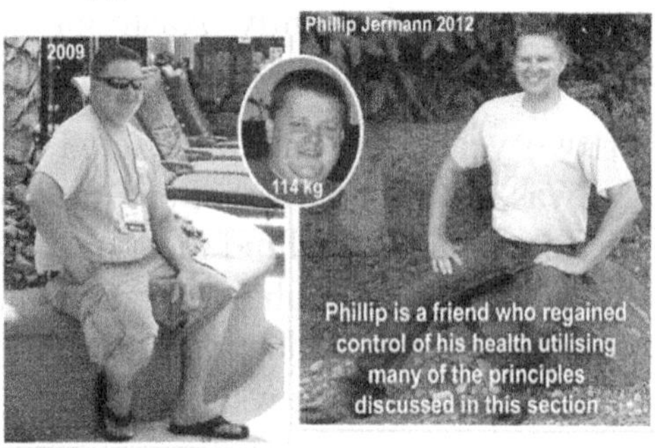
2009
Phillip Jermann 2012
114 kg
Phillip is a friend who regained control of his health utilising many of the principles discussed in this section

I have found several core aspects of life that, if pursued consistently, will make a considerable impact on your health and wealth. Most of these principles are detailed later in this book. I have purposely repeated just a few points because it's the same basic foundations again and again and often, if you read the ideas in a different context, finally the penny might drop.

1. Firstly, gain control over your thoughts and reduce **stress**. Your level of **stress impacts your body negatively, more than your actions or what you eat or drink.** Stress, worry and fear leads to poor cognitive choices, further compounding most situations. If you are continually stressed, your adrenal glands will constantly produce cortisol, an extremely acid hormone (2.4 pH), and cancer thrives in an acid environment. Stress alone causes disease.

How Does STRESS Impact Physically on the Body?

Making up each strand of DNA in every cell of the body are **chromosomes** and at the end of each chromosome are **telomeres**. Every time cells divide during their natural attrition-growth process, chromosomes divide, and they break off at the telomeres, slightly shortening them. Telomeres are meant to repeatedly replenish to full length again, given the right conditions.

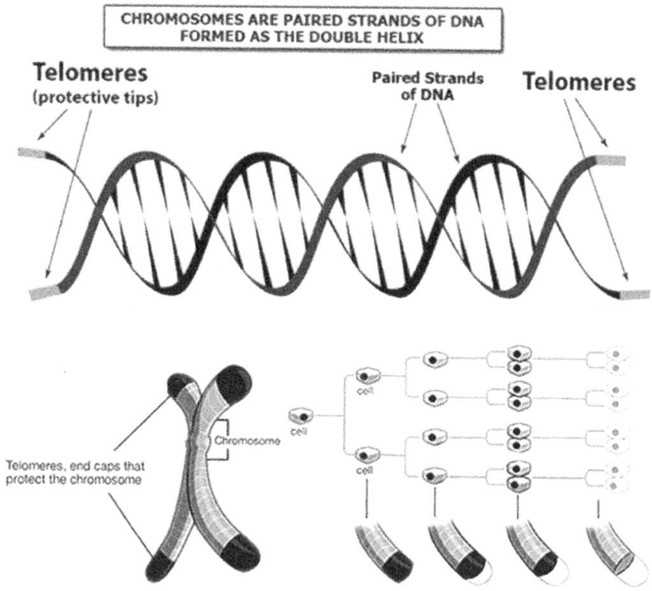

As cells divide over time...telomeres shorten, and eventually cell division stops.

The length of the telomeres governs wellbeing and how long a person lives. When the telomeres shorten to 50%, you will feel unwell, foggy-brained and chronically fatigued. When they shorten to 10% you will feel ill (diseased) and on your deathbed, and at zero you will be dead.

We call this aging, but you are not a victim of your telomeres. You have control over the length of your telomeres and can even lengthen them by providing your body with the right conditions. You can actually stop and reverse the aging process as I feel I have – *please see my photos on the first page of this book.*

The replenishment process is carried out by an enzyme called **telomerase** and its role is to heal, rejuvenate and lengthen the telomeres after it breaks away.

Guess **what activates the telomerase** enzyme and therefore rebuild telomeres?... good nutrition, exercise, stem cell circulation, supplements and heart-brain coherence (peace and happiness).

Behaviours that **fail to activate the telomerase** enzyme, therefore allow telomeres to shorten and increase aging are sugar, caffeine, stress through acidic stress hormones, alcohol, sedentary lifestyle, etc ~ all listed on the previous *'How you Create Your Own Reality" staircase diagram.*

Heart-brain coherence relates to the connect between what you do and how you experience day-to-day living, relative to where your heart really wants to be (your passion) and the direction your life is actually heading. Any conflict between your passion and purpose verses your actual life will provide chronic stress and progressive shortening of telomeres.

Fear, anger, frustration, bitterness, anxiety and conflict will cause stress and shorten telomeres. Love, consideration, kindness, compassion, empathy, gratitude, appreciation, happiness, laughter and harmony will lengthen telomeres. It's really that simple ☺

Recent research at the HeartMath Institute in California (www.heartmath.org) has shown that the heart contains about 40,000 neuro cells which have the ability to think independent of the brain. The brain receives most of its overall instructions from the heart (via the vagus nerve), and those signals are directed by your emotions, feelings and beliefs.

Connecting to Your Heart for a Happier (Stress-free) Life

Ask a question and your independently thinking heart will give you an instant answer on how it feels about a particular issue; if you stop and listen. For centuries, this has been called **intuition** and is generally an indication of the correct way to proceed, "follow your heart". Ask your brain the same question and it will go through a much slower, lengthy process of telling a story about your previous experiences, fears and doubts, logic, ego, justification, etc, before it answers.

How to Connect to Your Heart

Sit and access an extremely low vibration of 0.1 hertz for 3 minutes by:

1. **Shift your awareness from your brain to your heart.** Physically touching the heart area with your hands or place your hands in the traditional prayer position whilst touching your heart area.
2. **Slow your breathing** ~ 5 seconds in, 5 seconds out.
3. **Think about positive feelings** and/or memories that connect you to anything or anyone relating to:

- Appreciation
- Gratitude
- Care
- Compassion

You can strengthen and build your new heart-brain neuro network over about 72 hours of focus. So, do this first thing in the morning, repeatedly during the day, and at night. When you feel frustrated, angry or anxious, stop and do the above. It works instantly; you can't be angry and appreciative at the same time. You have control over your emotions. Soon you will be running your life via your heart neurons and have a far less stressful, happier life.

Taking the supplement CoQ10 daily also supports the heart and is good for a relaxed metabolism. *See 'Statins' and 'Stress and Adrenal Fatigue' later.*

Heart-Brain information is based on information presented by Gregg Braden

Stress and Sleep

Stress and a mind that is always thinking will interfere with **sleep** and if you have inadequate sleep, you compromise your immune system leaving you vulnerable to the next bug that comes along, further compounding stress. If you don't get between 7-9 hours' sleep per night, your metabolic rate may be 20% lower the next day, making you prone to store more fat. *see 'Sleep' later*

Stress can also tighten your gut and essentially screw the bowel causing **constipation** which allows your body to leach toxins continuously into your bloodstream. This is called autointoxication and is a precursor to liver disease and more.

Meanwhile, one of the **most effective stress-relieving moves** you can make today is to assess the friends and family you hang out with and ask yourself if their situation and how they relate/communicate to others is what you want to aspire towards. In five years' time, your health and prosperity (and therefore happiness) will reflect your **five closest friends and family** (even your partner), so if your current friends and family don't meet your vision for your future, stretch yourself and find more supportive people to be around.

"Before you diagnose yourself with depression or low self-esteem, first make sure you are not in fact surrounded by mundane, ego-driven idiots."

Also, consider resolving anything in your health/body that may provide chronic infections or inflammation, continually placing physical stress on the body. Issues such as teeth infections, joint inflammation, skeletal misalignment, vision and hearing issues, food intolerances, allergies, etc.

Stress and Money (your Abundance Heart Set)

Financial issues can be a major source of stress. You relationship with money and wealth is best summed up by Kyle Cease kylecease.com in his book, 'The Illusion of Money'

"Your relationship to money is just a mirror of your relationship to yourself. In fact, you don't really have a relationship to money – you only have a relationship to your thoughts about money. How you feel about money is just one expression of habitual thoughts, beliefs and stagnant emotions that you have been carrying around in your body and nervous system for years.

Fear around money is the belief that money equals security. Money has nothing to do with security. Seeing money as your only source of security is what is cutting you off from the infinite creative amazing inventive being that you are. Real security is being present in this moment – an open heart and acceptance of yourself – your awareness, appreciation for life and unconditional love – these are the real assets that make you invincible.

If you have total access to your open heart, you're already accessing the kind of internal security that most of the world is trying to achieve through money.

There is a space inside you that can't be touched by anything external. This is where you have access to true security.

You will never be able to change your feeling of insecurity by having more money. Money is never the cause of the way you feel – it's an effect. If you're broke and feel unsafe, it's more likely that you're broke because you have a deeply held belief that you are unsafe. Your business and income will almost always match what you are feeling inside. You have to find the foundation inside first."

2. Beyond the stress factor, two important issues are at the foundation of your health...

1. Most diseases are a result of chronic **toxicity and/or deficiency.**
2. Every organ and tissue in your body is made up of a series of **tubes/streams**, and if blocked (even partially), will slow circulation and may cause illness over time.

Therefore, starting with your body's largest tube, **cleaning out your bowel** should reduce the impact of toxins on your **liver**. As your liver filters all your body's blood every three minutes, it is critical that you detox consistently and there are numerous natural ways to do this, *as discussed later.*

3. Around 40 billion body cells die every day and are naturally replaced with fresh molecules whose quality depends on the number of stem cells in circulation, food, water, thoughts and absorption of nutrition. Supply quality thoughts, supplements, food and water, and you may slow down the aging process and reverse disease.

4. Everything you eat is digested by your bowel. If you eat too much **sugar**, your food will be **fermented internally** rather than digested, leading to constipation, disease, fatigue and even depression. Half the **sugar** you eat **turns to fat** within minutes of ingesting. Sugar also stimulates adrenalin and cortisol, leading to cravings and building an acid body. Sugar's fine particles of fat clog capillaries and contribute to macular degeneration, inflammation and circulation problems in the feet (diabetes).

Incidentally grain (bread, biscuits, cake and pasta) and starchy food (white potatoes) are converted into sugar by your body and is generally stored as fat too, especially if you are over 50 years.

5. Generally, an average person will absorb less than 20% of the nutrients from food ingested. The remaining 80% rots and passes through the bowel as waste. Eating **fermented food** with your meals (e.g. sauerkraut, etc.) may increase your absorption rate four-fold.

6. 80% of your immune system is within your digestive and elimination tract. Most prominent is gut bacteria and if unbalanced, will allow unfriendly bacteria to thrive and support viruses in taking over your body, often leaving you regularly ill. You can only introduce about **12-15 friendly gut bacteria** to your body through food - mostly fermented food.

7. Water quality is critical. Like our planet Earth, your body is made up of 70% water and contrary to the government line; **tap water is <u>not</u> supportive** to your health.

Tap water contains chemicals such as chlorine (which kills gut bacteria) and fluoride (which denigrates magnesium levels in the blood leading to mineral imbalances throughout the body, especially the brain and nervous system).

Most of the population are severely dehydrated and therefore circulation suffers, clogging your tubes and leaving debris behind instead of carrying waste to the kidneys and bowl. You should drink <u>at least</u> 8-10 glasses (2 litres) of quality, alkaline balanced water every day.

8. Adding significantly to your body's **acid** levels are excessive **dairy products**. Since we were children, we have been brainwashed with the notion that, *"1+1=2 and milk is good for you."* Sorry, but they lied... Dairy contains a protein called **casein** which makes up 87% of milk. Casein has been shown in repeated studies to consistently be a **trigger for cancer** genes to activate in people who are genetically inclined. Prostate cancer is four times higher in men who have consumed a lot of milk all their life.

Basically, all animal products are acid and contain zero fibre, but assist by stimulating bile production in the liver. Most vegetables are alkaline and contain lots of fibre. Changing to a more **wholefood plant-based diet with some animal protein and fat** has repeatedly been shown to unclog your tubes (arteries and capillaries) and repair illnesses such as heart disease and diabetes. Surgery may not be your first option. Having adequate **fibre** each day is essential to good health, lowering cholesterol and blood sugar levels, disease reduction and for the release of toxins and waste from your body.

9. Likewise, vegetable oils (which are actually seed oils and are used in nearly all packaged food and baked goods) generally have an extreme overabundance of Omega-6. When eaten in excess, **Omega-6 becomes a free radical** causing inflammation, disease, blockages and early aging.

It is critical that you **ingest sufficient, quality Omega-3 daily** to offer your body a better alternative to Omega-6. Your body can't store or make Essential Fatty Acids (EFAs) and if insufficient Omega-3 is ingested, your body will utilise Omega-6 in lieu - contributing to macular degeneration and circulation blockages (diabetes).

Omega-3 is highest in fish oils, but most commonly available cheap supermarket fish oils are high in heavy metal toxins. It is important to source quality fish oil like **Nordic Naturals** brand that are **toxin-free** and have 30% better absorption.

10. Daily **exercise is critically important**, for all age groups. Your heart can easily pump oxygenated blood to the smallest capillaries in your feet. However, the return up-hill journey of the dark de-oxygenated, waste-ladened blood to the heart is supported by movement (such as walking) to assist the pumping action. You are moving blood from the smallest tubes (capillaries) to larger veins, therefore the returning blood pressure drops as you go, so your heart needs help to pump. Walking also gently massages the bowel, stimulating a natural, daily motion.

11. 95% of **serotonin** (the brain's neuron transmitter and a precursor to melatonin – the sleep hormone) is **produced in the bowel** and sent to the brain. A clogged toxic bowel may contribute to insomnia, depression, dementia and other mental diseases.

12. Having insufficient magnesium in your diet can also contribute to mental illnesses, fatigue, moodiness, inflammation and muscle and joint pain. **Magnesium is a master-mineral** that other minerals rely upon to organise order within the body. Your body absorbs magnesium **through the skin** much more readily than if ingested. If ingested, combine with Bicarbonate Soda to form Magnesium Bicarbonate which is incredibly beneficial. *read more later*

13. Vitamin D is another essential part of your health puzzle. Getting about **20 minutes sunshine** directly on your skin produces natural **vitamin D** which is 1,000 times more active than ingested vitamin D.

14. **Glutathione** is made by every cell of your body and is the most important antioxidant used to protect every cell and which the body naturally relies upon to clean up toxins, supply energy, support the immune system and reduce inflammation. Eat cruciferous vegetables every day.

In Summary

Reduce contact with people and situations that cause stress and choose happiness, find your purpose and gain some direction for a meaningful life. Clean out your bowel and detox your liver. Supplement where needed until you improve your habits. Eat/drink less sugar, dairy, grain, packet food and alcohol. Ingest more vegetables, fermented food and quality water. Get plenty of sunshine, quality Omega-3 and transdermal magnesium daily. Stimulate your glutathione production and exercise for 30-40 minutes every day.

Other than that, there is not much to it — just joking☺. The complexity of the big picture can seem overwhelming at first, but it matters and that's why I strongly recommend starting with just three things you can handle for now and as you progress, and your wellness begins to improve (and those things become supportive habits), add on another activity, supplement or change. Small progressive steps, over a few years – simple really.

Why Supplement and Detox?

Eating more wholefood veggies, animal protein and fat is a step in the right direction; however, since World War Two (WWII), our soils have been depleted of many vitamins, minerals and micronutrients due to over-farming and lack of crop rotation and we're not getting what we paid for when we purchase fresh fruit and vegetables today. Tomatoes, lettuce, carrots, peas, cabbage, etc still look great, but they just don't taste the same as when I was a boy. For decades, most farmers have been fertilising using mainly nitrogen, potassium and phosphorus (originally from left-over material used in bomb making in WWII) and have forgotten about other base minerals like selenium, iodine, zinc, magnesium, manganese, etc.

Australian soils are deficient in such minerals and eating imported produce is not a good solution either, as **all imported fruit and vegetables are potentially toxic** because they are required by law to be fumigated with **methyl bromide** by Australian quarantine. To quote a Material Safety Data Sheet (MSDS) for methyl bromide, *"Toxic liquid or gas, may be fatal if* *inhaled, harmful if absorbed through the skin, can cause nervous system, lung, kidney and liver damage".*

Added to this, 95% of the average western diet comes from sugar-ladened, convenient, processed, packaged food (not fresh produce), so the need for supplementation becomes obvious.

Toxic Chemicals

World-wide, industry produces around 80,000 different herbicides, fungicides, pesticides and household chemicals every year, with about 1,000 new synthetic chemicals introduced each year. Added to this mix are genetically modified (GMOs) foods where there have been no long-term studies for toxic mutations of cells in humans. The gut can't digest GMOs because the gut bacteria don't recognise what GMOs need for digestion.

There are also hidden pollutants like **tyre rubber dust**, which is evident when you observe planes landing at airports. However, most hidden rubber toxins come from car tyres. Every revolution of a car tyre wears the tyre by one billionth of a metre. Every tyre releases about 2.5kg (5.5 lbs) of rubber dust over the tyre's life (x 4 per car). The particles released are around 10-25 microns in size and when inhaled, directly enter the bloodstream.

The rubber released contains known carcinogens like lead and sulphur compounds. Once airborne the rubber dust can blow up to 50km from the road and settle throughout the suburbs and in paddocks, pastures and streams. Some dust settles on roads and is eventually washed into the waterways as sediment where it enters the food chain. And there is no escape or solution to this!

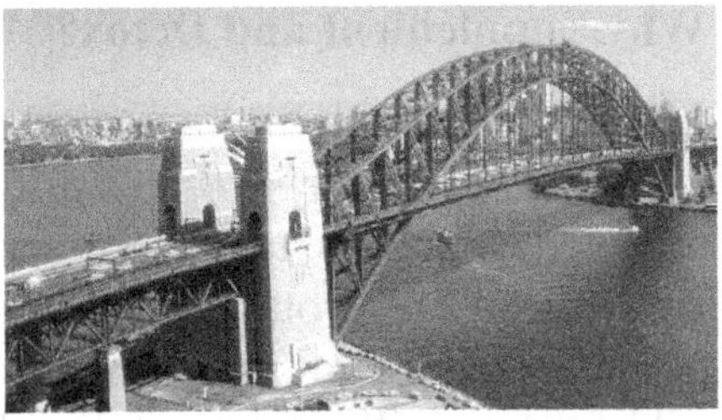

With 100,000 cars crossing the 1km (0.6 mile) long Sydney Harbour Bridge every day, 36kg (80 lbs) of toxic rubber dust is released daily.

You might be thinking, "I don't live in Sydney, so I'm alright." But open your mind — how many one-kilometre stretches of highway are within 50km of you and feed our major cities and arterial roads between Cairns and Melbourne with similar levels of traffic every day? Tens-of-thousands; extrapolating to thousands of kilograms of toxic rubber dust being breathed in (or consumed by) an unsuspecting public every day.

Added to the rubber dust toxic load, the average adult carries about 700 industrial chemicals in their body. Recent testing for 148 different industrial chemicals in 2,500 adults found significant quantities of toxic chemicals in

every adult tested. The Columbia School of Public Health estimates that 95% of all cancers are caused by a standard western diet and excessive toxins in the body.

As the liver becomes overloaded trying to deal with daily ingestion of sugar, processed food and alcohol (along with trying to metabolise fat) it can no longer deal with toxins, so toxins are stored which increases free- radical formation and impact.

The average cell in your body receives between 1,000 toxic hits (healthy lifestyle habits) and 1,000,000 hits (smoker, drinker, junk food) from free-radicals per cell, every day 24/7. Therefore, regular ingestion of antioxidants is important along with keeping your available stem cell levels high.

Fukushima

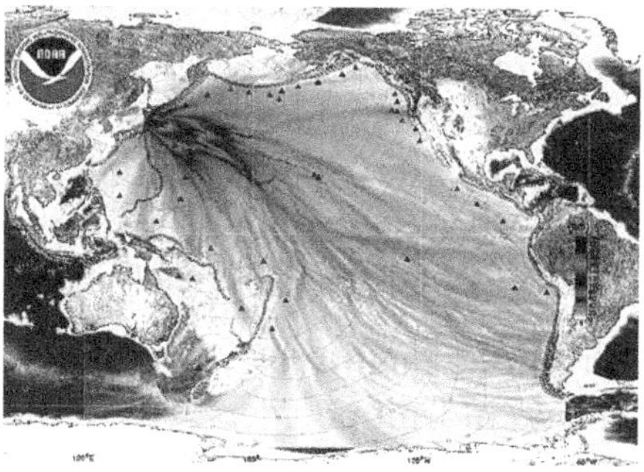

For several years following the Japan Fukushima Nuclear Power Plant melt-down, after an earthquake and tsunami in April 2011, the damaged plant leaked radioactive water into the Pacific Ocean at a rate of **300 tonnes per day**. This waste is now being stored in tanks, but they're running out of storage space.

Currents carried waste directly towards the west coast of Alaska, Canada, USA and South America.

This matters to us down-under too, and further promotes the need to regularly detox. Eventually radioactive toxins will circulate around the whole of the earth's oceans. This is one reason to make seafood a minimal part of your diet and supplement with quality fish oil.

There were numerous accounts of lies and deliberate deception by the plant operating company TEPCO, who have been caught using radiation detectors that max-out at 100 mSv per hour, when the actual rate measured was 1,800 mSv. That's 95% inaccurate or 18 times more toxic than previously thought.

You simply can't trust industry to self-regulate their self-interest, money is too important to them.

The Role of Stem Cells for Initiation

Stem cells identify injuries and requirements throughout the body, then initiates nutrients from food, juice and supplement for repair and replacement of old, dead and damaged cells. With enough stem cells in circulation, we can mitigate disease, repair injuries and slow down the aging process.

Fruit juice contains too much fructose and (often) high concentrations of chemicals, which are unsupportive. When a container of fruit juice boasts, "no added sugar" it doesn't mean there is no sugar contained, some fruit juices have as much sugar as soft drinks due to high levels of fructose — the worst kind of sugar *(see 'Sugar' later).*

Vegetable juices are one of the most beneficial, nutrient-dense supplements on the planet. Continuing to eat solid vegetables is important too for additional synergistic nutrients, fibre, enzymes and stomach acid stimulation. Though I eat a mostly wholefood, plant-based diet with meat protein and fat, because of the lack of proper nutrients in most of today's food, I supplement and detox daily utilising vegetable powders by simply adding quality water.

When I don't have time to juice vegetables (which is basically all the time), I use convenient wholefood powders and nutraceuticals. I supplement daily and leave our $1000 juicer sitting in the cupboard – in fact we've since given it away to an opp-shop charity. Powders are more convenient, easily affordable and less waste. Supplementing through wholefood powders also means that I receive peak nutrition every day, no matter what my schedule or location. If I know if I had to juice each day, I wouldn't.

Check the quality of your supplements and don't mix fruit with vegetables. Sugars in fruit powders will ferment vegetable juice, rather than digest.

Barley grass was selected as one of the 'Top 10 Super Foods' on Oprah.com, but not all barley grasses are equal. Some companies grind-up waste leaves and stems after harvesting the barley grain (creating chaff), which is mostly fibre with very few bio-available nutrients.

However, companies like AIM harvest (at night – when nutrients are at their peak), young barley grass shoots before they develop grain then juice and simply dehydrate (at low temperature) giving you maximum bioavailability. So, you actually get **dehydrated juice**, not chaff. AIM uses natural growing methods with organic standards with no added chemicals *(see resources).*

Wholefood Synergy

Food presented to us by nature is whole in its structure and has synergistic micronutrients to allow full-supportive uptake of nutrients. Nothing in nature is made of just one component, for example vitamin C, or E or zinc only. Natural food is a complex combination of millions of components and when eaten whole, provides a synergy that the body recognises and can readily use. It's good to eat most vegetables in combination with other foods, like a mixed salad with broccoli, nuts and meat. However, different fruit should not be mixed together or with other types of food *(see 'Sugar' later).*

If you take a calcium tablet for example, the body may find calcium difficult to absorb because it can't be utilised by the kidneys without vitamin D. Any excess calcium (consumed but not used, known as free calcium excess) can cause gallstones and kidney stones in the long term *(see 'Kidneys' later)*.

However, when you eat wholefoods in combination, like the mixed salad with spinach leaves, broccoli and mushrooms, you will find that the spinach and mushrooms contain both calcium and vitamin D to help absorption of calcium in the kidneys. The broccoli also contains large amounts of vitamins A, C and K1 along with calcium. All you should do is expose your skin to 15–30 minutes of sunlight a day to create activated vitamin D and support calcium uptake even more.

Food companies know this, that's why dairy companies fortify their pasteurised products with vitamin D (which by the way, they no longer call 'milk'— instead various brand names are often used — read the carton), because without vitamin D, only about 8% of the calcium is absorbed through the kidneys.

Timing of Supplementation

Upon rising each morning, after going to the loo, I drink a glass of water with a ¼ teaspoon of Magnesium Chloride plus one level teaspoon of Bicarbonate Soda (pharmaceutical grade) *see resources*. As you will read later, this combination in water creates Magnesium Bicarbonate which is highly beneficial for alkalising and mitochondrial cell energy.

If I'm eating breakfast, 20 mins after is a good time to have fibre supplements if you are taking any. Fibre is best taken around 20 mins before eating for reasons you will read later.

If you are eating breakfast, I strongly recommend eating an animal protein-based breakfast (e.g. meat and eggs with mushrooms, avocado, spinach, etc) within an hour of waking, because it's desirable to stimulate the liver to produce bile daily. I prefer animal protein rather than drinking apple cider vinegar or lemon juice to stimulate bile flow. Such acid-based drinks don't necessarily exercise the liver to sustainably produce bile. Above all, avoid carbs for breakfast; cereals, toast, oats, pancakes, sugar, fruit, etc.

Bile is the body's natural alkaliser and cleanser. Animal protein is acidic and stimulates a lot of bile production to neutralise the acid and is slow to digest, giving you a feeling of satiety all morning, reducing cravings for carbs.

If you're vegetarian, sorry – our whole family tried to be "veggies" for three years based on information provided by the author of 'The China Study', Colin Campbell, but it didn't suit us. Many vegetarians look to refined carbs (bread, pasta, dairy, sugar, potato chips, soy, etc.) to replace their protein urges and vegetable proteins have different reactions in the body to animal proteins. We found ourselves depleted in energy, unwell and carrying weight.

Feel free to conduct your own research and form your own opinions at: www.catalystathletics.com/article/50/The-Protein-Debate-Dr-Loren-Cordain-T-Colin-Campbell/

Timing of supplementation is not critical. If you can't meet the following criteria, you are best to take them whenever you can, rather than miss out.

- **Maximum absorption time** is with your first meal of the day, but also consider the following…
- **Vitamin B complex and C** (water soluble) – anytime
- **Vitamin A, B1, D, E, K** (fat soluble) – with food or fat
- **Iodine** – with meals containing fat
- **Essential Fatty Acids** (fish oil, etc) – with meals
- **Enzymes or Acid** (e.g. apple cyder vinegar) – just before meals
- **Electrolytes** (minerals) or **Alkaliser** (Bicarb Soda) – empty stomach, 20-30 mins before anything else
- **Green and Vegie Powders** – best with fat for absorption, but also okay other times
- **Herbs** – anytime
- **Fibre** – 20 mins before meals
- **Probiotics** – best before bed, otherwise with meals
- **Chelators** (EDTA, IP-6, etc) – empty stomach, 1.5 hours away from anything else

The above information is subject to recommendations on each container or your healthcare provider.

Full Disclosure

Our family gained so much benefit from taking certain products. We believe some products helped save our lives and we're certainly doing much better than many of our friends and family of a similar age. Details of such products can be found in the resources section at the back of this book and feel free to phone and ask more.

With our results, we decided to become members of various companies that manufacture such products and have regularly purchased products at wholesale prices and introduced others to receive the same benefits. This means I gain a small income from any products I recommend, and you purchase. This contributes to our income which assists in keeping our family supported and out-of-the-system, allowing time (over two decades) for valuable research and writing whilst ethically helping people with their lifestyle changes — my passion☺

You may choose to purchase products I recommend, or not — the choice is yours to consider. I have already made changes and improved my health utilising the products I recommend, and I can only offer this information freely to you. If you choose to purchase products recommended in this book, I would appreciate your support for my investment in time and resources, and you will gain by being supported through our (non-intrusive) follow-up system, so you gain the ongoing information you will need on your journey. Alternatively, feel free to contact the person who provided this book to you, they may be part of our alliance of knowledgeable friends.

I am a Justice of the Peace *(Qual.)* (JP) and have sat on several management boards for charities and schools. I hold my ethics and integrity high in my priorities. I ran for Queensland Parliament in 2009 in the seat of Gaven on the Gold Coast to stop fluoridisation of our water and to try and change things as an honest politician, but I didn't play the game well enough and failed to gain enough votes. In other words; I take action; I walk my talk.

Rebuilding My Body

I have worked on rebuilding my body cell-by-cell, repeatedly since 2003. Through my research I found that the body replaces most of its 100 trillion cells through its normal process of attrition and replacement. According to Deepak Chopra MD, 98% of our body cells are replaced each year, 25% are replaced every five to six weeks and some cells are replaced daily or less. Cells involved in the digestion process replace themselves every five minutes.

There are a few neurons in the cerebral cortex that are never replaced, some of the cardiomyocyte heart cells are replaced over a lifetime and fat cells are replaced over ten years.

Our body is like a river. You can easily observe a river flowing between its banks. The water you see passing under a bridge today will be different water to what you will observe tomorrow, but it is still the same river. If someone upstream contaminates the river with toxins, the fish will die. If someone builds a dam and blocks the river, the river will stagnate, putrefy, and become diseased. If the river is not flushed out regularly, it will become toxic with weed overgrowth. However, if a constant flow of supportive nutrients is maintained, the river will maintain its health forever. The river is in a constant state of change and renewal, as is your body.

It's logical to think that if I have sufficient stem cells in circulation and put the highest quality nutrients into my body every day through food, supplements, water, air and thoughts, when my cells replicate, they should be an equal or better cell than the cell I replaced. At the very least, I should provide the building blocks to create better cells than before, which should result in slowing the aging or disease process.

Over the course of one year, I can rebuild my body, cell-by-cell three times. Do this year after year and I am on the way to stopping or reversing disease, slowing down the aging process and creating a healthier body. I believe I have already begun this process with my body.

Consistently providing synergistic building materials for my cells has allowed my body, ultimately improving my health.

My Current Health

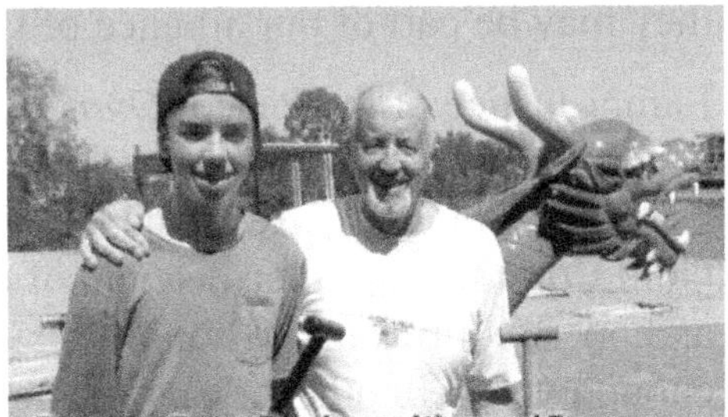

Dragon Boat Racing with my 15 y.o. son

At 64 years old, I am on no medication, I no longer wear glasses; I interact regularly with my 21-year-old son and 22-year-old daughter and still have energy for my wife and business.

Early in 2012 and again in 2015, I had a full medical check-up, and blood, urine and faeces tests showed I was extremely healthy. Remember, at the age of 48, my father had already had his double bypass heart surgery and retired.

Terminology Used in this Book – Can, May, Might and Could

You will find terms like *can, may, might, could, should and possible* used to describe many points. This is because Australia is one of the most litigious countries in the world and current laws prohibit me saying what I truly believe the products (or solutions) can do. Legally, if I was to write that something "will" achieve a result, I'd have to prove it scientifically through studies and research (costing hundreds of thousands or even millions of dollars).

Such are the tactics of Big Pharma's lobbyists who encourage laws and policy to keep their companies extremely profitable and in control whilst donating to both political parties. Such laws are designed to subdue new competition with products that may work better and to discourage research.

After each testimonial, you will also read words to the effect, "results may not be typical and may be different for each individual', 'consult your healthcare practitioner", etc. Again, this is legally required, and what you do is up to you.

Chapter 3

The Digestive System

Understanding Acid and Alkaline

What is 'pH'?

The measure of acid and alkaline is known as 'pH'. Many go through life using pH levels to regulate their pool or fish tank water, never really understanding what pH means. pH is an acronym for '**p**otential of **H**ydrogen', which translates to how much potential an oxygen atom has (in water) to engage with a hydrogen atom. That is, if the oxygen atom has unused receptors for a hydrogen atom (or 'free radical'), then it has a higher potential to connect with hydrogen, thus a higher pH number up to14 pH (most alkaline). For example, Baking Soda (Bicarbonate of Soda) has a pH of 8.

Acid has an abundance of hydrogen atoms (or few oxygen atoms), therefore has a low potential for more hydrogen to connect to other molecules and is noted on the low end of the scale as zero pH (for example, hydrochloric acid is 0 to 2.4 pH). Incidentally, Coca Cola has a pH of around 2 to 4 pH.

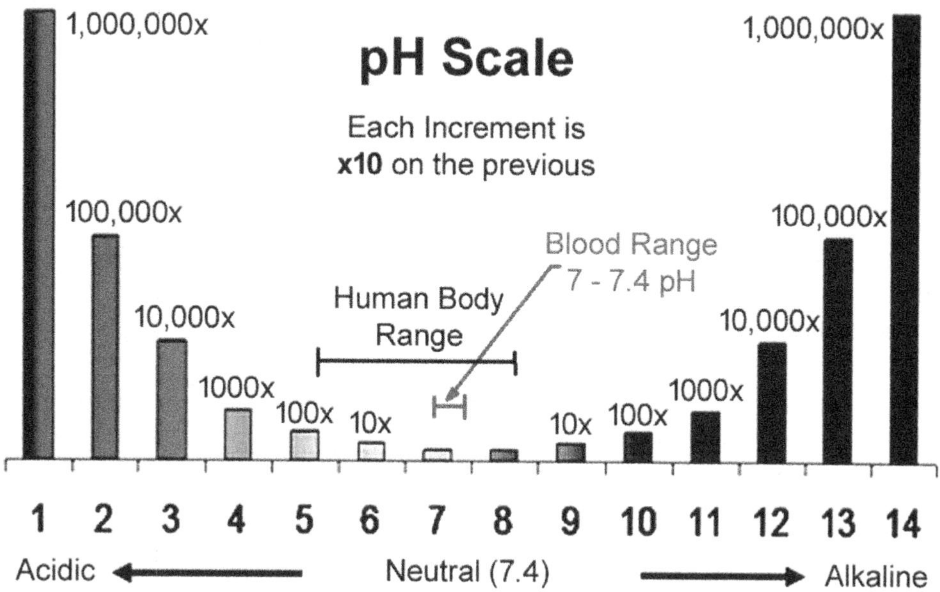

You might recall from high school that the formula for water is H_2O; because there are two hydrogen atoms to every one oxygen atom. Highly acidic water will have extra hydrogen atoms floating around (creating acid) whereas alkalised water will have fewer hydrogen atoms and more oxygen atoms. We balance pool water by adding either hydrochloric acid or Bicarbonate of Soda to water. Pools lined with rock pebbles tend to be more alkaline as minerals like calcium and lime leach from the pebbles into the water.

Different pH Levels

Different parts of the body have different optimum pH levels. Because of the digestive acid it contains, the **stomach** operates between 1.0–3.5 pH. The **colon** operates best when it is slightly acidic between 5.5–6.5 pH. **Blood** pH operates best between 7.3–7.45 (more alkaline). Of course, nature is always trying to create balance, therefore the **body** (overall) works best somewhere around the neutral range at around 6.8-7.4 pH, where it is virtually impossible for a serious health disorder or disease (like cancer) to sustain itself.

The 0-14 pH scale is also misread by most people and healthcare professionals alike. Each graduation on the pH scale is **10 times more potent than the previous number** (logarithmic). So, someone with a saliva pH of 5.4, may be around **110 times more acidic** than what is optimal at 7.4 pH.

Diseases of Affluence

Saliva generally measures up to 0.8 pH lower than the body's extracellular fluid. Extracellular fluid transports particles from the blood to cells.

Most people's **saliva** pH measures between 5.5 and 6.5 pH, which is up to 10 times more acidic than what it should ideally be at around 6.6 pH *(6.6 pH saliva + 0.8 = 7.4 ideal pH of the extracellular fluid).*

The body's **blood must maintain a pH between 7.0—7.4 pH** to keep you alive. Below 7.0 pH and you are most likely dead or in a coma.

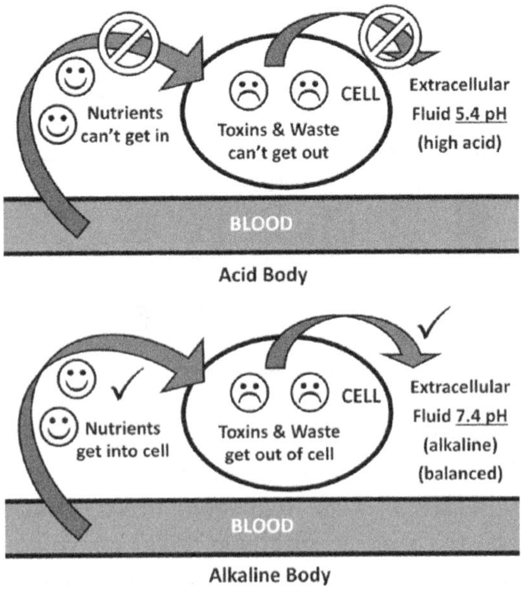

To achieve this, your blood may extract alkalising minerals from other parts of the body (via the extracellular fluid); like calcium from the bones (causing osteoporosis), magnesium from the cells (causing chronic fatigue) and sodium & potassium from the nervous system and brain (causing depression, anxiety, insomnia, etc.), which results in an acidic body pH and chronic illness over the long-term.

Outside the blood, the body utilises '**extracellular fluid**' to transport vital signals as well as nutrients and minerals into and out of each cell. Before this can happen, and at the same time, the extracellular fluid is supposed to extract toxins and dead body waste out of each cell. However, if your extracellular fluid is too acid the transfer won't happen, because the cells will hold onto their toxins and waste due to the pH ratios inside and outside the cells not supporting this process.

This is the body's safeguard so as not to over-burden the blood by releasing too many toxins (making the blood more acid). If the body's extracellular fluid is too acid for too long, the body will build-up toxins and waste in the cells which will ultimately manifest as disease. Remember – you create disease, through your choices – *Chapter 2*

Therefore, if you can raise the pH of your extracellular fluid, toxins and waste will be properly extracted from the cells, which allows for fresh nutrients and minerals to replace the old and positively replenish the cells (therefore the body – over time).

Research indicates that **excess STRESS, SUGAR and FLOUR** products (refined carbs) are the major factors that create acid within the body. Other factors include **inadequate water intake, alcohol, caffeine and lack of sleep and exercise**. Many types of bacteria, fungi and viruses actually use excess sugar to create more acid. Stress, caffeine and sugar also trigger acidic hormones; the major stress hormone being Cortisol (2.4 pH). Combined, they have a major impact on the body and contribute to many chronic diseases.

You don't just "catch" chronic disease; you accumulate acidic toxins over decades which make you feel unwell = dis-ease.

When left unchecked for several years, the above factors are probably why we have a dramatic increase in diseases such as autism, Asperger's, dementia, Alzheimer's, depression, bipolar, ADD, lactose intolerance, gluten intolerance, food allergies, diabetes, tooth decay, gout, arthritis, macular degeneration, cancer, eczema, psoriasis, etc.

That's part of the reason there is so much 'western disease' or 'diseases of affluence' not seen in poorer countries. With low oxygen supply from dehydration, little exercise, alcohol, drugs, stress and crappy, sugar-filled food, cells begin to die, and we age and deteriorate more quickly, becoming more susceptible to illness. *See Stress and Adrenal Fatigue later.*

Too much acid (**acidosis**) causes muscles to constrict and inhibit the exchange of nutrients and waste products in muscle cells, causing fatigue, soreness and pain. High acid in the body can also block vitamin absorption, create toxic build up in clogged cells, slow organ function, prevent proper digestion through enzyme dysfunction, create excess gas and bloating, cause unhealthy weight gain, and speed up the ageing process.

Symptoms of Being Too Acid
Initially an acidic body may display skin eruptions, headaches, allergies, colds, flu and sinus symptoms. You may also find yourself coughing, have an irregular or increased heartbeat, feel weak, feeling sleepy but highly-strung and irritable, sigh often, feel anxious and can't hold your breath for long.

Smelly Belly
The more acidic the food eaten (especially flour and sugar), the more acidic the body and therefore the more flatulence created (hydrogen sulphide and methane gas — the smelly ones) from food **fermenting** in the gut ~ creating gas, rather than digesting. The more alkaline the food eaten, the better the digestion and uptake of nutrients and the less flatulence and the fewer and sweeter our 'pop offs'. How nicely put is that?☺

Raising the Body's pH with Sodium Bicarbonate
Many doctors and naturopaths believe that pH and alkalinity are the same thing. They are closely related, but somewhat different.

Alkalinity is the capacity of water to neutralise acid, generally depending on the amount of minerals (carbonate, bicarbonate, hydroxide, borate, silicate and phosphate) that are dissolved in the water. **pH** is the expression (measure) of the acid or alkalinity of the water, depending on the amount of Hydrogen ions that are in the water.

Alkaline foods (e.g. green, leafy vegetables) are certainly good to eat for nutrition, enzyme and amino acid reasons. Alkaline foods might contribute towards **not increasing** acidity but **won't change** the body's current acidity significantly in the sort-term. Many vegans and vegetarians measure a low pH (acid) due to other factors mentioned previously (especially carb/sugar consumption and stress – fear-based); in spite of eating mostly plants.

Drinking alkaline water (8.5 pH+) won't change the body's alkalinity either, but it will cost you more. Water is absorbed by the liver within minutes of ingestion, thus temporarily (and falsely) signalling to the liver that your pH is alkaline, therefore the liver is less likely to produce as much alkalising bile. Like nature intended, we're best to drink **balanced water** at around 7 pH. The quality of the water (free from chemicals, toxins, bacteria, chlorine and fluoride levels) are far more important. *See Water later.*

For decades, healthcare professionals have promoted ingesting "alkaline-forming" foods like apple cider vinegar. The facts shown by this simple experiment, demonstrates that they have minimal impact on the body's alkalinity. Continually ingesting high-acid foods can contribute negatively towards the body having increasing acidity over time.

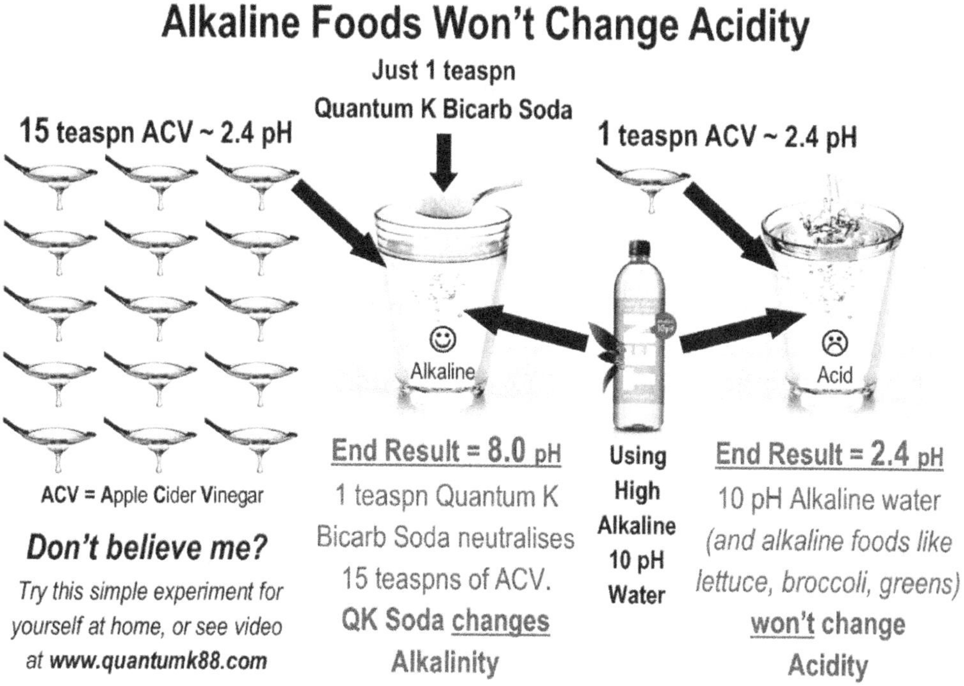

It takes a "**pH buffer**" like **Sodium Bicarbonate** to actually change the body's pH and encourage the body to become more alkaline. When Sodium

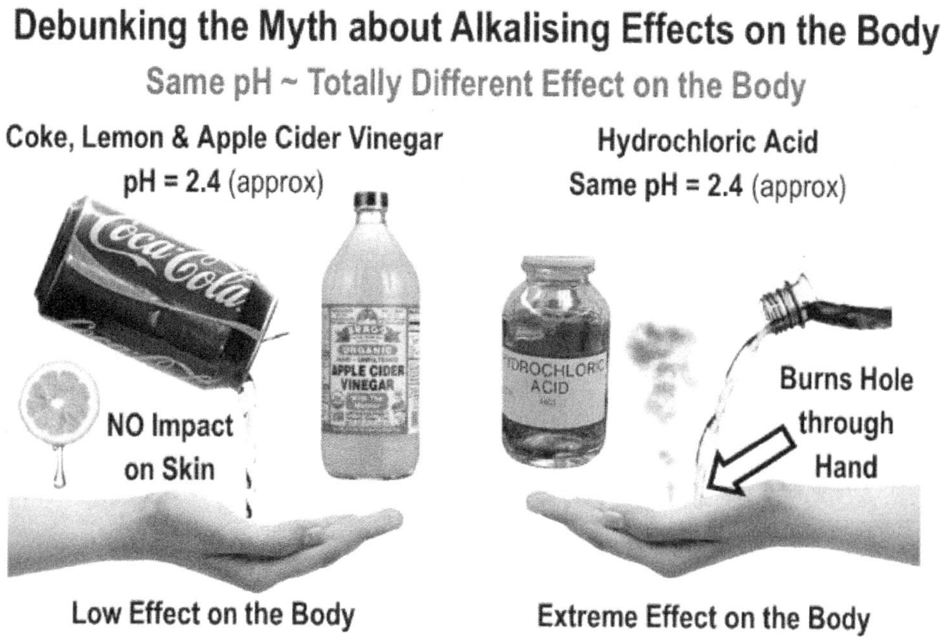

Bicarbonate enters the body (via ingestion or skin), it holds firm at 8 pH and forces the body to change and become more alkaline.

It takes 98 glasses of water to neutralise one glass of Coke, however just one teaspoon of Bicarb in one glass of water will do the same job.

The body creates its own Sodium Bicarbonate naturally to do just that – counteract and neutralise acid. No other natural mineral does it better.

Sodium Bicarbonate is naturally produced in the pancreas (especially), and in every part of your body via the interconversion of carbon dioxide and water through the **Carbonic Anhydrases enzyme**; how body regulates acid levels.

Sodium Bicarbonate is also known as Baking Soda (**not** Baking Powder), Bicarbonate of Soda, Bicarb, Bicarbonate Soda and Soda (not to be confused with unhealthy, acidic, sugary soft drinks Americans call Soda☹, or the healthy, alkalising soda-water with Carbon Dioxide bubbles☺).

It's important when using Bicarb orally or for soaking, that you **use high quality pharmaceutical (or practitioner/medical) grade**, organic and aluminium-free. *See resources section.* Food grade Bicarb (common supermarket brands) are okay for cooking but may contain fillers and don't completely dissolve in water. They are basically granules simply suspended in the water, therefore won't fully absorb into the body. In fact, the granules may contribute to blocking the smallest capillaries and filters of the body; feet, eyes, kidneys, liver and lymph systems.

A popular health food store brand is Bob's Red Mill Bicarb which is organic and aluminium-free. However, it is still food grade and granular.

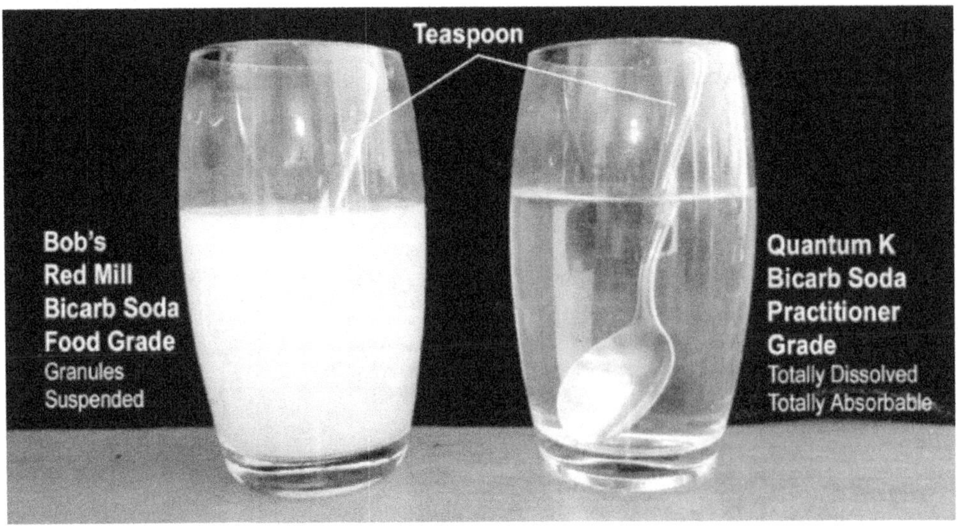

Practitioner grade Bicarb dissolves completely in water and turns clear within 20 seconds of stirring, to become completely absorbable within minutes of ingesting or soaking. *See resources section for details.*

The sickness industrial complex uses cartridges of Bicarb to filter the body's blood for Kidney Dialysis. The dialysis machine is simply a glorified pump; the Bicarb does all the filtering and cleanses the blood ready to return into the patient.

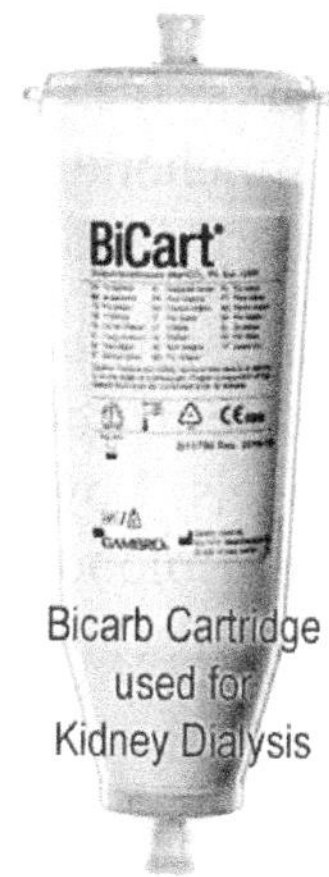

Bicarb Cartridge used for Kidney Dialysis

Bicarb is also commonly used in chemotherapy (to detoxify), for cardiac arrests, renal diseases, diabetes, dehydration, flu, radiation exposure, etc.

When to take Bicarb?

It's important to **only take Bicarb on an empty stomach**, and <u>not</u> with other supplements as Bicarb will neutralise stomach acid which plays a major role in digestion. Contrary to popular belief, your stomach doesn't always contain Hydrochloric Acid. Stomach acid is only formed when you chew, think about or smell food, so the best time to ingest Bicarb with water is around 30 minutes before meals and 2 hours after eating your previous meal, **if** your stomach feels empty.

Generally, **fluids** (on their own) pass through the stomach within 10-15 minutes of drinking, so when you drink a glass of water containing Bicarb Soda, allowing double that time (30 mins) before eating should not interfere with acid creation when eating later.

Initially you can take 1 level teaspoon (4g) in a glass of water, up to 4 times a day until the saliva pH averages around 6.6 pH over 5 days, then step back to 1-2 teaspoons, depending on your lifestyle, weight and health. Continue to regularly check your pH levels, especially after a big night out, which will give you excellent feedback on the acidic impact of your lifestyle choices. The best time to test your saliva pH levels with test strips or litmus paper is first thing in the morning before you ingest anything.

Bicarb is absorbed brilliantly through the skin via baths or foot baths.

Supercharge your Bicarb with Magnesium Bicarbonate

When you mix Bicarbonate Soda with Magnesium Chloride ($MgCl_2$) in water, you create Magnesium Bicarbonate ($Mg(HCO_3)_2$), which only exists as a solution in water.

According to Dr Mark Sircus, Ac, OMD, author of 'Sodium Bicarbonate - Full Medical Review' and 'Transdermal Magnesium Therapy', *"Magnesium Chloride and Sodium Bicarbonate work together seamlessly making a dynamic duo that one day will tear down a great part of the pharmaceutical empire."*

Magnesium is vital for over 300 functions within the body; however, Magnesium does not readily reach the cell's mitochondrion (energy centres of each cell). *See Magnesium later.* With plenty of Sodium Bicarbonate on hand, the Bicarbonate will act as a transporter of Magnesium into the mitochondrion, thus providing the body with better cell communication, more energy and more efficient detoxing.

Ingesting or bathing in Magnesium Bicarbonate increases **albumin** (the main protein produced by the liver) and **creatinine** (a para**thyroid** hormone (PTH)) levels. Low levels of both are associated with arthritis, asthma, migraines, high blood pressure, stroke, heart disease, osteoarthritis, osteoporosis and atherosclerosis (hardening of the arteries).

A study involving 1.7 million people with high albumin levels, showed that they lived longer and had a higher survival rate if they had serious diseases.

Sodium Levels

If you're worried about your Sodium levels because your doctor has put you on a low salt diet, Sodium Bicarbonate is safe. To quote Dr Sircus, *"sodium bicarbonate as well as citrate and phosphate salts* ***do not raise blood pressure*** *to the same extent as do the corresponding amounts of sodium chloride."*

Ingesting Magnesium Chloride with Bicarb

Ingested Magnesium Chloride must be of the highest quality and seawater-evaporated magnesium is not appropriate for this type of application.

According to Dr Sircus, *"Ancient Minerals Bath Flakes are pure enough for oral consumption, even though they are not sold for oral use."* Magnesium Chloride (flakes) are extremely bitter, however when just a few flakes are added to drinking water, it enhances the texture and flavour. 'Food-grade' more reflects the conditions in which a product is packaged, i.e. stainless steel, dust-proof processes, etc.

The brand of 'Ancient Minerals' Magnesium Chloride is from the Netherlands, 2000 metres below sea level from the old Zechstein Sea, laid down 250 million years ago and independently tested to contain around 32% Magnesium Chloride and to be free of heavy metals. Most other brands contain around 16%.

If you choose to take Ancient Minerals Magnesium Chloride **orally**:

- **With Soda:** follow the pack instructions and add 3-6 flakes per glass.
- **Drinking water:** for every litre, add 1/8th teaspoon of Soda and 3-4 flakes of Magnesium Chloride. This should simply balance your

regular drinking water and have little impact on digestion.

Transdermal use (on the skin) *see resource section*:

- **Skin:** apply Magnesium Chloride via a Lotion or Spray daily.
- **Bath:** add 2 tablespoons or more (each) of Soda and Magnesium Chloride Bath Flakes. Soak for around 20-30 minutes.
- **Foot Bath:** add 1 tablespoon or more (each) of Soda and Magnesium Chloride Bath Flakes. Soak for around 20-30 mins.

Molasses & Bicarb Treatment

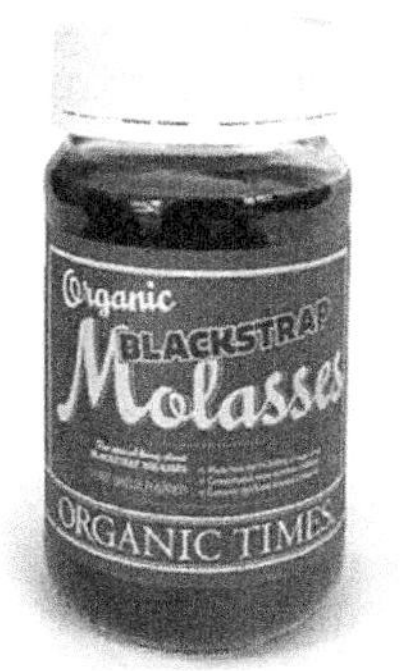

Blackstrap Molasses (also known as treacle) is made from the third boiling of sugar syrup and contains a range of significant, concentrated vitamins and minerals. It is black in colour, opaque, strong and sweet in flavour with the consistency of honey.

Official Queensland government documents informs us that, "cancer prefers to use sugar for fuel". So, if you have cancer and are on a low carb, low sugar diet, any cancer should readily absorb sugar as its main food.

If you mix Blackstrap Molasses with Bicarb Soda in a glass of water and drink it 2-3 times a day; in a Trojan horse effect, the sugar should be drawn into the cancer (for food) and covertly release the Bicarb inside any cancer, causing the area to be alkalised, therefore less supportive of cancer growth.

Dr Sircus notes in his book, an example of a man who had bone and prostate cancer who took varying amounts of this sweet mixture over 10 days. His results quoted medical reports afterwards stating, *"No convincing evidence of an osseous metastatic process."* And his PSA count was 0.1, where previously it measured 22.3. In other words, there was no sign of his bone or prostate cancer after just 10 day's use.

The treatment is 2 teaspoons of Soda and 2 teaspoons Blackstrap Molasses in a glass of water. Drink twice daily for 2 weeks. Reduce to 1 teaspoon if detox symptoms become unbearable.

I don't claim this as a cure for cancer, but wouldn't it make sense to have all the measurements done by your doctor first, then try this sweet process using just two natural products for 10 days and then get measured again afterwards, before you commit to surgery or toxic chemotherapy treatment where there is a 98% failure rate. I strongly recommend you fully read Dr Sircus' eBook prior to commencement of any treatment.

Acid and Alkaline Foods

Dieticians recommend eating low-acid food, which is generally correct. However, that's not the whole story — it's more about the effect the food has on the body after ingestion.

So rather than looking at a food's pH level to improve your eating, it's also good to look at the PRAL (Potential Renal Acid Load), where zero is neutral, negative (-) is more alkalising and positive (+) has a more acidic impact.

Food with high protein and phosphorous levels contribute to higher levels of acid in the body. Conversely, higher levels of potassium, magnesium and calcium decrease the acid in the body, giving an alkalising effect to the body.

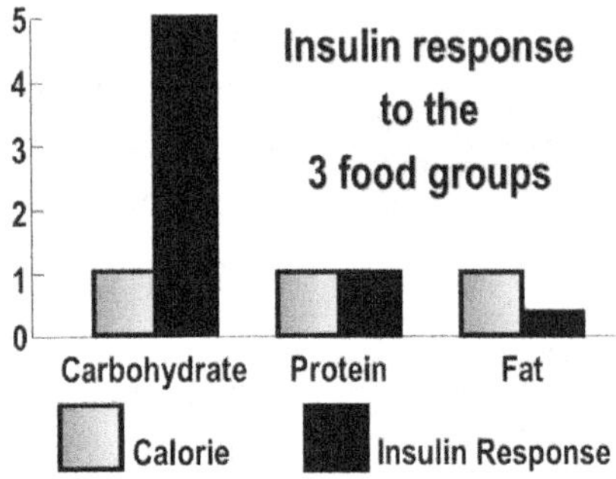

Not all protein is equal and animal protein may raise acid levels but initiates supportive bile activity (exercises and flushes the liver and gall bladder) and lowers insulin response. *Also see Detoxing later.* Whereas green plant protein may lower acid levels because green plant proteins increase the kidney's ability to remove acid from blood. However, complex carbohydrates are plants, but are acid and significantly increase insulin response and insulin's major signal is to store fat.

Basically, grains, most nuts and nearly all animal products (meat, poultry, seafood, dairy, eggs), have positive PRAL values (acidic impact), however are supportive for bile production, whilst some fruit and most vegetables and vinegars have negative PRAL values (alkalising impact, or at least won't contribute to increasing acid).

PRAL of Food (100 grams)		
	Food	PRAL
Alkalinzing Effect on Body	AIM BarleyLife®	-56.43
	Dates	-13.67
	Bananas	-6.93
	Carrots	-4.10
	Broccoli	-3.57
	~~Oranges~~	-2.70
	Lemons	-2.31
	Blueberries	-1.04
	Black Beans	-0.10
Neutral		
Acid Effect on Body	Milk	0.13
	Yogurt	0.16
	Eggs	8.81
	Cashews	8.93
	Salmon	11.55
	Tuna	12.70
	Chicken	15.60
	Tiger Prawns	18.20
	Cheddar	19.98

Sugar (Fructose) and Acid

Just to complicate things a little further, the sugar content (especially fructose) in food may also designate its acidic effect on the body too, regardless of PRAL values. For example, orange has a more alkaline value (-2.7 PRAL) than lemons (-2.31), but oranges are higher in fructose content (4.5% fructose) compared to lemon's 1% fructose, therefore oranges may contribute to higher acid levels in the body because of sugar.

Likewise, dried fruit has one of the most alkaline PRAL values, e.g. dates at -13.67. However, dates contain 32% fructose because dates are dehydrated and fructose is super concentrated, increasing insulin.

Excess sugar has a highly acidic effect on the body and is one of the major causes of cancer! *(You can read more on sugar and cancer later)*

I've personally found one of the **best alkalising supplements** is AIM BarleyLife®. As you can see from the table above, AIM BarleyLife® is 5–7 times more alkalising than most other foods. *See resources later.*

An added tip to help with your body's acid levels; don't drink water immediately after or during meals. Water will dilute the acid your stomach creates for digestion and food may travel through the intestines undigested and putrefy rather than digesting, turning the body more acidic. If you're thirsty, drink a glass of water five to ten minutes before you eat. Eat slowly, chew well and the body's saliva will wash down the food and aid with digestion.

Meat and Acid

Meat can be acidic to the body (depending on your liver's ability to create bile). If you choose to eat meat, a serving no larger than the back of your hand of free- range (grass fed), hormone-free meat is best.

There are ethical issues surrounding the negative impact on the environment and the inhumane treatment of animals through beef, lamb, pig, poultry and fish production and processing. Avoid grain-fed beef — cattle are meant to eat grass. Grass-fed meat should be high in omega-3 which is supportive. Grain fed to cattle is mixed with GMO soy pellets. Pellet-fed meat is high in omega-6 which is inflammatory to the body.

One meat that should be avoided or limited to 50 g (1.8 oz.) per week is processed meat like ham, prosciutto, bacon, salami, pepperoni, frankfurts (hot dogs), corned beef, sausages and luncheon meats.

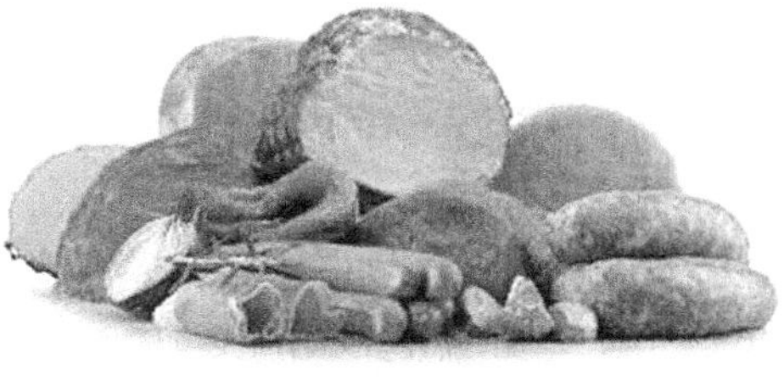

Processed meat is often high unhealthy salt and often made of tongue, snouts, hoofs and offal tissue from animals. Many are cured using smoke, chemicals and salt and contain preservatives to extend shelf life. Fifty grams equates to one sausage, two slices of ham, one hotdog, two rashes of bacon, 1 cm (½ in) thick slice of salami or two slices of luncheon meat.

A recent Swedish report found that consuming more than 150g (5.3 oz.) (approximately three sausages) of processed meat introduces chemicals, colouring and preservatives which the body converts to carcinogenic nitrosamines and can increase your pancreatic cancer risk to 57%.

Consuming red meat, and (in particular processed meat), has also been associated with an increased risk of bowel, oesophageal, stomach, prostate and lung cancer, possibly due to the lower vegetable fibre intake of meat-eaters. We also don't know what else the meat-eaters were consuming (potato chips, pastries, pasta, etc) or if the meat-eaters in the studies also drank alcohol, smoked, etc.

So, What Should You Eat?

Bottom line, when it comes to eating and drinking (especially processed and packaged foods and drinks), companies are always trying to sell you their products, and their product's negative impact on your health is not high on their agenda. To win you over, they will point you to a possibly biased, supportive study or video (like drinking red wine, gluten-free, etc) that has the best chance of increasing their profits.

Don't stress-out over this issue. Simply eat as close to nature as possible, sparingly, and in moderation. Drink plenty of quality water, have moderate, regular exercise and be happy (avoid stress). Simples really ☺

Mouth

When chewing food, the length of time food stays in the mouth and the size of the food particles you swallow matters. During the chewing process, the body adds two digestive enzymes that are not introduced anywhere else in the body, which begins the digestive process. It's also important to macerate the food into a paste-like material, which allows the next stage of digestion to work more efficiently in the stomach.

Tooth Decay

An acid body can encourage tooth decay internally, as well as from external sugars/acid contacting tooth enamel.

Teeth have thousands of minute tubes that leach fluid through the bone and enamel, supplying nutrients and keeping your teeth alive. If your body is too acid, these tubes can be corroded by your body acid from the inside out, giving external sugars a passage into your teeth, causing decay.

The obvious solution is to have a more alkaline body; however, you can assist your teeth externally by washing the following mix around your mouth for one minute, twice a day after brushing, then spitting it out. Swallowing the mix would be unsupportive as it will neutralise stomach acid.

Mix half a teaspoon of Baking Powder in 250ml (1 cup) of water. This mix should last several days and may assist in positive chemical reactions with your tooth enamel which can stop, prevent or reverse decay progression. The Baking Powder combines with substances in the mouth and teeth to form Calcium Phosphate which assists in re-mineralising tooth enamel and decayed areas.

It is important to use Baking Powder, **not** Baking Soda. Baking Soda has a more cleansing-sterilising reaction, than rebuilding attributes.

This requires an ongoing, long term commitment that may take 3-6 months to show positive effects that you may not even notice, but it's happening.

Root Canals and Implants

As mentioned previously in *'My Own Health'*, I sustained a significant injury in 1985 when hit in the lower jaw with a hockey stick which caused a horizontal fracture below my front teeth and culminated in a root canal procedure.

One of my front teeth was broken off just above the gum line, so after straightening my front teeth back upright and bracing for months, my dentist removed the nerve of the broken tooth and replaced the void with Gutta Percha (a wax-type material), then capped the top of the tooth with plastic resin (root canal).

I was doing okay for about 15-20 years, when I began to have regular lower jaw swelling and infections every 12 months initially, then 2-3 times a year. I had X-rays, tests and antibiotics, but then I started having seizures.

My gum and Gutta Percha at the base of the root shrank over time leaving a void that was filled by anaerobic bacteria (thrives in the absence of oxygen) which continuously leached toxic bacteria into the body for 30+ years.

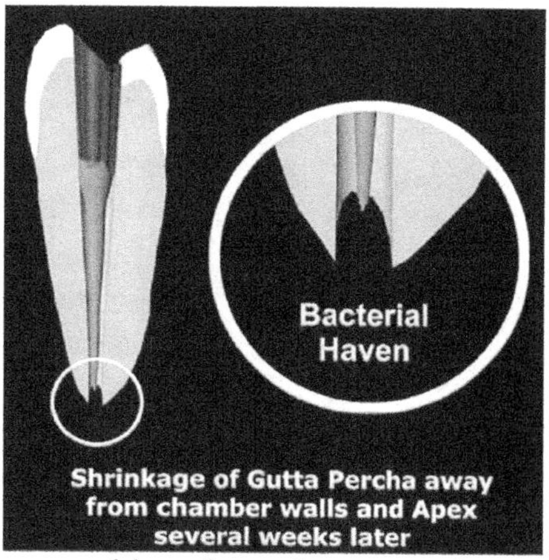

Shrinkage of Gutta Percha away from chamber walls and Apex several weeks later

In 2015, I had the root canal removed along with five other teeth, revealing a pool of **green puss** which lead along my jaw-fracture line to two molars, where I had another pool of **white puss**.

My dental surgeon said, "It's like I've been sucking through a straw into a sewage pipe 24/7 for 30 years, compromising my endocrine and lymph systems, putting extreme strain on my liver and kidneys to continually clean up the mess". Of course, my liver couldn't keep up with my continual barrage of contamination, therefore (I feel) leading to my seizures 20 years later. Thankfully I had my amalgam removed some 10 years prior, or I would have been in a much bigger bind.

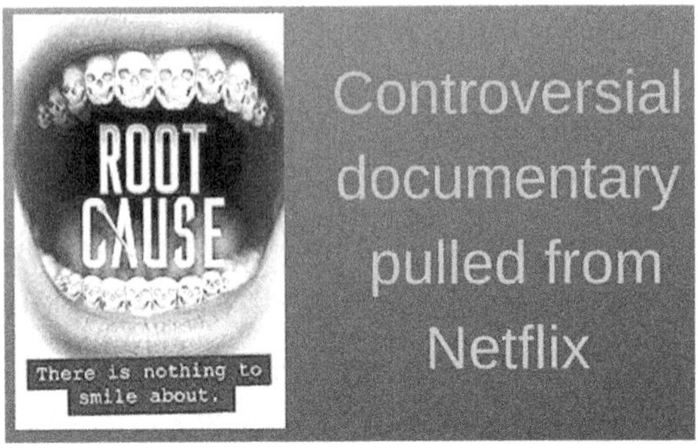
ROOT CAUSE
There is nothing to smile about.
Controversial documentary pulled from Netflix

The current trend for implants has similar long-term negative impacts too, as there is always shrinkage, leaving a void that will be filled by anaerobic bacteria. The sickness industry doesn't want to spoil one of its primary money-spinners *(chapter 10)*, so informative documentaries like the Australian produced "Root Cause" won't be found easily on Google and has been quietly pulled from Netflix but can be found on Vimeo. Also search for *"Dr Hal Huggins root canals"*.

My Recovery

Because my immune system had to work excessively for three decades to continuously combat my anaerobic bacterial infections, my immune system didn't realise it could now slow down. For 30 years, my immune system had to perform like a Ferrari to just keep me alive, now it could simply run like it should, a Mazda☺. Combined with over-production of Superantigens from bacteria, this caused serious inflammation and skin rashes (on and off) around both eyes, temples, ankles and left hand for two years *(see photos)*.

I visited a doctor for pathology tests, and all was clear. The doctor could only prescribe steroid cream to relieve the itching – so I declined.

Other blood chemistry tests by a naturopath revealed my chronic bacteria-

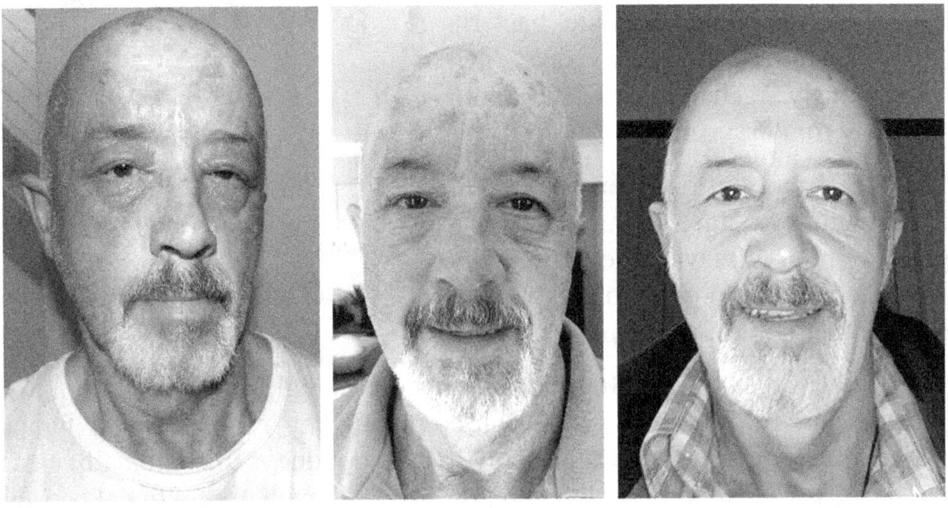

June 2016 — *9 months after root canal removal*

July 2017 — *1 year later*

Aug 2018 — *After 3 weeks of Stem Cell Nutrition*

leak ultimately produced early markers for future illnesses including heart disease and dementia – I was already noticing cognitive slowness and memory loss. How many elderly people do you know that are suffering from heart disease, memory-lapses and mental illness which may be caused by root canals and tooth decay creating chronic toxicity resulting in chronic disease?

My uncomfortable skin rash and inflammation was only slightly improved by eating better; meat, butter and vegetables and seriously limiting sugar, carbs and alcohol. The only thing that helped a little, was a fortnightly galvanic spa treatment, but if I didn't have the treatment, the irritation would return with a vengeance.

In July 2018, I was introduced to stem cell nutrition. *See 'Stem Cells are the Secret' and resources later.* Within a few weeks of taking just 4 capsules daily, my skin cleared up and there has been no reoccurrence. I'm so grateful; what a relief after two years of massive irritation and embarrassment.

Stomach

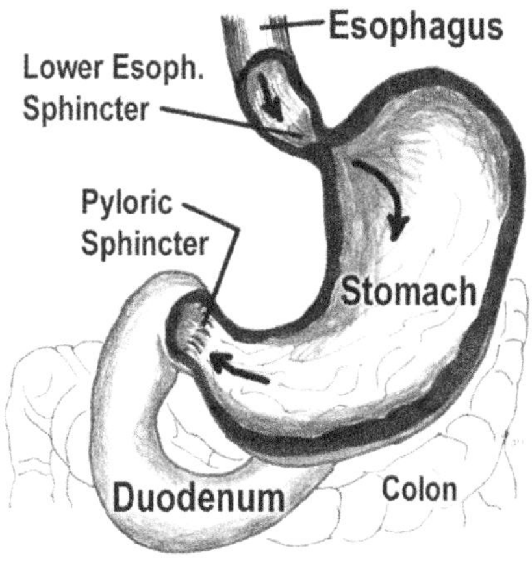

The body uses **hydrochloric acid** and salts (potassium chloride and sodium chloride) in the stomach to dissolve food into sludge, kill unsupportive bacteria and emulsify fat further on in the digestive process. Hydrochloric acid is an extremely strong acid and is often used in industry to burn through metal or clean concrete. However, the stomach and duodenum are the only parts of the anatomy that produces a thin mucus coating, preventing the acid from eating through the stomach wall — truly incredible! If undigested food remains too acidic further in the digestive process — into the small intestines and colon — it can lead to gastric ulcers and Crohn's disease.

One of the main functions of the stomach is to temporarily house food until dissolved enough to pass onto the duodenum. If not for this, you would have to eat continuously, but fortunately the stomach houses enough food for one to four hours and progressively allows enough food through to the bowel for digestion, leaving the remainder until later.

Approximate Times for Food to Exit the Stomach

Liquids

- Water – immediate to 10 mins, on an empty stomach
- Juices and Soups – 15-20 mins
- Smoothies – 20-30 mins

Fruits

- Watermelon – 20 mins
- Other Melons, Grapes, Citrus – 30 mins
- Apples, Pears, Stone Fruit – 40 mins

Vegetables

- Raw Salad – 30-40 mins
- Steamed – 40-45 mins
- Root Veggies: Carrots, Beetroot, Parsnips – 50 mins
- Starch Veggies: Pumpkin, Squash, Corn, Potatoes – 60 mins

Grains, Nuts and Beans

- Rice, Wheat, Millet, Oats, Lentils, Chickpeas, Beans, Peas – 1.5 hrs
- Soy, Sunflower, Sesame and other Seeds – 2 hrs
- Nuts – 3 hrs

Dairy

- Whole Milk Cheese – 2-4 hrs

Animal Protein

- Eggs and Seafood – 30-45 mins
- Poultry – 1.5-2.5 hrs
- Beef and Lamb – 3-4 hrs
- Pork – 5 hrs

Simply seeing, smelling, chewing and tasting food triggers cells on the stomach wall to release hydrochloric acid and digestive salts so the digestive process can start immediately, therefore be careful of fast food advertising around mealtime which designed to stimulate such a response. The stomach produces a little over 1 litre (2.2 pints) of hydrochloric acid every day. That's why you need to ingest quality salt daily.

It takes around 20 minutes for receptors in the stomach to signal the brain that you have eaten enough food. Therefore, eat slowly and you should eat less. The stomach has receptors for feeling stretched (bulk) and this is where fibre and plant proteins are helpful to fill the stomach without adding many calories. The stomach does not need to be filled every time you eat. If you can become used to eating less and less often, your stomach will shrink, and you'll automatically eat less — positive habitual drifting.

Another receptor will signal the brain when the food you are eating is too rich, e.g. chocolate mud cake, small in bulk, but high in sugars/calories. And yet another receptor will signal when you have eaten enough food to gain enough nutrition, but nowadays we are basically numb to this signal and keep eating.

Acid Food and Reflux

If you eat acidic food like sugar, soft drink, alcohol, coffee, dairy and refined/packet food (biscuits, pasta, bread, white flour or rice), the stomach will add its own acid to break down this food. Often people who eat this way may have 'heartburn' or acid reflux and take an antacid to dilute the acid, which fixes the symptoms, but not the cause. Heartburn is mainly caused from a relaxed oesophageal sphincter and an over-acidic diet.

It's unsupportive to take antacids to relieve heartburn or reflux in the longer term. My father always had a packet of 'Quick-Eze' (antacid tablets) in his pocket and took them several times daily; he eventually passed with cancer of the bowel and liver. Antacids neutralise the acid content in the stomach, leading to undigested food passing through the small intestine and colon, which inhibits nutrient uptake and creates excess gas, acid and body waste.

Acidic Food + Stomach Acid = High-Acid Chyme

(Chyme is the brown sludge produced after dissolved food from the stomach enters the duodenum and bile is added to the mix – looks like gravy).

High-acid chyme may have a **negative impact** on the remainder of your digestive process.

Peptic Ulcers

If the food we eat is too acidic and/or the protective mucus is not produced correctly, it can lead to the acid eating into the walls of the stomach and duodenum creating 'peptic ulcers' or other gastric ulcers along the way.

Alkaline Food

If you eat alkaline food (like most vegetables and some low-sugar fruit), then the acid will still do its work of breaking down the food into chyme, but the end chyme will be less acidic and better for your body.

Alkaline Food + Stomach Acid = Neutral Chyme (or low acid)

Neutral chyme should have a **positive impact** on the remainder of your digestive process.

Gastritis

A common complaint of the stomach is gastritis, where people experience discomfort after eating (usually unsupportive, high-acid food). The main acute causes are excessive alcohol consumption or prolonged use of non-steroidal anti-inflammatory drugs (NSAIDs) such as aspirin. Sometimes gastritis develops after major surgery, traumatic injury, burns or severe infections. Bacteria, chronic bile reflux, stress and certain autoimmune disorders can also cause gastritis.

Quality Salt is Better for You

Contrary to the mainstream message, quality salt assists in the production of hydrochloric acid. The government recommends an intake of six grams of salt per day for an adult and less for children. Most people take double that amount through unsupportive table salt and junk (or packaged) food, rather than quality salt like Canning and Pickling salt, sea salt or Himalayan salt.

Common Table Salt is Not So Good

Table salt is a by-product of sea salt with all the important trace minerals extracted (the minerals are used for the supplement industry) through chemical cleansing and heat treatment, leaving it 97.5% sodium chloride. The other 2.5% are chemicals, toxins and anti-caking agents. Therefore, common table salt is nutrient deficient, and can draw minerals from the body, harden the arteries and collect in body tissue causing fluid retention, inflammation, toxicity and circulation problems.

Sea Salt

Sea salt is preferred by many people and is certainly better than table salt, however (depending where the seawater is collected for evaporation), it may be polluted from oil rigs, shipping, industry, decaying Russian nuclear submarines or nuclear power plant leaks and pesticide run-off.

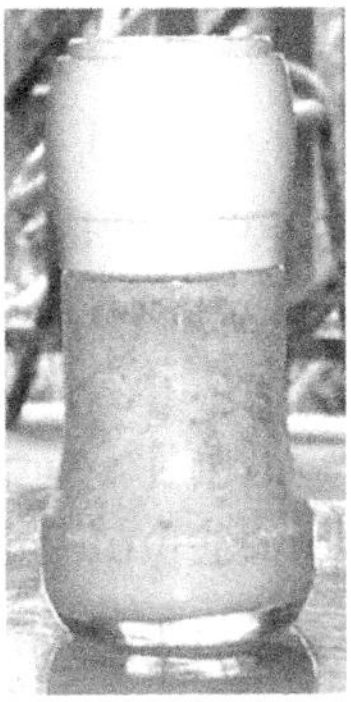

Himalayan Salt

Himalayan salt (pink in colour) was laid down 250 million years ago when our planet was being formed and contains all 84 trace minerals the body needs. According to mercola.com, Himalayan salt enhances the flavour of food and is 85% sodium chloride and 15% trace minerals.

Canning and Pickling Salt

Is 100% Sodium Chloride with no risk of toxic contamination. You can use as much as your taste buds desire and your body will adjust your taste when proper levels of sodium are restored by the kidneys.

Quality salt may draw excess water from body tissue and have an alkalising effect on the body because minerals mostly have a high pH around 10–12pH *(see 'Understanding Acid/Alkaline' previously).*

Salt is Necessary to Function

The human body needs sodium, potassium, chloride, zinc, magnesium, manganese, bicarbonate and other minerals to act as electrolytes (message carriers) for communication within the nervous system and brain. The kidneys endeavour to hold the sodium to potassium ratio at 15:1, but if salt intake is insufficient, or you use table salt, the adrenals may suffer exhaustion trying to supply the hormones to create this balance. Quality salt also helps regulate blood pressure and there are several vitamins that also require minerals to facilitate absorption into the body and vice versa.

Many doctors and nutritionists may tell you to reduce salt, and I believe this is true of table salt and salt in processed/junk food only. Have as much quality salt as your body craves and you should adjust your thirst to balance and automatically eliminate excess minerals through urine.

Personally, I've found by adding Himalayan salt to meals (sodium chloride + trace minerals), having medical-grade Bicarbonate Soda *(see resources)* each morning (carbon and sodium) and Diatomaceous Earth daily (silica), my skin, nails and hair (what's left of it ☺), feels amazing and calluses on my finger and toe joints have been replaced with smooth, flexible skin.

Generally, the beneficial minerals within salt are harnessed by plants (from the soil) as they grow. Animals eat these plants (grass) and minerals are passed through the meat and are easily absorbed and readily bio-available to the human body.

Salt in its granular form is more difficult to digest, absorb and utilise. The best way to add salt to your cooking is by **adding a quarter of a teaspoon to water and steam your vegetables**. This way the minerals are absorbed into the vegetables at a cellular level and are easily utilised by the body.

Fulvic Minerals

Fulvic minerals were absorbed by prehistoric plants 40 million years ago and preserved in soil sediment in isolated areas of southern USA. Fulvic minerals have the advantage of already being absorbed into plants, therefore being readily bioavailable.

Combined with small amounts of acid (apple cider vinegar, kombucha, vinegar, etc), fulvic minerals are commonly known as 'Fulvic Acid'. Fulvic molecules can carry up to 60 times its own weight in minerals and nutrients directly into cells, thus significantly increasing nutrient absorption.

This makes fulvic acid one of the best electrolytes available today and an extremely powerful antioxidant and detoxifier. Fulvic minerals can be obtained from: www.fulvicminerals.com.au/

Duodenum

When the food is adequately liquefied by the mouth and stomach acid, a valve called the pyloric sphincter at the bottom of the stomach lets the acid/food mix through to the duodenum, the first of three stages of the small intestine. The duodenum is about 23 cm long (9”) and is horse-shoe shaped, cradling the pancreas.

Much of the **iron and calcium** in food is absorbed through the duodenum, which also regulates the rate of emptying of the stomach through hormonal pathways.

Here the highly acidic mix is blended with sodium bicarbonate released from the wall of the duodenum and bile from the liver and gall bladder, as well as bicarbonate salts and enzymes from the pancreas. The pancreas also releases insulin depending on the blood-sugar levels and digestive enzymes from activity and food eaten 15–60 minutes ago.

Chyme

This mix of food, acid, bile, bicarbonate, enzymes and insulin is churned around in the duodenum to form a light caramel-brown liquid called ‘chyme’. Chyme has the colour and consistency of gravy. The brown colour comes from the greenish-yellow bile, which gives faeces its darker-brown colour when mixed with dead and discarded blood cells from the spleen. Bile also gives urine its yellow tinge.

Bicarbonate Neutralises Acid

If you know much about basic chemistry, you’ll understand that bicarbonate neutralises acid. You may have seen car batteries with white or green growth (acid) on the terminals. When you add liquid bicarbonate of soda, the growth fizzes and dissolves (neutralises) and is rendered harmless. The same happens when bicarbonate is added to the acid mix from the stomach — it neutralises the acid so the chyme can advance further without being too acidic and burning into body tissue.

If your liver or pancreas are diseased or dysfunctional, or you’ve had your gall bladder surgically removed, your body is likely to add less bicarbonate, therefore allowing the chyme to remain more acidic, creating a more acidic environment for your organs to function.

It’s been shown that **cancer thrives in an acidic environment**. Cancer has been shown to regress and sometimes disappear when the body is made more alkaline through better food, water, thought (stress reduction and attitude) and supplementation choices.

Small Intestine

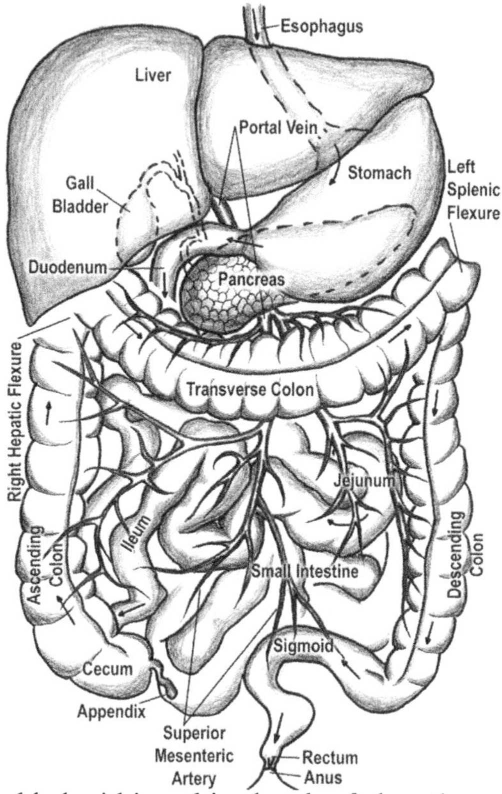

The next two sections, the **jejunum** and the **ileum** are commonly known as the small intestine; however, coupled with the **duodenum**, all three parts officially make up the small intestine.

Overall, the small intestine is around 5.4 to 6.4 metres (21 ft) in length and is about 38mm in diameter (1½").

It's in the small intestine where most of the uptake of oil and fat-based vitamins and minerals are absorbed and transferred via a series of blood vessels that lead to the **portal vein** and then into the liver for conversion into energy the body can use (gluten and ATP). These smaller blood vessels are imbedded within a thin sheath of clear tissue called the **superior mesenteric artery**. This sheath also contains visceral fat (also known as omentum), and it's in this area that, if we are going to put on weight, (belly) fat accumulates which is an indicator of future disease *(see 'Fat' later).*

Fibre passes through the small intestine undigested and becomes fermented when it reaches the large colon.

Intestine Functions

Each section of the small intestine has a specific role. The duodenum introduces bicarbonate and mixes this with food to form chyme, while the jejunum is where 90% of the vitamin and mineral uptake happens, especially any carbohydrates and protein, and the ileum is where the fats and oils are treated and dispersed into the bloodstream via the liver. Minerals like phosphorous, calcium, iron, copper, zinc, magnesium etc, and fat- soluble vitamins A, D, E and K1 are absorbed into the body via the small intestine. Vitamin **K1 is plant-based** and **K2 is produced by gut flora in the colon** later in the process, however some K1 is converted into K2 in the small intestine too. Vitamin K is needed to transport magnesium and calcium into the bones. Without Vitamin K, anyone taking oral magnesium and calcium supplements may find plaque building up in their arteries causing hardening of the arteries, therefore high blood pressure.

Normally the intestines process up to 11 litres (2.5gal) of liquid, food and body waste daily.

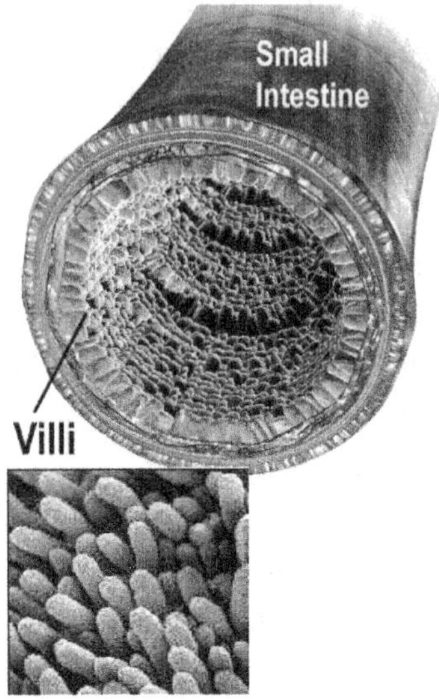

Jejunum

As chyme enters the jejunum from the duodenum, small finger-like extensions (villi) on the wall of the small intestine, absorb the nutrients from the food/beverage ingested (with the assistance of friendly gut bacteria and enzymes) where they are then transported directly to the liver to be converted to energy. There are around 20,000 villi per square inch on the inside wall of the small intestine that increase the surface area to about 19m^2 (200 sq ft) for maximum absorption.

Ileum

The second half of the small intestine (ileum) is where vitamin B12 is absorbed and bile salts (from the liver/gall bladder/stomach/pancreas) act like detergent and partially breaks down fat and oil particles which are transported via the blood vessels into the body's blood stream, which eventually travels through the liver to be filtered and metabolised as energy or stored as fat (in the liver initially).

If you eat more sugar and refined carbohydrates (white flour, pasta, etc) than the bile salts and insulin can deal with, then you may literally have fat particles floating around your blood and (like in a river), fat particles can gather on the inside of bends and joints, causing partial blockages of the arteries, eventually leading to heart disease or stroke. Studies conducted by Dr Lester Morrison and Dr Caldwell Esselstyn Jnr have shown that this situation can be reversed through improved diet alone.

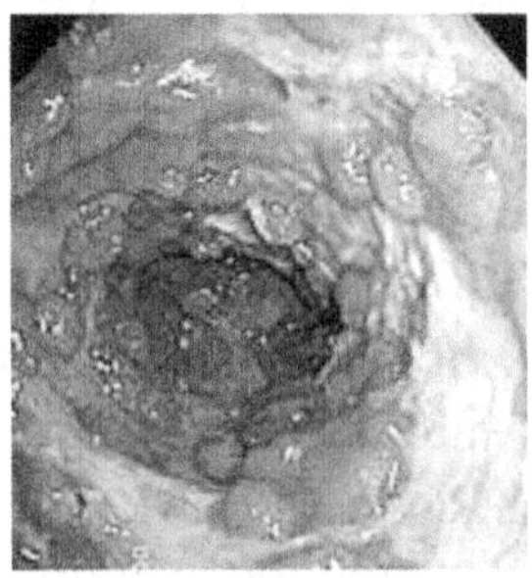

Crohn's disease inside the small intestine

Colitis, Crohn's Disease and IBD

Inflammatory bowel disease (IBD) is a term used to describe two diseases: ulcerative colitis and Crohn's disease, which cause inflammation of the bowel. IBD can mutate into bowel cancer.

The medical industrial complex may tell you that there is no known cause for these diseases and they often speculate that they are caused by a virus or bacteria.

Doctors will often speculate 'viruses' as a cause when they don't know the actual reason.

The symptoms of Crohn's disease are varied, but mostly consist of abdominal pain in the lower right area, diarrhoea, rectal bleeding, weight loss, arthritis, skin rashes, boils and fever. Colitis has similar symptoms, though the pain may be elsewhere in the abdomen. Children with the disease may appear to have delayed or stunted growth, basically caused by malnourishment (lack of nutrient absorption).

Doctors may prescribe steroids, immunomodulators (which cause the immune system to be less active), anti-inflammatories, anti-depressants or a low-fibre diet, to relieve the symptoms.

Dietary changes to include some meat and a more wholefood, high-fibre, alkaline intake with increased quality water along with probiotic supplementation may make a significant difference. I know several people who have taken medical-grade bicarbonate soda and eaten increased amounts of green leafy vegetables or supplements and cleaned out their bowel with extra fibre supplements to help alkalise the chyme, relieving the irritation whilst improving their 'alkalising' diet and eating more meat and fat.

Let food be your medicine.

It's interesting to note that the symptoms of a dysfunctional digestion and elimination system are similar for most bowel disorders; because they are all ailments of the bowel. Overall, if you don't uptake the nutrients from the food you eat, similar symptoms are the result. They can all mostly be eased or resolved by cleaning out the colon, detoxing the liver, alkalising the diet and supporting friendly gut bacteria and enzyme activity.

(Colitis, Crohn's disease and IBD are also discussed further in 'Conditions Caused by Constipation'.)

Celiac Disease

Celiac Disease is an allergic reaction to gluten (contained within certain grains (carbs) and MSG), causing inflammation in the small intestine. The inflammation swells, damages and flattens the villi (like worn carpet), reducing the uptake of nutrients (especially from fat and oil), so the body is malnourished, no matter what is eaten. As a result, food doesn't get digested properly causing diarrhoea, flatulence and ultimately vitamin and mineral deficiencies, which accelerates aging and organ degeneration.

Other Things that Damage Villi

Studies (for example, one conducted in the Netherlands by Nieuwenhuizen, Pieters, Knippels, Jansen and Koppelmanin 2003) indicate that repeated exposure to antibiotics (prescribed by doctors and in nearly all dairy products) creates an imbalance of bacteria in the intestines allowing a chronic yeast infection called 'candida albicans' to take hold, causing inflammation. Yeast, grain and sugar love to party together (as in making bread and beer) and they ferment in the bowel rather than digest, producing gas and increasing acidity in the intestines, damaging villi.

Normally, good bacteria flourishes in the small intestine. It's only when an imbalance occurs that unsupportive bacteria, yeast and fungi can begin to dominate. This usually occurs due to antibiotic medications, a junk-food diet and poor lifestyle choices.

Absorption and Celiac

A very fit Olympian only absorbs about 24% of the food they ingest. People who are less fit and eat less supportively, absorb far less. The remaining undigested food passes through the bowel as waste, putrefying, requiring us to eat more than we need to gain adequate nutrition, resulting in weight gain.

Adding fermented food (sauerkraut, etc.) to your meal may increase the absorption rate significantly.

Your bowel needs the right balance of (what is commonly known as) friendly (probiotics) and unfriendly bacteria. With unsupportive diets, unfriendly bacteria predominate causing bowel and mental disorders like depression and anxiety, supporting virus infections to spread and therefore lowering the immune system (80% of which is in the bowel controlled via friendly gut bacteria and enzymes).

The bowel produces some of its own friendly bacteria; however, you can introduce about 12-15 strains of friendly bacteria via ingestion. Most commonly advertised probiotics only introduce two or three strains commonly known as acidophilus and bifida.

Balanced gut bacteria and enzymes are **amazingly important for food absorption** and are key to ongoing wellness.

One third of your normal stool should be food waste (fibre), one third body waste (dead cells and toxins) and the remaining third; gut bacteria – friendly and unfriendly.

If you are not eating enough fibre or absorbing good nutrition to replace dead cells and don't have balanced gut bacteria, your stools may be about a quarter of what they're meant to be, leading to constipation, toxic build up, autointoxication and bowel disorders - that may progress to cancer.

If you don't like sauerkraut or don't feel you could possibly ingest fermented vegetables every day, there are a few supplements that adequately supply 12-

15 strains of probiotics. Combining such probiotic intakewith your daily food or nutrition supplements further enhances your wellbeing by allowing more nutrition to be absorbed. If your nutrient absorption is diminished through Celiac Disease, then increasing absorption of nutrients is vitally important.

There's no known cure for celiac disease; however, symptoms can be reduced by eating a completely gluten-free diet and it's most helpful to reduce dairy, sugar, caffeine and alcohol. Enzyme supplementation assists people with celiac issues greatly, as it's enzymes normally utilised by friendly gut bacteria that breaks down proteins for absorption.

Ginger and turmeric tea acts as an anti-inflammatory and may support the villi in the small intestine too.

Liver

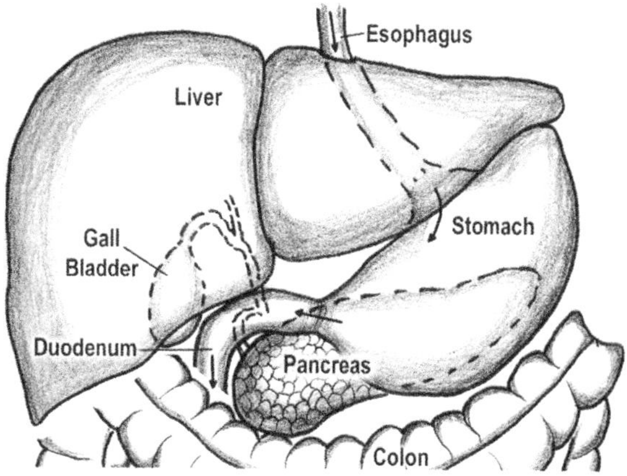

Located under the right ribcage for protection, the liver is the largest single organ in the body, apart from the skin, (weighing 1.5–2kg (3– 4lbs)) and is a vital and magical organ which, along with the colon, governs the long-term health of every other organ in the body. If there is an ailment elsewhere in the body, it's likely that the origins can be traced back to the colon which may be blocked (to some degree), constipated, diseased, or toxic; therefore, the liver may be diseased, toxic and dysfunctional as a result.

The 'Lifer'

The aptly named 'liver' is derived from the Old-English word 'lifer' because a properly functioning liver gives life and if the liver is diseased or dysfunctional, life is bound to be shortened and lower quality.

Liver Function

Fat-soluble vitamins A, D, E and K1 (absorbed from the small intestine) are stored in the liver if not used immediately. Water-soluble vitamins B complex and vitamin C (from the colon) are **not** stored and require ingestion regularly. The liver also receives oxygenated blood from the lungs before it is passed onto the heart for distribution around the body.

Generally, the liver deactivates toxins like ammonia, rendering it to a more harmless chemical called 'urea', which is excreted through the kidneys. Toxins introduced from external sources (e.g. lead, mercury, fluoride) that can't be eliminated or processed immediately are passed through the liver and generally imbed themselves in fat, muscles, bones and other organs. In this way, the liver becomes as toxic as the rest of the body. Toxins produced through stress, negative thoughts and emotions (electro-chemical reactions in the brain) tend to be stored in specific organs or parts of the body, depending on the body's overall health and stress level at the time. This is how worry and anger can cause ulcers, high blood pressure, and other problems.

If a segment of the liver is cut out through surgery, the liver can regenerate that segment. The liver is the only organ in the body to have this regenerative ability — that's why I call it magical — along with the amazing chemical and filtration work it does.

The liver converts ALL the food we eat (presuming the bowel correctly digest that food) into energy that our muscles use and, while it's doing that, it's filtering toxins and discarding them through the bile it creates every day, which also includes cholesterol for lubricating the blood. The liver also breaks down fatty acids and produces blood plasma proteins used for clotting blood. However, the liver will also store toxins that it can't breakdown, therefore over the longer term can become diseased if not cleansed regularly.

Regular coffee enemas and eating beetroot and carrots (or juice/powder) will support the liver significantly. *See resources.*

Little Stress Feedback

Because of its regenerative ability, the liver often doesn't show signs of stress until it is truly overwhelmed. Even when 75–90% of the liver is diseased or damaged, the liver can continue to function in an apparent, normal way with little indication of the stress it's under. By the time feedback is felt, it's often too late. Because of the lack of problem-signalling feedback (pain), the liver needs ongoing daily maintenance and care.

Blood Filter

The entire body's blood is filtered through the liver every three minutes, which gives an indication of how vital the liver is. If the liver is toxic and dysfunctional, the resultant blood may carry small toxic particles, which can become trapped within other organs, joints and the lymph glands. Do this around 500 times a day with 1.4 litres (3 pints) of blood passing through the liver every minute and you can easily see how cancer can spread from the bowel or liver to other areas of the body.

The liver also filters used, dead cells, waste and toxins from the body which are carried by bile and blood for elimination through the colon and kidneys in the form of faeces and urine. If the liver, colon or kidneys are dysfunctional, the body will pass some of the burden onto other normal elimination systems like mucus (sinuses, lungs and throat), skin (rashes, pimples, boils) or eyes (red eyes, irritation, tears).

The Liver Converts Food to Energy

The liver metabolises the vitamins and minerals absorbed from the small intestine and colon into energy molecules (generally glucose) that are transported to every organ and muscle in the body via the blood. This effectively gives us the energy to breathe, create heartbeats, walk, move, and think. If you supply your body with junk or low-energy food, you will have less energy and more waste, fat and toxins, therefore, you can feel chronically fatigued most of the time and eventually diseased. It's pretty simple really — input creates outcome (karma or consequences for actions).

However, if you decide to **clean up your act** and begin to eat well or exercise (or both), this may give permission for the liver and body to begin detoxing and you can often feel worse in the short term. Over the longer term however, you may be dispersing toxins that could potentially be the seeds of your future chronic or fatal diseases, shorter health span, low quality of life and premature passing *(see 'Detoxing' later).*

Cirrhosis

One of the main chronic liver diseases is cirrhosis, which is a broad diagnosis of a permanently damaged (yellowish in colour) or scarred liver, usually leading to cancer. Cirrhosis is mostly caused by excessive alcohol, hepatitis or an inflamed/fatty liver, but can have other causes like excessive levels of toxins and fat from an unsupportive lifestyle.

Cirrhosis can cause internal bleeding, kidney failure, mental confusion, coma, body fluid accumulation, and frequent infections. Symptoms include yellowing of the skin (jaundice), itching, and fatigue. Basically, the liver becomes overwhelmed and blocked with toxins and fat, and blood flow stops to parts of the liver. The liver is the first-place fat and toxins are stored in the body, and once the liver is overloaded, fat and toxins may be stored elsewhere.

Generally, people who have cirrhosis also have gallstones, which can be an indication of poor diet and exercise regimes.

Fatty Liver Disease

If you drink too much alcohol, the liver will be distracted for 2 hours for each standard drink to process the toxins delivered. Meanwhile the liver won't metabolise the body's fat, therefore storing fat in the liver (firstly), then elsewhere in the body once the liver is full. You may then be diagnosed with Fatty Liver Disease which may lead to cirrhosis as discussed previously.

Similarly, when you eat too many carbs and sugar (packaged food), the liver will store the excess energy as fat. As mentioned later, fat stores toxins, leading eventually to a cancerous liver and/or liver failure.

That's why avoiding a fatty liver matters!

If you're overweight, it's extremely likely (for the reasons mentioned) that you have a fatty liver and that's why such people are more stressed, have a shorter, low-quality or life and a higher rate of cancer and diabetes.

If you've been diagnosed with Non-Alcoholic Fatty Liver Disease (NAFLD) or Non-Alcoholic Steatohepatitis (NASH) which is an inflammatory version of the same disease, you may want to take note…

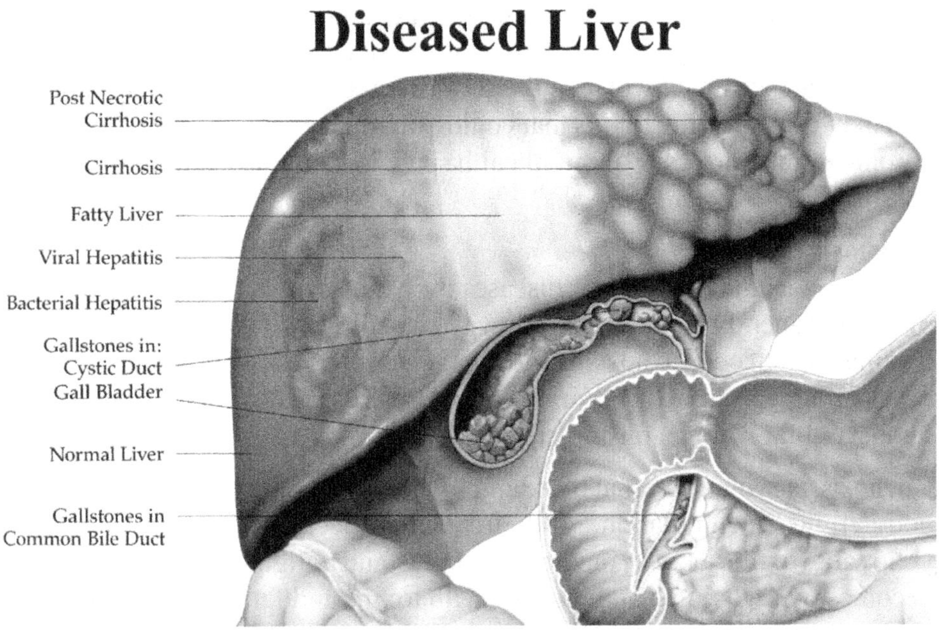

Don't ingest alcohol, paracetamol (pain reliever and fever reducer), fruit juice, seed oils (canola, sunflower, etc) and stop snacking. Significantly reduce (or eliminate) your carb (grain) and sugar intake. Ingesting these places more stress on the liver, reducing the metabolisation of liver/body fat.

Eat more healthy fat, animal protein and green leafy, cruciferous and fermented vegetables. Cook in coconut oil, olive oil, lard or butter. Drink more quality water and moderately exercise. Minimise eating fruit. Essentially the 'Keto Diet' mentioned in the *'Losing It' section later.*

If it's not too late, fat in the liver will progressively be metabolised and your liver should return to its normal, functional state. This could take three years.

We've found taking a supplement called 'Phosphatidyl Choline' very supportive to have in conjunction with the above. When we did our last liver and gall bladder flush, there were very few 'gallies' present; meaning fat from my liver was being dissolved and released and not stored.

Cleaning Out your Liver

Regular gall bladder and liver flushes *(as detailed in 'Gall Bladder' later)* will help support the liver.

My experience has shown that the liver can be cleansed through products listed in the resources section of this book. Some products contain sulforaphane (broccoli sprouts) which has been scientifically proven to remove toxins that have the potential to be carcinogenic. Beetroot has been used for centuries to support the liver, especially after hepatitis. Cleaning out the colon with herbal bowel cleansers and extra fibre will take some load off the liver as the colon begins to function correctly. As noted by the Gerson therapy, one of the most effective ways to detox the liver by having **regular coffee enemas** as detailed in Chapter 9.

Jaundice

If the liver is holding toxins, is diseased and unable to filter waste and toxins from the blood, then the skin may take on a yellowish tinge. This is often seen in the last days of passing of liver cancer patients as we observed with my mother-in-law.

Babies can also be born with a toxic liver. Babies are essentially created from their mother's body (therefore the mother is also likely to have liver issues too). Within the sickness industrial complex, this is called **jaundice** and their solution is to cover the baby's eyes and place them under bright lights.

Our daughter was jaundice at birth and was given this treatment in hospital with little effect, so we took her to a naturopath-homeopath who prescribed herbal drops that helped clean her liver slowly. Occasionally she would break out in welts (lines on the skin that looked like scratch

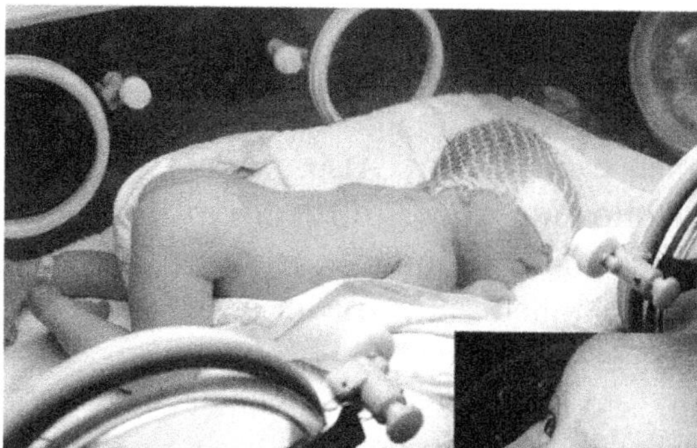

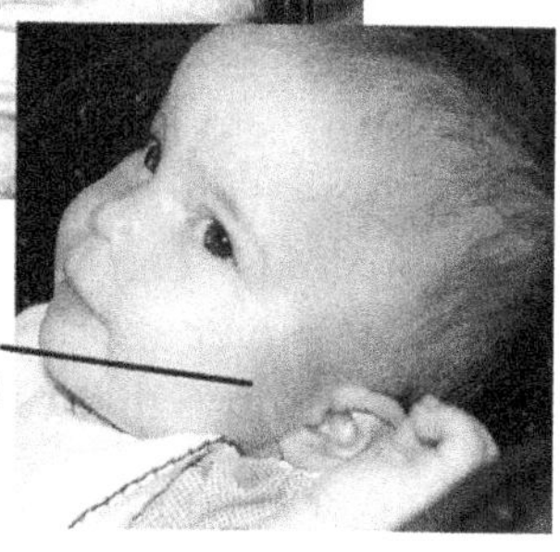

Above: Jaundice treatment in hospital.

Right: Jaundice treatment with herbs releasing toxins from the liver. Note the two welt marks near the left ear which appeared for about one hour as the toxins released through the skin.

marks) for just an hour. According to our naturopath, these were toxins clearing from the liver.

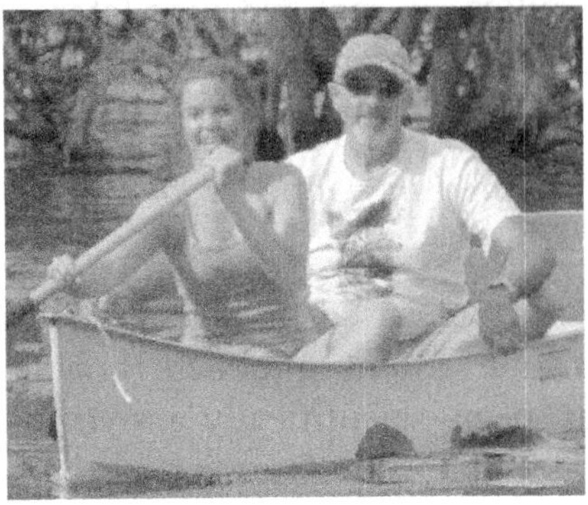

Now at 22 years old, my daughter is healthy, fit, slim and well and supports her body by supplementing daily, as she has since she was six years old.

A few times a week she has coffee enemas as she progressively cleanses her liver from her jaundice origins. She is determined not to pass on a diseased liver onto her children in the future.

Signs of a Struggling Liver

The first indication of a struggling liver is often chronic fatigue, skin rashes, yellow tinge in the whites of the eyes, darkness around the eyes, dark spots on the skin and/or a sharp pain (like stitches) behind the lower right ribs *(see photo)*. If you feel pain in the liver occasionally, try and recall what you ate or drank recently and reduce it from your diet. If you have liver pain constantly, then it may be supportive to act soon and detox your liver, or perhaps have a scan to see if there are any serious issues that may need attention.

A struggling liver can present pain behind lower-right ribs, right shoulder and/or knee, headaches, diarrhoea, light-coloured stools, dark urine, anxiety, depression, mental confusion, jaundice, food intolerances and allergies, chemical sensitivities, loss of appetite, exhaustion, fatigue, lethargy, and pre-menstrual tension. Also, if you find the following foods difficult to digest; radishes, onions, green capsicum, cucumbers and garlic or have a metal taste in the mouth, you may have a compromised liver. Varicose or spider veins on your legs or face and haemorrhoids can be a sign of a struggling liver as the blood struggles on its way through the liver back into the heart.

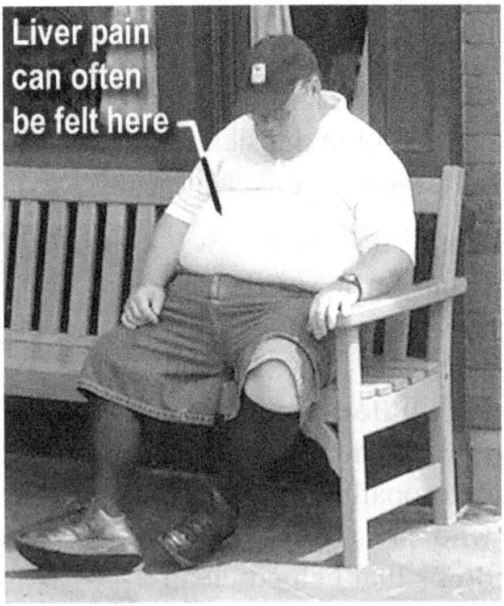

A struggling liver can make you feel chronically fatigued

If the liver is compromised, the kidneys, then skin will be the body's backup filter/elimination system, leading to sweaty, smelly feet and armpits.

I had liver pain constantly for many years, peaking when I ate or drank poorly. I didn't know what the pain was or what to do about it, but now you do... Isn't it great that you can learn from someone else's experience?

Anger and the Liver

In Chinese medicine the liver is related to anger. Anger will often impact negatively on the liver. I've often heard the term 'livid' (derived from the word 'liver') or 'SOL' (shit on the liver) to describe someone who is consistently grumpy, never happy or just plain angry most of the time. There is some truth to this, as anger excites the heartbeat and adrenal glands and whilst more blood and adrenaline is pumping around the body, most is going to the extremities (head, arms, fists, legs and feet) as the body prepares for fight or flight. The extra blood going to the extremities depletes the liver of the amount of blood necessary to function optimally, causing stress to the liver, and expressing in anger. I've met some people who can't let go of past issues and are just 'bloody angry' all the time. This can cause chronic blood depletion of the liver, high blood pressure and general inflammation throughout the body.

Conversely someone who has a struggling liver due to reasons of diet or disease may be angry, aggressive, anxious or obstinate most of the time too. A struggling liver can impact on most of the body's organs, making such a person feel chronically unwell, fatigued and generally miserable — and they'd love to share it with you. Unless such a person eats better and becomes more peaceful and happier in their heart, their anger may drain the liver of vital amounts of blood in a never-ending cycle. These people can often live short, unhappy lives and pass early through disease, injury or self-harm.

I tend to avoid such people unless they are genuine in asking for help, as they are vexatious to the spirit and don't add to my life. The greatest predictor of someone's future is their unresolved past and the people with whom they associate, so I choose not to associate with angry people. A happy life is easy!

Personally, I've found that through detoxing, my liver has become more efficient and I don't need to eat as much food to sustain myself during the day. Basically, my liver gains more energy from less food. If I eat like I used to, I put on weight. This is my challenge — to separate my habits from my needs relating to food, and I'm winning slowly.

Lymphatic System

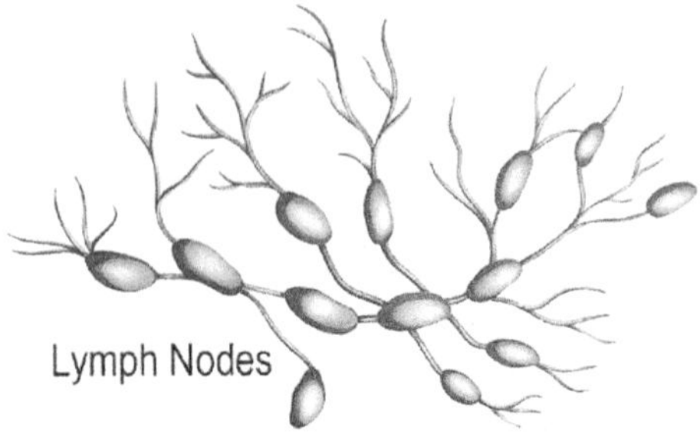

People can go all their life hearing about the 'lymphatic system', but never really know what it does. The lymphatic system is a vital part of the immune system and acts as a secondary blood filter after the liver and delivers nutrients, oxygen and hormones from the blood to the cells of body tissue via the blood circulatory system.

The lymphatic system includes **bone marrow, thymus, lymphatic vessels, lymph nodes, spleen, adenoids and tonsils.** Lymph organs are involved in the growth, development and deployment of white blood cells, which are key to the proper functioning of immune system.

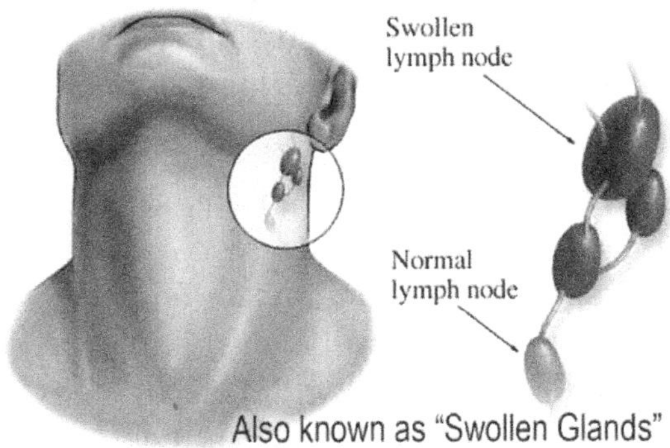

The lymphatic system rids the body of bacteria and viruses, filters the blood and removes toxins and dead cells as well as producing lymphocytes (part of white blood cells).

There are hundreds of lymph glands placed around the body (often around joints and between organs) which act as secondary filters. However, over years of unhealthy living, the lymph glands can become clogged and blocked, slowing the release of waste and distribution of nutrients, oxygen and hormones, making you feel lethargic, fatigued; impacting the immune system.

When detoxing especially, it's important to regularly clear clogged waste and toxins from the lymph glands for the lymphatic system to operate properly.

AIM Herbal Release® is a herbal lymphatic cleanser that has been specially developed using eleven herbs known for their ability to work with the lymphatic system and produce a positive cell environment. I use it regularly when feeling down physically. I know of several people suffering lupus (immunity and autoimmune problems) who have had great results from using this product. *See resources section later.*

Regular exercise is important to keep the lymphatic system working optimally. Exercise pumps blood through the lymph glands, clearing and cleansing as the blood passes through. If you can't or don't like walking, jogging, riding or outside exercise, you can use a mini trampoline.

Fat

You are What You Eat (Because of Your Thoughts)

If you eat a hamburger, chips and a dairy shake, the carbs and sugar consumed can be physically measured as fat in the blood just one hour after consumption by letting it settle in a test tube!

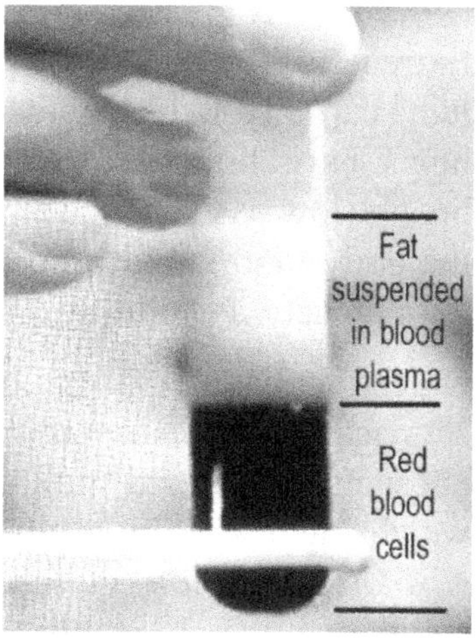

The thick, white suspended fat in this photo should normally be clear, yellowish liquid called plasma

It takes around four hours for the liver to process and store fat from the above meal and if we eat a similar sweet, hi-carb meal three times a day, the liver is constantly occupied processing sugar and carbs, let alone trying to perform its other vital functions. Do this day after day, year after year… there's little wonder why our society has become overweight, malnourished, unhealthy and diseased.

Fat and Blood Supply

Each kilogram (2 lb) of body fat grows an additional 640 km (400 miles) of arteries and veins to sustain its existence. This places extra stress on the heart to pump and return blood to and from these fatty deposits.

Fat Storage

When the liver's capacity to store fat is exceeded, the body will store fat in other areas of the body — often the midsection, around the hips, thighs, buttocks and belly areas.

We store fat around our midsection as part of our evolution when we used to hunt and kill a beast, feast for a day before the meat decayed, then eat less for the rest of the week. The body is designed to store fat close to the liver so the fat can be easily transferred via the portal vein to the liver and used for energy for the next few days until another beast is killed. Nowadays the most hunting we do is in the back shelf of the pantry.☺

Visceral Fat or Omentum

Belly fat is called 'visceral fat' or 'omentum' and if present, is an indicator of future disease. Visceral fat is different to normal fat, in that the toxins stored within are absorbed through the portal vein and go directly to the liver, increasing toxins in the liver, therefore essentially poisoning the liver. As mentioned previously, these toxins are then spread throughout the body and end up in other organs, creating disease.

The extra bulk tends to leverage and place pressure on the spine and lower back, push against and place pressure on the kidneys, liver, gall bladder, pancreas, lungs and heart, resulting in irritations, creating mucus and inflammation which contributes to high blood pressure and heart disease.

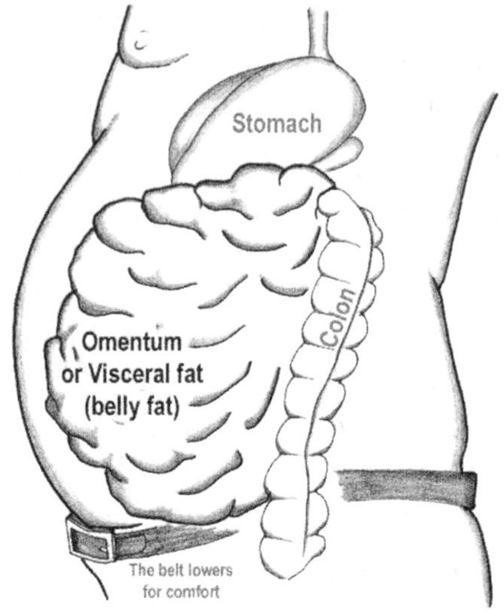

Extremely obese people can have their lung capacity halved and because their lungs have limited depth, shortness of breath (low oxygen) occurs which makes the body more acidic and is detrimental to brain activity.

Omentum hangs off the bottom of the stomach and transverse colon and the constant downward pull of the extra weight can lead to a prolapsed colon *(see 'Prolapsed Colon' later)*. The extra weight can weigh as much as 20 kg (44 lbs), equivalent to carrying four or five bags of potatoes around your waist. As the colon also hangs off the back of the ribcage, omentum can also cause lower back pain as the body's centre of gravity shifts forward.

Reduce Your Life by 15 years

The measurement around your waist at the navel (belly button) should measure no more than half your height. For example 183cm (6') tall = 91cm (3' or 36") waist. According to Dr Mehmet Oz, if you have excess belly fat, **you may reduce your life by 15 years** on average — that's the difference between living to **65 years or 80** years. And the last five to ten years may present a low quality of life, requiring dependence upon others (often your partner or children). Is this fair to yourself or them?

Omentum is most effectively burnt through aerobic exercise like swimming, running, brisk walking, cycling, or any other activity that raises the heartbeat and makes the lungs work harder, as opposed to resistance exercise like gym workouts, weights or push-ups. Aerobic training burns around 67% more kilojoules than resistance exercise; however, resistance exercise is still important for muscle strength and toning and should be included in your weekly exercise regime *(see 'Exercise' later)*.

Sugar, Refined Carbohydrates and Insulin

Excessive amounts of mainstream refined carbohydrate-based diets (processed flour, potato and sugar) are converted directly into fat by insulin.

The body treats all the above foods as sugars.

Any meal high in refined carbohydrates (carbs) initiates a rapid rise in blood sugar, triggering an insulin release from the pancreas. Insulin decreases blood sugar levels and directs fat and protein into the cells. Insulin also converts glucose into energy, but any sugar and fructose that can't be utilised immediately is turned into fat and stored — evolution's way of dealing with feast or famine as mentioned previously. The main signal from insulin is 'storage' (fat) rather than burn (use).

High insulin production also **suppresses** glucagons (releases blood sugar and fat from the liver) and growth hormones which are responsible for burning fat and promoting muscle development, therefore reducing the body's ability to utilise fat.

On top of this, the body is designed to burn ingested sugars and alcohol prior to burning the body's stored fat. Therefore, eating too many carbs, then exercising will mostly burn the ingested sugars, rather than burning body fat, thus little weight loss and the body's natural cell attrition will replace dead cells with lower quality DNA built from your lower quality food choices. You are what you eat – almost instant karma☺

Fat Cells

Fat cells are mainly built until puberty. Except for about 10% of fat cells, which die each year and are replaced with new fat cells, the number of fat cells remains the about the same throughout life. Fat cells can dramatically increase or decrease in size, depending on how much sugar and carbs you are eating relative to your energy expenditure through exercise or work.

Therefore, if adolescents eat excessively in relation to their energy output, they may create an excess of fat cells during this period. This is a particular problem for **obese children** who will carry this burden into their adult lives and often onto their own children.

It would be supportive for parents to inform their children about nutrition and exercise or they may lead them towards a future of illness, failing eyesight, medication, strict diets, low confidence and the need for excessive exercise.

However, it's difficult to convince teenagers about anything they don't want to do. Usually by 25 years they become more aware to their personal responsibilities. Best you can do is lead by example from an early age.

Calorie Quality

The golden rule with eating: **it's not the number of calories you eat; it's the quality of the calories**. Many rural Asians eat more calories per day than the average Australian or American, but their calories are mostly meat and natural, unrefined, wholefoods like wholegrain rice, vegetables and a little fruit, which are utilised by the body for energy and metabolism functions. Because of the fibre content, such foods naturally signal to the body "I'm full" when you have eaten enough.

The low-quality, refined carbohydrates like white flour, rice and sugar are typical in the Australian diet can contain fewer calories, but the food ingested is of low nutrient value. Such foods signal to the body the body "I'm unfulfilled — nutrition wise. I want more", and when more is consumed, it's mostly stored as fat.

A chocolate 'Tam-tam' biscuit and a banana each has around 100 Calories. Guess which one is of greater quality and better for you? It's simple, common sense.

Detox to Reduce Body Fat

Toxins are mostly stored in fat to protect body organs from damage. Therefore, in order to reduce weight, it's supportive to detox first so the body can let go of the fat that is no longer needed. Detoxing can be done through deep tissue massage, a high alkaline diet and exercise coupled with detoxing herbs or homeopathics. *See 'Detoxing' later.*

Feedback on Choices

Look at body fat (or the lack of) as a means of learning about yourself; as a scoreboard for change. Fat is actual physical feedback for your choices in life — emotional choices, resulting in physical actions. It's a type of 'instant karma' resulting from your actions.

As your emotions rule your thoughts and initiate action, **your body distorts** and compensates to house the effects of your actions. Over many years, the results of your choices impact on your body because of emotions, personal issues not dealt with, fear, laziness, anxiety, habits, food and exercise. Work on controlling your emotions, feelings, beliefs, habits and triggers as well as improving lifestyle issues like food and exercise. Emotion Code and Body Code therapies (as mentioned in Chapter 2) are an excellent way to eliminate habitual actions caused by trapped emotions. *See resources later too.*

Cholesterol

There are 100,000 km (60,000 miles) of blood arteries and veins in the human body and 25 trillion red blood cells. Envisage your blood vessels as vehicle tunnels and if blocked, result in major traffic jams, backing up traffic causing inflammation and irritation of drivers; just like when you're caught in a traffic jam – emotional, angry, inflamed and irritated.

For decades it's all been about LDL, the "bad" cholesterol. High or low LDL is no longer a reliable indication. Recent research indicates that it's more about ratios and artery health.

"Good" cholesterol, **HDL** (high-density lipoproteins) is produced in the liver at about one litre per day (2.2 pints) to help build cell walls and lubricate the blood. HDL takes cholesterol from arteries and cells back to the liver for processing and excretion as body waste.

"Bad" cholesterol, **LDL** (low-density lipoproteins) is mostly added to blood by ingesting refined carbohydrates, sugar and excessive dairy. LDL takes cholesterol from the liver and delivers it to cells where it is needed. Too much LDL can build up in the arteries, causing blockages (clots) and circulation problems leading to heart disease, stroke and diabetes. With plenty of HDL, excessive LDL is returned to the liver for processing; that's why HDL is the "good guy".

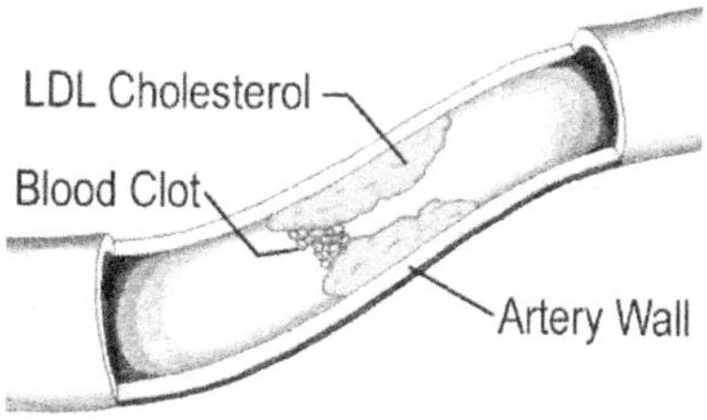

Eating protein, fat, sugar and carbs together (e.g. ice cream, custard, cappuccino/latte and cake, burger, chips and soft drink), will cause LDL to become very sticky and is therefore more inclined to stick to artery walls, causing blockages.

Triglycerides are a type of fat found in the blood. When you eat, the body converts any calories it can't use immediately into triglycerides that are stored in fat cells. When needed, hormones release triglycerides for energy.

Cholesterol is vital for hormone, vitamin-D and bile production, along with cell-membrane support and blood functions.

What's good:

- **Low triglyceride over HDL ratio** = less insulin resistance *(see later),* lower insulin and glucose levels (target <4.5 mg/dL)
- **Low total cholesterol over HDL ratio** = less risk of coronary disease (target <2.0 mg/dL)
- Measuring the number of **particles** of LDL (LDLp)
- **Flexible** arteries = less risk of LDL build-up (+ good blood pressure)
- Healthy LDL particles from a low-carb diet
- Healthy HDL removes more built-up LDL from artery walls

What's bad:

- **<u>High</u> triglyceride over HDL ratio** = twice the insulin resistance, higher insulin and glucose levels
- **<u>High</u> total cholesterol over HDL ratio** = twice the risk of coronary disease
- Measuring the **concentration** (size) of LDL (LDLc)
- **Hardened** or inflamed arteries allow LDL to build up more readily
- HDL and LDL oxidisation and damage from poor diet, smoking, etc

Search YouTube for "Ivor Cummins" or www.thefatemperor.com

Strokes and Heart Attacks
LDL build-up on artery walls forms a crust over the top which, if the cap of the crust is dislodged, can hinge up like a valve and block blood flow suddenly causing strokes and heart attacks. This is the cause of most heart attack and stroke sufferers who were never previously diagnosed with potential coronary problems.

B Vitamins are Essential
The June 2005 issue of the *Canadian Medical Association Journal* showed that inadequate consumption of vitamin B6, B12 and folic acid (B-group vitamins) caused plaque to form in the arteries, leading to cell damage and hardening of the arteries (arteriosclerosis), causing high blood pressure and blood clots leading to stroke and heart attack.

If the body does not have enough B vitamins (usually because of ingesting too much processed food and not enough wholefood), it forms an amino acid homocysteine (HCY), which leads to arterial plaque, altering artery walls. B vitamins have direct control over the levels of HCY in the blood, relieving arteriosclerosis. Either eat a diet high in leafy green vegetables, meat and fat or supplement to avoid the possibilities mentioned above.

Correcting Cholesterol Through Diet
It has been scientifically proven though many studies that incorrect ratios of cholesterol to triglyceride in the body can be reversed through the correction of diet alone. There is often little need for expensive statins (cholesterol-lowering drugs).

According to the Expert Review of Clinical Pharmacology, Vol 8-2, 2015, "Statins stimulate atherosclerosis (artery thickening/hardening) and heart failure." This is due to statins reducing cholesterol levels, therefore disabling the return of LDL to the liver for processing and excretion as waste.

Statins

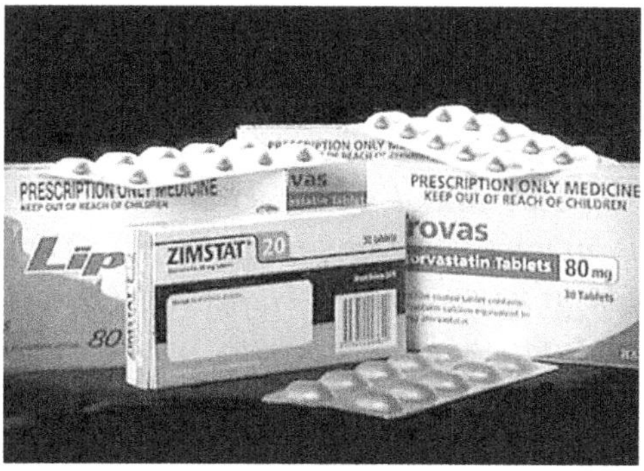

Statins (such as Lipitor – $12 billion annually) are the world's highest-prescribed category of drugs with total sales of $39+ billion annually. Statins block the enzyme pathway involved in the synthesis of cholesterol and Coenzyme Q10 (**CoQ10**) and can reduce levels of CoQ10 by 50%. The heart, liver and skeletal muscle cells have a high requirement for CoQ10.

The side-effects of taking statins are primarily liver problems which can also include muscle pain and fatigue, stomach upsets, sleep reduction, headache, dizziness, blurred vision, a decrease in energy levels, mood swings, cognitive impairment, diarrhoea, skin rashes and increased risk of diabetes.

Tissue levels of CoQ10 decline with age and CoQ10 is an essential co-factor for energy production through stabilising cell membranes and providing antioxidant protection.

Studies have shown statins to add zero longevity to life, whereas walking for just two hours a week will add two years to your life with no ugly side effects.

If you feel you should follow your doctor's advice and take statins, you should take a CoQ10 supplement as well.

You may not have heard of the NNT (Number Needed to Treat) which is a medical term for the number of people who need to be treated (drugs, surgery, etc.) before one person gains benefit; the lower the number – the better.

Big Pharma giant GlaxoSmithKline (GSK) themselves calculate that 90% of all drugs only work in 50% of the people. The NNT for one brand of statin is 300. Side-effects for this drug occur in 5% of patients. This means you are 15 times more likely to be harmed by statins than helped. Simple math☺

The overall message is that consuming animal protein and fat as part of a plant-based diet is fine, just make sure it is the right type and quality fat, grass-fed meat and poultry, avocados, olives and mostly leafy green vegetables. It is mainly sugar and excessive Omega-6 (seed oils - commonly known as vegetable oils) consumption that causes most chronic inflammation and disease.

With numerous exposés on the actual effectiveness of Statins, Big Pharma have hit back through their doctors. It seems $39 billion per year is not enough; they really need $80 billion a year to keep their corporate jets flying.

Big Pharma are cranking up the machinery to double their profits through doubling sales of Statins. Here is an excerpt from the LA Times, Nov 2013...

"Under the new guidelines, physicians should prescribe statin medications to all patients with high odds of suffering a heart attack or stroke in the short-term — that is, those who have had such an event already, patients with Type 2 diabetes, and those with exceptionally high levels of LDL cholesterol linked to familial risk. But the guidelines also recommend that patients with a 7.5% risk of suffering a stroke or heart attack over the next decade be prescribed statin medication as well.

Until now, treatment with cholesterol-lowering drugs in the United States has generally been limited to patients judged to have a 20% probability of heart attack — roughly 36 million Americans. The new, expanded treatment guidelines would roughly double that figure."

Make your own choice, zero extended life with side-effects from taking Statins, or extend your life by 2 years through moderate exercise with only beneficial effects.

Losing It (Shhhh… Top Secret – it's the Cabs!) ☺

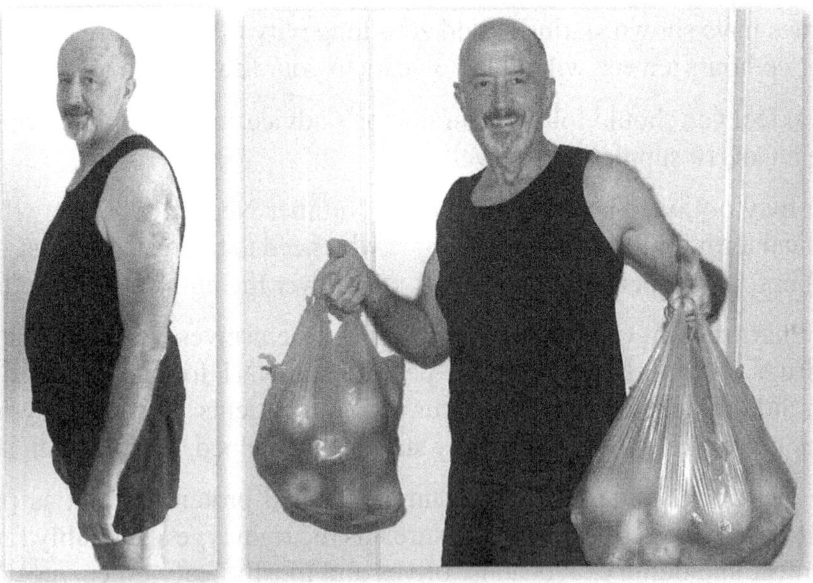

Recently I took action to reduce my weight from 87 kg (192 lbs) back to my correct weight of around 76 kg (168 lbs). The 11 kg (24 lbs) lost was equivalent in weight to the two bags of fruit and vegies I am holding. Can you imagine carrying this extra weight around with you all day? No wonder I had back pain. Find out what I did...

Middle-Age Spread

In a similar way to how hormones affect teenagers at around 12-13 years of age, the body changes its metabolism at around 50 years too and begins to store food as fat differently. In fact, your metabolism burns 2-5% fewer kilojoules every decade after the age of 40, but regular exercise can help counter this.

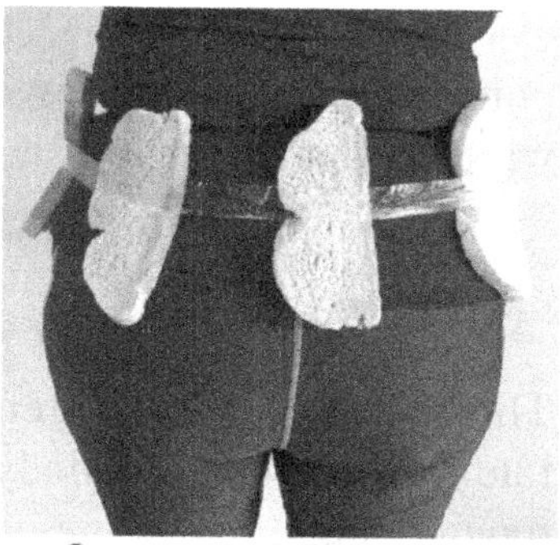

Once you reach 50, your body produces more enzymes that turn **Bread, Potatoes and Sugar into fat.** If you eat such food, you may as well simply tape them to your hips!

According to Dr Mercola *www.mercola.com,* middle-age spread (belly fat) tends to increase as your fat cells produces the hormone **leptin,** which signals the body to stop eating. This may seem counter-intuitive, but overweight people have an overload of fat, and therefore an overload of leptin and the brain becomes less receptive (numbed by continual, insistent bombardment) of leptin's signals, so the body disregards the signal leading to overeating.

Fat cells also produce another hormone called **adiponectin,** which improves the body's insulin sensitivity. Larger fat cells naturally produce less adiponectin; therefore, obese people's insulin sensitivity is lowered and doesn't perform as intended, which may increase blood sugar levels.

Finally, your fat cells also produce **more** of an enzyme called **glycerol-3-phosphate dehydrogenase,** which converts starch and sugar into fat, making the body more efficient at turning potatoes, grains and sugar into fat.

Thermodynamics

Controlling weight is basic thermodynamics, however there's much, much more to it. Basically, if the energy you put in is more than the energy you're burning, the excess energy (food) will be stored as fat. To reduce or burn stored fat, you need to reduce the quantity and type of energy input (less carbs), increase your energy usage (exercise) or both. It is really that simple!

However, emotions initiated in childhood, ongoing habits, hormones, relationships, stress, sleep and self-worth all come into the equation.

The unit generally used to measure food energy is the **kilojoule** or **Calorie** (which, when spelled with a capital 'C', represents the kiloCalorie). Calories are generally used in the US and UK, with most of the rest of the world using kilojoules, including Australia (officially), however, 'Calorie' is widely used in Australia too.

In the food industry, a 'joule' is the measure of potential energy that food possesses to raise the temperature of one *kilogram* of water by one degree Celsius (1.8 degrees F). A 'calorie' (with a small 'c') is the measure of potential energy that food possesses to raise the temperature of one *gram* of water by one degree Celsius (the prefix 'kilo' means '1,000').

1kj = 239 Calories or transposed: 1 Calorie = 4.185kj

Sorry if I confused you, I didn't make the rules — I'm just the messenger☺

The body has two requirements for energy. The first is the basal metabolic rate (BMR) when the body is at rest – about 40-70% of the body's energy requirements, depending on your age, sex, size, heritage and activity. This is the underlying energy used to simply keep the body functioning; like the heart, lungs, brain, liver, temperature and digestion. There are numerous BMR calculators online; search and calculate your own BMR.

Building muscle increases the BMR and therefore burns more Calories without exercise. A person with a lower BMR is more likely to gain weight because they don't burn as much energy to appease their BMR, therefore requiring more exercise, which should increase muscle and consequentially their BMR, supporting weight loss.

The remaining energy requirement, on top of BMR, is energy required to take action such as sport, working, walking, running or carrying something.

The amount of energy the body requires varies depending on sex, age, height, weight, health, fitness and lifestyle. For example, a 180 cm (5'11") tall, 76 kg (168 lb) male, over 50 years who exercises moderately uses around 6,720 kj (1,600 Calories) per day for the BMR and a further 2,520–3,780 kj (600–900 Calories) for effort, a total requirement of 9,240–10,500 kj (2,200–2,500 Calories) per day.

A 160 cm (5'3") tall, 58 kg (128 lb) female in a similar situation uses around 4,620 kj (1,100 Calories) BMR and 2,100–2,940 kj (500–700 Calories) for effort, totalling 6,720–7,560 kj (1,600–1,800 Calories).

In general, the typical energy requirement for **women** is around 7,560 kj (**1,800 Calories**) and for **men** around 8,400 kj (**2,000 Calories**) per day.

In 2014 the average American consumed 15,770 kj (3,770 Calories) per day. Remember, these are average figures, not considering sex, age, height, weight, health, or exercise. The primary source of extra kilojoules was from the increased consumption of carbs in the form of sugar hidden within soft drinks (soda), which accounts for 25% of daily Calories in young adults.

Requirement vs Intake

'Requirement' is different to 'intake'. 'Requirement' is what a body needs to maintain a healthy weight and 'intake' is what is actually eaten, most often too much and/or unsupportive food.

Some individual fast food **meal** servings alone are more than the daily average requirement. For example, a McDonald's Double Quarter Pounder, large chips (fries), Coke and caramel sundae equals 8,777 kj (2,090 Calories).

Also, the recommended daily average energy intake for a six-year-old is 6,700 kj (1,600 Calories), and 7,600 kj (1,810 Calories) for a ten-year-old. A Happy Meal can contain up to 2,800 kj (667 Calories), 36–41% of their daily requirements. Partly because of the low cost and ease of fast food, the US, Australia and the UK hold the world record for the world's three most overweight populations (as a percentage of population).

Any food that is eaten over the total daily requirement is stored as fat. Even if it's only 25 g (0.9 oz) over the requirement, it's still stored as fat. If you do this daily — 25 g x 7 days = 0.175 kg (6 oz) weight gain in one week. That extrapolates to 0.75 kg (1.6 lb) per month or 9 kg (20 lb) over one year. Do this year after year and you can easily put on an extra 20–30 kg (44–66 lb) over two or three decades.

Control your Emotions

Scientific studies (and personal experience) have shown that Calorie-counting and extreme exercise simply don't work in the long-term. Rigorous and expensive regimes are difficult to maintain, and people revert to old habits.

The solution is to resolve emotional triggers that engage cravings for short-term pleasure – like unsupportive food. Over time, you will naturally develop new supportive habits - lifestyle (positive hypnotic drifting).

Resolving emotions is surprisingly easily done through the Emotion Code and Body Code work by Dr Bradley Nelson www.drbradleynelson.com *see resources section for practitioners who can conduct sessions via phone, etc.*

Alcohol

Alcohol contains 29 kj (7 Calories) per gram. The problem with alcohol is that the body metabolises alcohol and sugars **ahead** of burning fat, which isn't desirable. On top of the Calories alcohol contains, you often consume extra Calories from the carrier or mixer (Coke, tonic, ale, etc). Alcohol also stimulates hunger and reduces self-control, encouraging you to munch on unsupportive food and eat more than you intended. Alcohol is mostly consumed during the evening, when the body should be slowing down to metabolise the day's ingestion.

A 375 ml (12 oz) stubby of beer contains around 609 kj (145 Calories), whilst a glass of red wine or a gin and tonic, contains 500 kj (119 Calories).

Every standard drink of alcohol (glass of beer, wine, or one shot of spirits) distracts the liver from performing its normal functions for **two hours**. The outcome of the liver's processing of alcohol is a very toxic mix of free radicals, which provide your hangover the next day.

If you drink alcohol daily, you will continually supply your body with a toxic mix which will contribute to degenerative diseases over time and increase your weight. Search YouTube for *"Is Binge Drinking Really That Bad?"*

Each time you drink alcohol, the intestines trigger production of mucus for protection. This mucus accumulates toxins and impedes nutrition and waste transfer. On top of this, alcohol also kills friendly gut bacteria.

So, if you're having a few drinks, before you go to bed, take AIM Herbal FiberBlend™ (HFB) which has insoluble fibre that 'scrapes' the colon wall to clear mucus. Also ensure you take probiotics which works brilliantly with HFB in this situation. Also add a couple of capsules of stem cell nutrition to rebuild damaged cells whilst you sleep. *See resource section*

Kombucha – an Excellent Alternative to Alcohol

Kombucha is a great tasting, refreshing and healthy **alternative to alcohol**. Personally, we only moderately drink alcohol socially on weekends. The rest of the week, we carbonate our filtered water using SodaStream and combine with a quarter glass of kombucha.

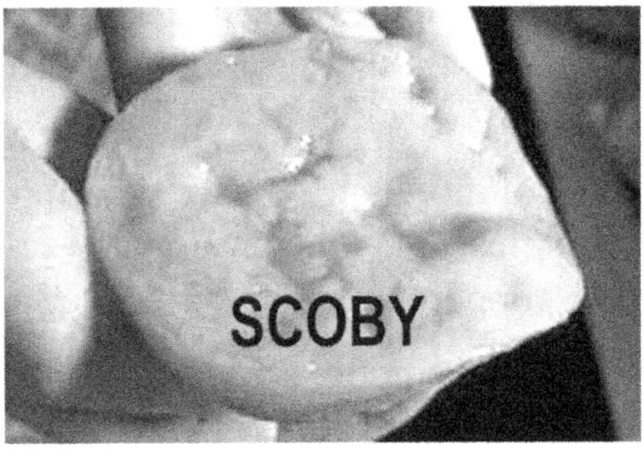

Kombucha uses a 'SCOBY' (Symbiotic Culture of Bacteria and Yeast) that is grown in sweetened black tea and provides healthy gut bacteria to your gut. The sugar is converted into acid/vinegar so is good for your gut.

Making Kombucha

- Allow 20 mins
- Obtain a SCOBY and 750 ml of mature Kombucha from a friend or call us and we may have one spare
- Make a large pot of normal black tea (containing caffeine) with 2 tablespoons of tea leaves and let cool to ambient temperature
- Once cooled, pour into a bowl and stir in 150g of sugar

Into a 4-5 litre jar (available at K-Mart, etc) …

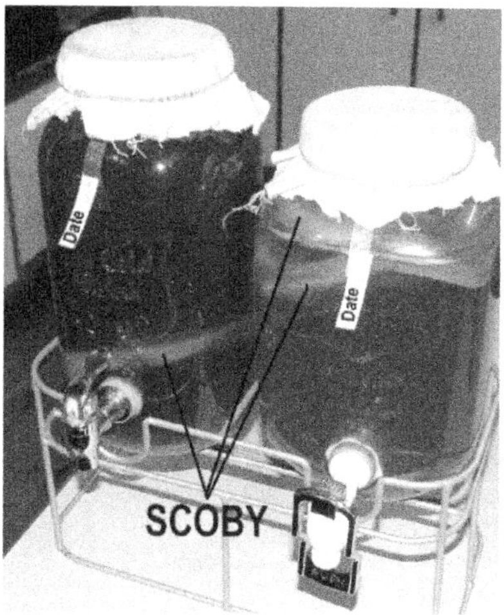

- Add about 750 ml of previously matured Kombucha
- Add the cooled, sweetened black tea
- Top up with filtered water (not tap water – no fluoride or chlorine)
- Add the SCOBY
- Place cloth and rubber band over the top of the jar
- Label and date the jar

Then…

- Wait 7-10 days and drink as desired. The longer you leave a batch sit, the more vinegar/acid will be formed which will taste more bitter and better for gut bacteria
- Retain the SCOBY and about 750 ml of this matured batch for the next batch
- If an extra SCOBY grows, share it with a friend and spread the love. Share this book with them so they know how to make their own batch.

Separate Calories from Nutrition

All nutrition contains Calories, however, not all Calories are nutritious.

For example, a refreshing glass of half a freshly squeezed lemon with soda water contains 16-32 kj (4-8 Calories) and supportive nutrition that the body can utilise.

Alternatively drinking a lemon soft drink (soda) with its nine teaspoons of sugar, artificial flavours and colours contains 525 kj (125 Calories) and almost no nutrition – basically most of the Calories will be stored as fat.

Energy in Food Information

On the next page, I have presented just one page from an extensive list of Calorie, kilojoule, sugar and omega-3 levels for food that is typically eaten in a western diet.

I've also included more supportive choices (vegetables) for comparison with refined carbohydrates, for example.

Omega-3 ratings are based on the higher the number, the more benefit. Lower omega numbers (especially minus [-] numbers) indicate a predominance of inflammatory omega-6 over essential omega-3 oils. *See 'EFAs' later.*

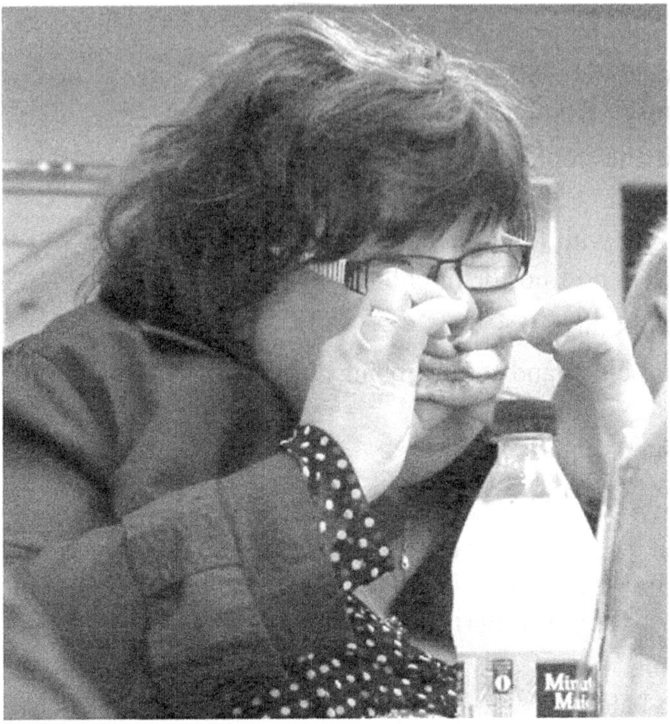

How you feel about every-day events in your life triggers emotions that lead to thoughts, producing activity which creates habits that create your life.

To change your life, you have to do something different.

Taking responsibility gives you the ability to respond.

Priority should be given to low calorie, low sugar, high fibre and high Omega-3 content foods. And no prizes for guessing what food fits this category best: vegetables, especially leafy green vegetables.

I tried to source such a document but was unsuccessful. I focused for many weeks to compile this valuable resource for my readers. You won't find such a list anywhere else.

You can download a complete list of over 130 common foods from:

www.cleanup-your-act.com

Our website is the only place you will find such a useful, extensive list!

Energy, Sugar and Omega-3 Levels in Food

Food	Comparative Metric	Comparative Imperial	Energy kj	Energy Cal	Sugar %	Omega-3 High in?	Typical Serving Size Metric	Typical Serving Size Imperial	Energy kj	Energy Cal
Chips – McDonald's large serve (fries)	NA				0	-12	1 serve		1900	455
Pizza – Pizza Hut Meat Lovers thick	100 g	3.5 oz	1148	275	4.2	-5	3 slices		3099	744
Quarter pounder – McDonald's	NA				*6.2 g	-6	1 burger		2300	550
Shake – McDonald's (chocolate)	NA				8.5	-2	1 large cup (470 ml, 16 fl oz)		2110	503
Subway – 6" chick. teri. no dressing	100 g	3.5 oz	538	129	4	-3	1 Sub with basic salad		1280	306
Sushi – chicken and avocado roll	100 g	3.5 oz	700	167	6.5	-2	1 roll (110 g, 3.9 oz)		770	184
Chicken – breast (grilled)	100 g	3.5 oz	690	165	0	-4	200 g	7 oz	1380	330
Fish – barramundi (grilled)	100 g	3.5 oz	505	121	0	41	200 g	7 oz	1010	242
Ham – leg (lean)	100 g	3.5 oz	453	108	0	-5	100 g	3.5 oz	453	108
Steak – rump (grilled)	100 g	3.5 oz	740	177	0	-2	210 g	7.4 oz	1554	372
Bread – white	100 g	3.5 oz	986	236	4	-2	2 slices		690	165
Cereal – muesli (toasted)	100 g	3.5 oz	1692	405	19.7	-5	55 g	1.9 oz	931	223
Cereal – oats	100 g	3.5 oz	1590	380	1	-6	30 g	1 oz	477	114
Flour – white	100 g	3.5 oz	1484	355	0	-2	140 g	1 cup	2087	497
Noodles – egg	100 g	3.5 oz	1179	282	0	-4	⅓ pack (70 g, 2.5 oz)		825	197
Pasta – plain	100 g	3.5 oz	584	140	0	-3	150 g	5.3 oz	876	210
Rice – white (boiled)	100 g	3.5 oz	671	161	0.1	0	80 g	2.8 oz	537	129
Sugar – white or raw	100 g	3.5 Oz	1600	383	100	0	1 rounded teaspoon		80	19
Sardine – canned	100 g	3.5 oz	946	226	0.5	44	1 can (110 g, 3.9 oz)		710	170
Butter	100 g	3.5 oz	3000	718	0.5	-3	1 tablespoon		600	144
Cheese – cheddar	100 g	3.5 oz	1700	407	0.5	-1	25 g	0.9 oz	425	102
Cheese – cottage (low fat)	100 g	3.5 oz	375	90	0.3	0	1 tablespoon		75	18
Ice cream – full cream 10% fat	100 g	3.5 oz	815	195	21.4	0	1 litre (500 g, 17.6 oz)		4075	975
Milk – full cream 3.6% fat	100 ml	3.4 fl oz	280	67	*4.7 g	-1	250 ml	1 cup	700	168
Yoghurt – 2% fat with strawberries	100 g	3.5 oz	405	97	15	0	1 tub (170 g, 6 oz)		689	165
Biscuits chocolate – Tim Tams (orig.)	100 g	3.5 oz	2180	522	44	-2	1 biscuit		410	98
Biscuits – plain	100 g	3.5 oz	1895	453	2.2	-15	1 biscuit		190	45
Potato chips	100 g	3.5 oz	2180	522	1.7	-16	1 packet (175 g, 6.2 oz)		3815	914
Snickers chocolate bar	100 g	3.5 oz	2113	506	50	-6	1 bar (53 g, 1.9 oz)		1120	268
Jam – strawberry (jelly)	100 g	3.5 oz	1123	269	64.4	0	1 tablespoon		168	40
Peanut butter	100 g	3.5 oz	2521	603	6.5	-19	1 tablespoon		504	121
Beer	100 ml	3.4 fl oz	152	36	*0.2 g	0	1 can (375 ml, 12.7 fl oz)		570	135
Rum and cola mix	100 ml	3.4 fl oz	282	67	*10 g	0	1 can (375 ml, 12.7 fl oz)		1058	253
Wine – red	100 ml	3.4 fl oz	285	68	0	0	1 glass (160 ml, 5.4 fl oz)		456	109
Coca Cola	100 ml	3.4 fl oz	180	43	*10.6 g	0	1 can (375 ml, 12.7 fl oz)		675	161
Energy drink (Red Bull)	100 ml	3.4 fl oz	192	46	*11 g	0	1 can (355 ml, 12 fl oz)		682	163
Egg – hard boiled	100 g	3.5 oz	545	130	0.3	-9	1 large egg		240	57
Peanuts – oil roasted with salt	100 g	3.5 oz	2635	630	4.7	-22	30 nuts		791	189
Broccolli	100 g	3.5 oz	124	30	0.4	3	2 florets (45 g, 1.6 oz)		56	14
Carrot	100 g	3.5 oz	132	32	5	-3	1 medium (140 g, 4.9 oz)		185	45
Lettuce	100 g	3.5 oz	40	10	0.4	4	3 leaves (30 g, 1.1 oz)		12	3
Peas	100 g	3.5 oz	246	59	2.7	0	80 g	½ cup	197	47
Potato (boiled)	100 g	3.5 oz	251	60	1.7	0	1 medium (100 g, 3.5 oz)		251	60
Pumpkin	100 g	3.5 oz	218	52	7.1	0	1 medium (100 g, 3.5 oz)		218	52
Sweet potato – orange (boiled)	100 g	3.5 oz	273	65	5.6	0	200 g	½ cup	502	220
Apple	100 g	3.5 oz	204	49	10.4	-1	1 medium (150 g, 5.3 oz)		282	68
Avocado	100 g	3.5 oz	862	206	0.5	-9	1/2 large (100 g, 3.5 oz)		862	206
Banana	100 g	3.5 oz	378	90	16.9	0	1 medium 20cm (8") long (200 g, 7 oz)		510	122
Orange	100 g	3.5 oz	175	42	8	0	1 medium (200 g, 7 oz)		285	68
Dried – sultanas	100 g	3.5 oz	1311	314	73.2	-1	40 g	1.4 oz	524	126

* grams (weight) of sugar contained within 100 ml (volume), rather than percentage of weight

Omega-3 ratings = high #, the more benefit. Lower # indicate a predominance of inflammatory Omega-6 over Omega-3 oils.

The average calorie intake per person is approx 7560-8400 kj (1800-2000 Cal) per day

Remember, it's about the quality of Calories consumed, not necessarily the quantity.

A banana at 122 Calories is better for you than one Tim Tam at 98 Calories.

<u>What I Did</u> to Reduce Weight

Importance of Animal Protein

I found this difficult to comprehend when I was recently introduced to the concept of eating more meat, fat, eggs, butter, cream and cheese during my recent detox program when I had my root canal removed.

Initially I was sceptical, however the more I followed the plan, the more weight I reduced and the better I felt. I continue to follow this strategy as part of my normal routine now and I'm feeling better, fitter and stronger than ever.

Eating should be based around one main meal per day with 60-70% fat, 20% protein, 15-20% steamed or raw veggies from the garden which includes carbohydrates. Included in the above carb intake – grains, fruit or sugar should be no more than 5%.

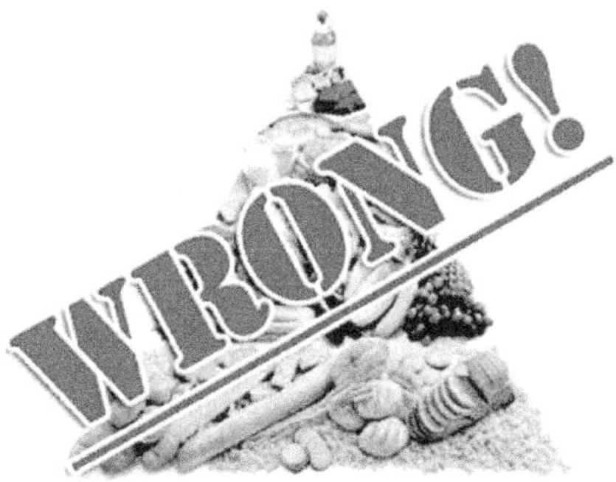

This concept goes against most popular nutrition advice and the mainstream food pyramid. We have been misled by US grain-grower lobbyists for 'Big Ag' who influenced congress in the 1950s to make grain and broad-acre farm products the main part of our western diet – **it was a big fat lie** and the truth is now being revealed through publications like this. If in doubt, do your own research and/or trust one who has been there (me☺). Be sceptical of someone who has read information out of a book, been taught in a class and repeated it – you should look at the original source of information.

Google, YouTube and Wikipedia

When researching, I've found that I **<u>can't trust</u> Google, YouTube or Wikipedia** as their algorithms have a bias towards mainstream medicine's views regarding health, left-leaning politics, etc. As much as possible, I use other search engines or video platforms like Brave, Firefox, DuckDuckGo, Bing, BitChute, BitTube.tv, Vimeo, Dailymotion and more.

One family in Silicon Valley controls around 90% of the world's internet search information and dictates what you see and therefore can manipulate what you believe and who you trust.

YouTube CEO, Susan Wojcicki and her husband **Dennis Troper** (Google exec) strongly influence what is recommended and you find when searching online. Susan's sister, **Anne Wojcicki is CEO of Wikipedia** and Anne was married to co-founder of Google, Russian immigrant **Sergey Brin**; they divorced in 2015. Sergey was **CEO of Alphabet**, Google and YouTube's parent company, until he stepped down in Dec 2019 when he was replaced by Indian immigrant Sunda Pichai who is currently CEO of Google too.

With their Polish and Russian heritage, is it any wonder why most of the "truth" we find online and in lamestream media/medicine is left-leaning, socialist, victim, hope, greater-good and system-controlled via this family's opinions? Their truth, beliefs and prejudices are what you to see when you search for facts. Alternative views and actual facts/truth are often purposely suppressed for control. **YouTube removes over 3 million videos every month** that don't match their version of the "truth" under the guise of "hate speech". They do this via AI and it's 10,000 employees dedicated to this function. At a basic level, this is propaganda or censorship and if it were a country, dictatorship or socialism. www.stopbitburning.com But I digress…

Animal Protein

Animal protein stimulates bile production and has a low insulin response; therefore, you store less as fat. The extra bile combined with fat, attaches to toxins as amino acids *(see '<u>Detoxing</u>' later)* and escorts them out the bowel, bladder, etc.

Animal protein is slow to digest but is a quality nutrient and is therefore offers plenty of nutrition for energy and provides a feeling of satiety (feeling satisfied) between meals, reducing cravings for carbs.

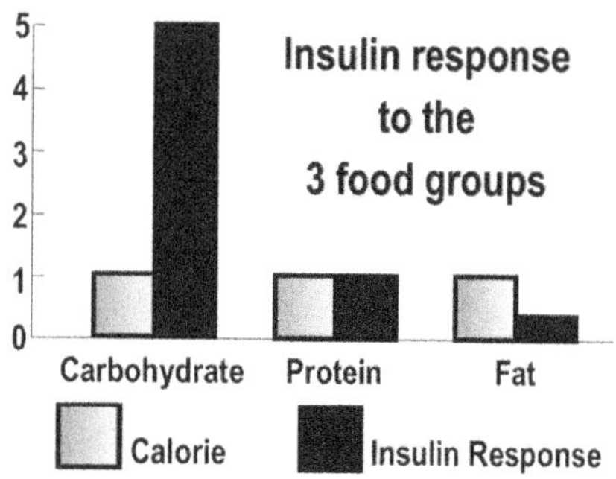

Combined with the elimination of unsupportive carbs like sugar, grain products, caffeine and alcohol the body has a real chance of repair. And the idea is entirely logical as carbs trigger a huge **insulin response, five times greater** than the carbs ingested and most people are in some way carb intolerant. Stimulants and alcohol distract the liver from metabolising fat, so the lack of such food allows more fat to be metabolised and toxins to be processed and discarded.

A minimum four-month commitment is necessary because it takes around 120 days for all the body's red blood cells to be fully replaced. Four months also breaks old habits and comfort reliances that may have previously been unsupportive. I found the first 2-3 weeks most challenging, and it took my bowel 6-8 weeks to adjust and pass normal stools again.

It's well-worth the effort! It's amazing how 'normal' some habits become (cake, biscuits, coffee, 1-2 beers or wine daily, snacking on chips at night, etc). Each of my previous 'normal' habits were contributing gram-by-gram to my weight-gain and potential long-term mental or other illnesses.

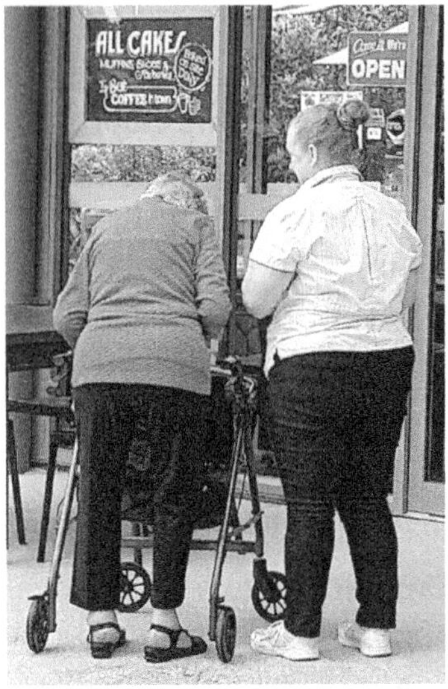

I observe so many people around my age in shopping centres on walking frames moving steadily to the nearest café with their carer in tow, ready to order another cappuccino and donut to support their carb addiction that has created their disability.

I'm so grateful I'm no longer one of them. I know my knowledge could help them, but I also know they probably won't listen. They perceive they've simply been unlucky and 'caught' their disease or disability and they fully expect the public health system and taxpayers to support them through their illness and nursing.

Stocking your Low-Carb Pantry

Flours

- Almond flour and meal
- Coconut flour
- Flaxseed meal
- Hazelnut meal
- Pecan meal
- All other ground nut meals

Thickeners / Binders

- Eggs
- Psyllium husk
- Ground flaxseed
- Chia seeds
- Xanthan gum

Sweeteners

- Monk fruit sweetener
- Erythritol
- Stevia
- Tagatose
- Xylitol

Fats

- Avocado
- Avocado oil
- Coconut oil
- Coconut cream or milk
- Almond milk
- Ghee
- Butter

Other

- Vanilla bean powder or extract
- All herbs and spices
- Baking powder (aluminium-free) or cream of tartar
- Baking soda

An excellent website is DrPompa.com for a free eBook featuring meals and recipes. Another is DrBerg.com who also has a YouTube channel.

My Program

I weighed myself after my first urination, before my shower, at 6am on the same day each week and followed my progress on a chart. Weighing weekly under the same circumstances is important as your weight can vary 1-2 kg each day, depending on what you've ingested, excreted and your activity. First thing in the morning is a consistent situation not affected by food, water or exercise (depending on activity in bed, of course ☺).

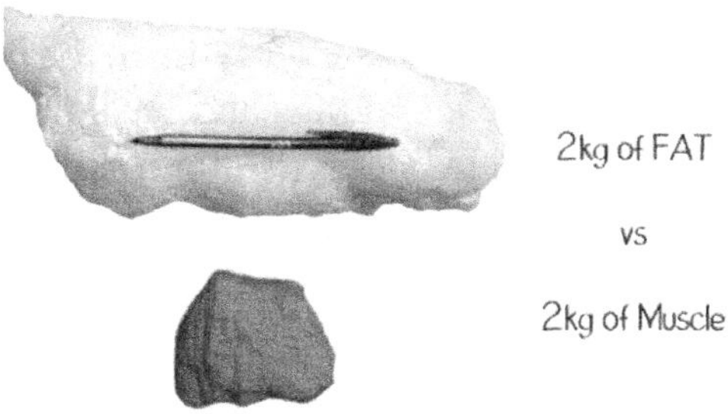

Incidentally, one kilo of fat has more mass than one kilo of muscle, so when you are reducing weight and building muscle through exercise, you may not find much change in your weight, but you should find your belt size reducing and your clothes fit better.

Guaranteed Weight Reduction Principles – the IMPORTANT PART

- Generally (through ignorance, conditioning and inherited habits), we eat way-more than we need.
- Insulin's chief message is to store fat, and body fat stores toxins.
- **Every time** you eat, the pancreas is triggered to produce insulin.
- **Carbs trigger five times more insulin** than protein or fat.

- When you eat, you store some of that energy (glycogen) in the liver which the body uses for energy for the next 10-hours or so.
- When you eat every 6 hours or so and snack in between, your body adapts to living of the energy produced by ingesting carbs.
- When you **don't eat** (i.e. fast) for periods of 12-18 hours, the body releases your body fat into the bloodstream. When the liver burns fat, it releases chemicals called 'ketones' (a state known as 'ketosis') which is highly advantageous to your health, especially the brain.
- This process of regular fasting is called Intermittent Fasting (IF) which has its most significant impact after 16-18 hours when ketones are increased up to 20-fold.
- Add to this, what is commonly known as a 'Ketogenic Diet' (next), which increases ketones 4-fold and you have a significant tactic to use and avoid your middle-age-spread and potential mental illness.
- Therefore, eat only during a 6-8-hour window, say between 12 noon and 6 pm. Avoid snacks, do your best to eat only one or two hearty meals. Over time, work on narrowing your eating window down to around 4 hours with only one meal.
- By skipping breakfast, you also reduce your daily Caloric intake by one third. It's desirable to extend your fasting window between 16-18 hours plus. The easiest option is utilising your previous evening, sleep time and morning to extend your fasting period until lunch. It takes a few weeks to adjust to this process and up to 6-9 months for your body systems to adapt and become normal and regulate the body's fat levels.
- Currently, your body is probably regulated to obtain its energy from the food you eat (esp. carbs), therefore you often have cravings and feel hungry. Over time, your body will adjust to obtain energy from its stores of fat (using less energy for digestion), only urging hunger when needed.
- If you like, once a week (say Sunday or on special occasions), eat and drink whenever and whatever you desire. This interrupts the body's automatic by-pass systems and reduce the feeling of missing out socially. Observe how your choices naturally improve to better choices over time.
- Meals should be 60-70% fat, 20% protein, 15-20% steamed or raw veggies from the garden which includes carbohydrates. Included in the above carb intake – grains, fruit or sugar should be no more than 5%.
- When you eat, make your one or two meals primarily animal protein (150-200g) plus vegetables and mushrooms with fat from coconut, avocado and olive products, butter, cream and a little cheese, etc.

- Make your vegetables primarily leafy-green and/or cruciferous, (cabbage, broccoli, cauliflower, kale, brussels sprouts, onion, garlic, bok choi, etc) and fermented (sauerkraut, kombucha, etc). Add mushrooms for variety.
- Make your animal products (meat, dairy, eggs, etc) primarily grass-fed and/or organic for the best nutrients and Omega-3 content.
- If you're taking supplements, you're best to take them with your first meal of the day for maximum absorption, however they can be taken at other times during your eating window.
- Take fibre supplements (like AIM Herbal FiberBlend *see resource section*) 30-mins before you eat. Because you are eating less, you will have less faeces to pass and extra fibre will assist with being regular.
- Avoid (or minimal) fruit. Fruits are carbs and contain fructose (sugar). Berries or Kiwi Fruit are best.
- Don't eat carbs, (grain products, rice, oats, bread, cake, biscuits, cereals, pasta, sugar, white potato, etc. – basically most packaged food).
- Avoid alcohol (at least 4-5 days a week). Kombucha or lemon with soda water is a fantastic, healthy alternative and satisfies habitual needs.
- Drink 2-4 litres of quality water each day (not tap water).
- Have herbal teas or a quality black coffee during your fasting period if desired. If you really must have your coffee white, add coconut cream, but drink only during your eating window.
- Add quality salt as desired.
- After several weeks, once a week (say Monday), fast for a 24-hour period for bonus ketones and benefits. Increase this to 36+ hours when ready.
- Follow the above principles long enough and they will become a normal way of life without burden.
- Search YouTube for Dr Nicholas Sudano DC and Dr Berg for excellent guidance on keto.

What else to do…

- Have daily coffee enemas to remove toxins. *See chapter 9*
- Apply magnesium chloride to the skin after your daily shower.
- Exercise for a minimum of 30-40 mins daily.
- Skin Brush once a week to remove a layer of skin and toxins.
- Allow for times when you feel tired from detoxing and need to rest. Look at what you are achieving, rather than what you avoid eating and drinking

Weight Loss Benefits

The benefits I've experienced by shedding my extra 11kg have been many:

- I've detoxed my liver and body substantially
- After my initial skin rashes on my face, my skin is now much clearer, liver spots are reduced and detox pimples under my arms have disappeared
- My thinking is clear, and I find I have better focus
- The minor pain in my lower back, upper thoracic, shoulders, hips and knees has disappeared
- The gout I was experiencing in my left big toe is gone
- I have more flexibility and find it easier to bend over and move
- My eyesight has improved and no longer wear glasses
- My sinuses are clearing with less mucus around my throat and nose
- My clothes fit and feel better
- Flatulence is almost non-existent and when it happens, there is little odour
- I sleep more soundly
- I have much more energy
- I am happier and more at peace
- My immune system is stronger. I rarely get sick.

My experience supports my original beliefs regarding how we create our own ailments and reality through our ignorance, habits and choices.

My experience also shows that you don't need expensive weight-loss programs to achieve your goals. Statistics show that a large majority of weight-loss program customers usually return to their original weight within two years, unless they continue to pay for the program.

Since the viral spread of the effective 'keto diet', **Weightwatchers** share price has plummeted by 83% from US$102 in June 2018 to just US$17 a year later.

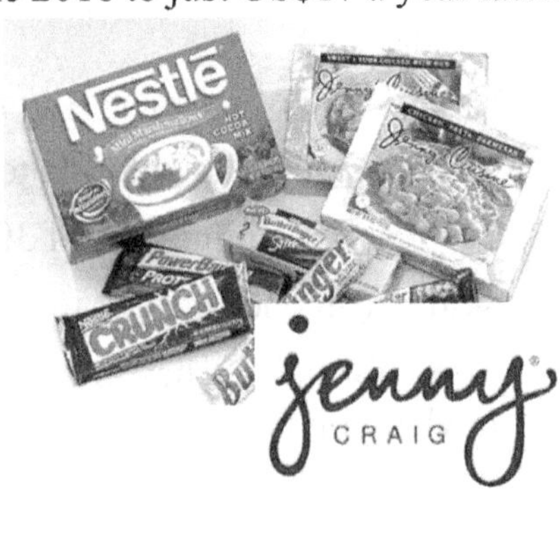

The largest weight-loss business in the world, **Jenny Craig, is owned by** the largest food company in the world — **Nestlé** — manufacturer of Mars Bars, Kit Kats and other junk food. So, whilst they're fattening you up on one end with sugar and chocolate, they're taking your weight loss dollars at the other. Nestlé also owns the Lean Cuisine frozen meal brand.

Weight Control Footnote

Having a good enough reason to control your weight is helpful to have the determination to carry through when times get tough. One reason that gave my wife and I the determination to follow-through and maintain our goal weights was the fact that we are older parents with 20-something children. When I'm over 70 years old, they will still be around 30ish and I want to be around to be part of their lives and a grandfather to their children. If I didn't make changes a decade ago, this may not happen. Sometimes you simply need a big enough reason to achieve your goals. What's yours?

Understanding High Blood Pressure

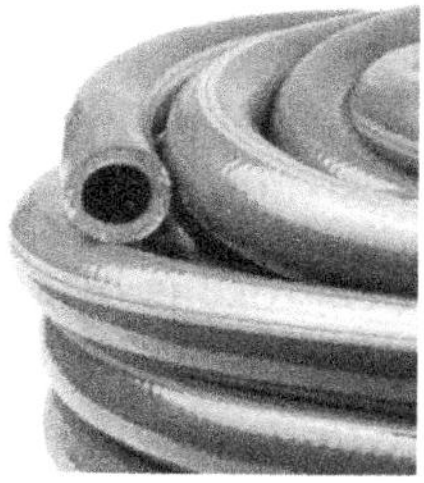

If you take a hard-walled garden hose and have a constant flow of water streaming through it, then the water pressure inside the hose is low. If you kink or block the end of the hose and continue streaming water through, the water pressure inside the hose will rise because the wall of the hose can't expand to take up the volume needed to hold the extra water. This creates high water pressure inside the hose.

If you do the same with a long sausage balloon, the soft walls of the balloon expand, taking up the water volume. This creates a constant, low water pressure inside the balloon.

That's what should happen with arteries. They should be more like the soft-walled balloon, expanding to take up the extra blood pressure created when we exercise, or we're stressed. Instead, because of medications like Statins and inadequate diet and exercise, our arteries become hardened (arteriosclerosis) and can't expand to take up the extra flow of blood, therefore, the heart keeps pumping and blood pressure rises which can lead to heart attacks, aneurisms and stroke.

Sugar

Sugar is extremely addictive, highly acid and one of the body's **major contributors of obesity, inflammation and cancer**. The cancer industry knows that sugar feeds cancer; however, your doctor will rarely tell you to ingest less sugar.

Since birth we've been programmed to eat grains and sugar daily for breakfast, enjoy sugar as a "treat", as a reward to celebrate an achievement or give as a gift. If we're feeling down, we've been taught to ingest sugar to help pick you up (i.e. chocolate) and make you feel better, and because we always want to feel better, sugar has become a daily habit to a point that the average person eats around 35kg annually in Australia and 46kg (101 lbs) in the USA.

Glucose and Fructose

Cane sugar is essentially made of two components, **glucose** which is captured in the blood by insulin and readily converted to energy in the liver. Glucose is not very sweet tasting on its own.

The other half of sugar is **fructose,** which **doesn't trigger insulin production** from the pancreas, leaving fructose to be absorbed directly into the bloodstream within minutes of ingestion without going through the liver. However, when fructose reaches the liver through its normal blood-filtering process, it is readily metabolised into fat. Fructose metabolised into fat in the liver can lead to non-alcoholic fatty liver disease (steatosis), as well as insulin resistance and type 2 diabetes.

Fructose is often represented in food ingredients as cane sugar, high fructose corn syrup (HFCS) or sucrose. Basically, most food-words with the suffix "ose" are sugars (e.g. sucrose, lactose, glucose, maltose, dextrose). There are a few commonly available sugars that don't contain fructose, like **dextrose, xylitol** (often branded as SweetLife) and herbs like **stevia**, which are better choices if you need something sweet in your life. Dextrose can be found in the home-brew section of most supermarkets.

According to *www.mercola.com,* fructose is the number one source of calories in the US.

Immune System Inhibitors

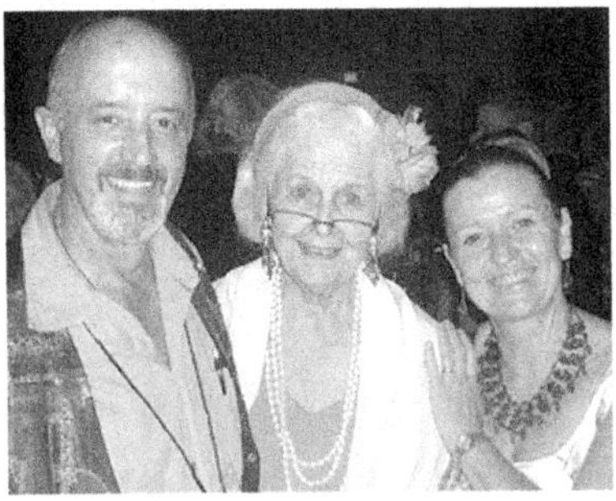

Ramiah & Shakti with
Dr Mary Ruth Swope 2009

According to Dr Mary Ruth Swope in her book, *Green Leaves of Barley*, sugar **inhibits the body's immune system** by redirecting the white blood cells (normally used to kill bacteria) and utilising them to deal with the impacts of sugar.

Normally a white blood cell will kill 14 bacteria every 30 minutes, however simply ingesting two cans of soft drink in one day (18 spoons of sugar), reduces the white blood cell's bacteria-killing capacity down to just two bacteria every 30 minutes.

The average Australian ingests 700g of sugar per week, which reduces the body's white blood cell killing capacity by around 70%, leaving bacteria and viruses to thrive. Is there any wonder there is so much sickness, infection and the perceived need for medication and treatment?

Every time you ingest sugar or carbs, you support unfriendly gut bacteria in the bowel, which in turn supresses the immune system and supports virus expansion. Unfriendly gut bacteria want to thrive in your bowel, therefore generate cravings for more sugar and carbs so they can continue to proliferate.

Adrenal Stimulant

Cortisol is produced in the adrenal glands which sit on top of the kidneys. Fructose and carbs stimulate the production of **cortisol** (an adrenaline hormone) to raise and stabilise blood sugar. Cortisol is acidic by nature and normally converts fat to sugar, but also causes water retention and is directly related to the accumulation of belly fat through its stimulation of insulin production.

If cortisol is produced and not used through exercise or work, it can accumulate and cause complications like heart disease. Ego-based thoughts and activity like vanity and narcissistic actions, and the ensuing stress derived, also produces cortisol and if not used physically, can be detrimental to health too.

Cortisol is an opiate (and gives a high for a short time), and consuming sugar stimulates cortisol production. The body craves more sugar in order to continue feeling high, which leads to addiction, even though the body is not addicted to the sugar, but rather to the high from cortisol.

Coffee (caffeine) reacts in a similar manner and can also be addictive. If you have a coffee and cake every day for morning tea, you may be keeping your cortisol levels artificially high, creating chronic stress and inflammation and eventually disease.

Appetite Control

Fructose tricks the body into gaining weight by fooling the body's metabolism, as it turns off the body's appetite-control system. Fructose does NOT appropriately stimulate insulin, which in turn does NOT suppress ghrelin (the 'hunger hormone') and does NOT stimulate leptin (the 'satiety hormone'). Together they result in eating more, gaining weight and developing insulin resistance.

Insulin Resistance

Insulin is like a key that allows glucose, amino acids and nutrients to enter cells. When we ingest sugar or carbs, insulin is released from the pancreas to capture glucose in the bloodstream and use it for energy.

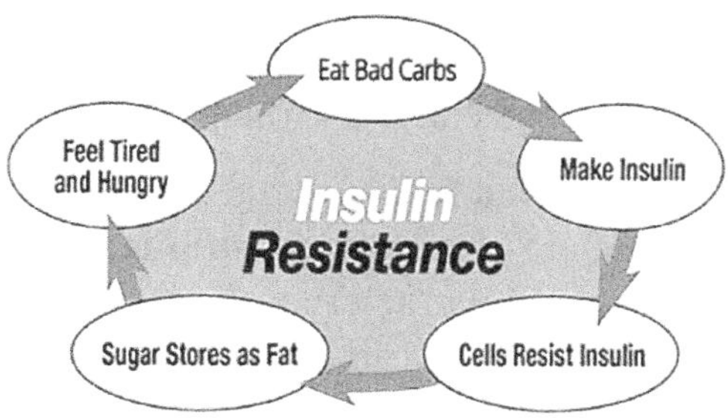

If we eat too much sugar too often, the pancreas becomes overworked and the insulin can't capture everything (the body becomes insulin-resistant), leaving the fructose and fat particles to settle in the arteries and capillaries in the body, causing disease as previously mentioned.

Also, cells no longer absorb insulin, which (incorrectly) signals to the pancreas that it needs to produce massive amounts or insulin in a denigrating feedback loop. The combination of not absorbing insulin in some areas (problems with brain, nerves and inflammation) with excess insulin in other areas (fatty liver, obesity, etc) causes major issues often related to diabetes.

Insulin resistance is the root-cause of most common health problems from heart disease, inflammation, arthritis, autoimmune diseases, high blood pressure, brain and mental illness, obesity, eyes, diabetes, bowel disorders, liver and kidney disease, hormone issues and ultimately cancer. Yet the sickness industrial complex treats each illness with a different drug, rather than fix the cause – eating too many carbs, too many times, every day. **Stress** also produces high levels of cortisol which breaks down protein, which in turn increases the production of insulin.

Fermentation Rather than Digestion

Sugar also acts as a catalyst for fermentation of food in the bowel. Rather than digesting, food tends to ferment, creating gas, increasing acidity, foggy brain and lack of concentration. The body uses fructose in the same way fructose is used to make alcohol. E.g. vodka is made by letting potatoes ferment by adding sugar and heat. Leave a batch sitting in warmth for a while and alcohol is formed then distilled to make vodka.

So, when eating a meal, avoid having dessert, fruit or soft drink immediately after or with your meal. Adding sugar, e.g. drinking soft drink with your chips, may initiate a vodka-like process in your gut, instead of digesting potato's starches.

Sugar in Fruit

In general, ***fru***it contains fructose (that's where ***fru***ctose derives its name) and when low sugar fruits are eaten as whole fruit in moderation (say one to two pieces a day), is beneficial to your diet because of the added synergy of fibre, vitamins and enzymes contained within.

Ripe or **dried fruit** contain more concentrated fructose. Dried fruit can also contain preservatives like **sulphur dioxide** (E220) used in dried apricots as a preservative and to retain the orange colour. E220 is used to preserve wine and beer too and can cause asthma, liver and gastric irritation and toxicity.

Fruit juice contains concentrated fructose and should be avoided — even if the label says, "no added sugar". Fruit juice can often contain more fructose than soft drink, so why would manufacturers need to add sugar?

Also, if you are eating fruit; eat it on its own, away from other food and eat just one type of fruit at a time. For example, it's best to eat a couple of apples or a couple of bananas on their own but avoid eating a banana and an apple together. Avoid mixing fruit or having a 'fruit salad'. Combining fruit mixes the sugars and has a similar fermenting effect as above.

Kidney Disease

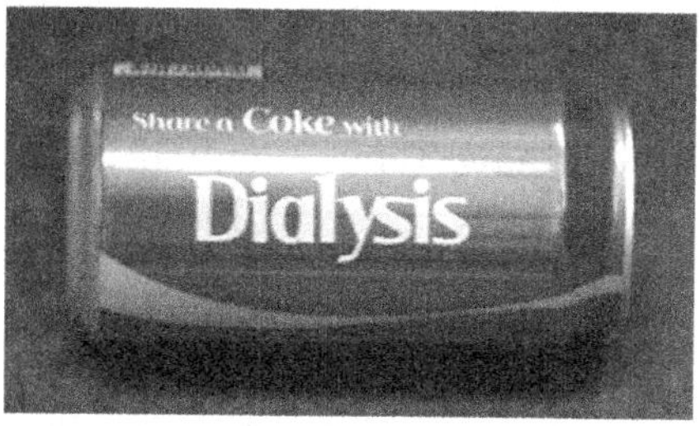

With a population of just 244,000 people, the Northern Territory in Australia has the highest per capita consumption of Coca Cola in the world. The Northern Territory also has the highest per capita incidence of kidney disease in Australia, extrapolating to kidney disease being the number one cause of hospitalisation in Australia. Hmmm... could there be a connection? One can of soft drink contains approximately nine teaspoons of sugar, plus caffeine…

Diabetes

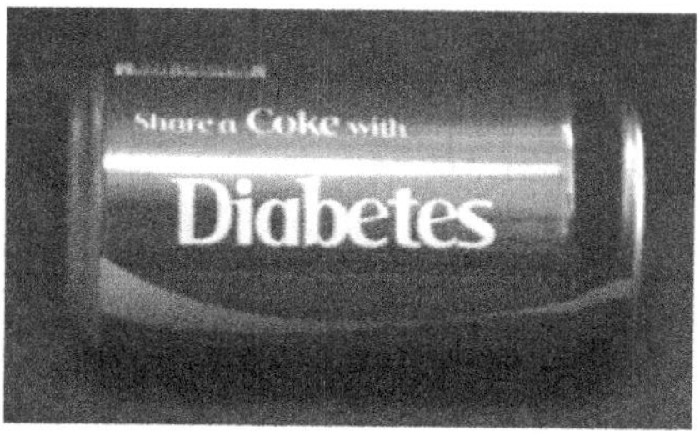

Diabetes is responsible for nine limb amputations per day in Australia, and at 63 a week, has an incredible impact on our health, rehabilitation and welfare resources. Diabetes can also lead to blindness, kidney failure, heart attack and stroke.

'Type 1 diabetes' was originally called 'child onset diabetes' and **'Type 2 Diabetes'** was called 'adult onset diabetes'. In general, both were given the name 'sugar diabetes' until the food industry had that changed in the 1960s. However, over the past few decades, sedentary, obese children have skipped right past child onset diabetes to adult onset diabetes, prompting the medical industry to rename the two types to avoid confusion.

What's the Difference?

Type 1 – the body's immune system destroys the cells that release insulin, eventually eliminating insulin production in the pancreas, progressing onto…

Type 2 – the body can't use insulin the right way and so becomes insulin resistant. As type 2 progresses, the pancreas makes less insulin. This is called insulin deficiency.

Go to YouTube and search for, "*diabetes explained simply*".

According to Dr Karl Kruszelnicki, "A study of indigenous Australians who returned to their traditional bush diet (away from the western refined-carbohydrate diet of flour and sugar) for just seven weeks found that even in that short time, they had both decreased weight and reversed metabolic abnormalities such as type 2 diabetes," saving potential dialysis, amputations and the above impact on the health system.

An 11-year study of 1300 people from the University of Western Australia showed that men between 55 and 84 years with type 2 diabetes had double the chance of developing bowel cancer.

If you have type 2 diabetes, it is particularly important to try to control it. Chronically raised blood sugar damages brain cells which may lead to depression and dementia.

The movie 'Forks Over Knives' demonstrates numerous examples of people reversing diabetes and heart disease through diet and lifestyle choices alone.

Working against this taking responsibility-based approach, in May 2012 Big Pharma *(see chapter 10)* were pushing for self-diagnostic diabetes kits to be released to the public with access to pharmaceutical drugs without visiting your doctor or obtaining a prescription.

Energy Drinks

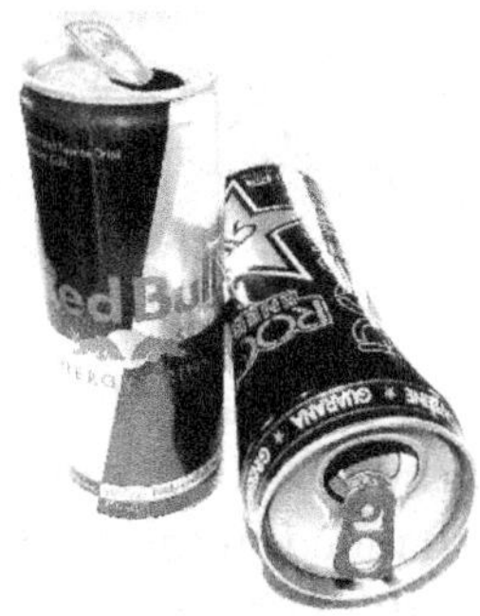

Concentrated sugar and caffeine (energy) drinks are waiting to unfold their long-term ugly side-effects on society. I observe on Friday and Saturday evenings numerous teenagers purchasing three or four cans of energy drinks at the local 'servo' as a legal alternative to alcohol. Though not marketed directly to children or teens, and displayed away from soft drinks, with health warnings clearly visible, a teenager can purchase one can for $3 or a four-pack for just $5, making it legal and affordable for teenagers. And the cans are getting bigger.

Drinks such as V, Mother, Red Bull, RockStar and Monster contain up to 14 teaspoons of sugar (compared to nine teaspoons in regular soft drink) and three times the caffeine content compared to Coke. Some also contain stimulants like guarana, ginseng, taurine, glucuronolactone, inositol and B vitamins. There can be significant problems if energy drinks are combined with sport, alcohol and recreational or pharmaceutical drugs.

Energy drinks can cause dehydration, headaches, diarrhoea, hyperactivity, dizziness, nausea, insomnia, aggression and can contribute to a 25% increase in heart rate maintained for twice as long as normal — increasing body stress.

Yet some school students, young teenagers and many twenty-somethings consume a can for breakfast and two to four cans per day to maintain their continuous hit of caffeine and sugar. They are addicted. Consuming this quantity is way above the recommended daily intake suggested on the can, but what child reads the small print on a can?

An article presented by the Royal Australian College of General Practitioners points out that a typical 250 ml mug of coffee contains about 85 mg of caffeine. Energy drinks contain about the same amount of caffeine per 100 milligrams (32 ml), but most energy drinks come in larger sizes and are drunk more often during the day or evening, often by children. Adults can consume the same amount during the day, on top of coffee. And remember, children eventually become adults bringing their addictive behaviours with them as they slowly develop their consequential chronic illnesses which will eventually overload the sickness industry.

Monster contains 160 mg of caffeine per 500 ml can. Drinking three to five cans per day can supply up to ten times the recommended daily limit of caffeine. Symptoms of caffeine overload include anxiety, jitteriness, nausea, diarrhoea, insomnia and increased heart rate. Withdrawal from caffeine can often cause the same symptoms but with increased headaches and moodiness. Do you know any millennials or Gen Ys' around you that fit these symptoms?

As a side note, sports drinks like Gatorade or PowerAde provide electrolytes and sugars and have been shown to be beneficial for elite sportspeople who strenuously exercise for many hours. Children drinking sports drinks are normally unable to fully utilise these sugars which are consequently converted to fat, contributing to childhood obesity. There are numerous healthy ATP enhancing energy drinks mentioned in the resources section.

What our younger society are really doing is exhausting their adrenals which may impact on the body in the longer term resulting in high blood pressure, anxiety, depression, kidney problems, diabetes, blindness and Alzheimer's.

Once addicted to caffeine and/or sugar, having a hit only brings you back to where you would have been (energy-wise) if you weren't addicted. Most need a morning 'hit' first up, to feel normal again and function in our world.

Recent research shows that ongoing consumption of energy drinks lowers the empathy level of the drinker, therefore they have less consideration of their impact on other people — they become self-centred and find it difficult to read other people's emotions and relate in a meaningful way. This has often been a stereotypical complaint about 'Gen Y' and millennials, but perhaps it's more about what they're consuming than how they were raised. Incidentally, drinking caffeinated soft drinks like Coke on its own had a similar effect on the empathy scale, whereas drinking water on its own improved empathy.

Health Foundations for Sale

Diabetes Australia and the Australian Heart Foundation (AHF) don't use sugar as a determinant for either diabetes or heart disease. That's why they give the AHF 'tick of approval' to Nestlé's sugar-ladened breakfast cereals — for a fee.

They use data supplied by the Dieticians Association of Australia (DAA) who issue our government-approved health guidelines for schools, defence forces, education and hospitals, and are linked to Glycaemic Index Ltd (who dish out the 'Low GI' ticks — also for a fee). The DAA receives money from the sugar industry, leading to conflicts of interest, which appear to be happening — how else does Milo cereal (29.7% sugar) obtain a tick of health from the AHF who use DAA data to justify their decision?

Likewise, governments in Australia have recently introduced laws requiring kilojoule (energy consumption) ratings to be displayed next to food signage at fast food outlets like McDonalds, Hungry Jacks, KFC and Pizza Hut. Because of sugar industry lobbying and DAA advice, sugar content was left off the signage, even though science proves that sugar consumption is directly related to increased weight and all its health complications.

There is a direct link between sugar consumption, obesity, diabetes and heart disease, the science proves it — but the various food and health foundations choose to use more convenient, selected data. Remember this next time they ask for your donation.

Despite what the diet industry might tell you, the only way to reduce weight is to detox, clean out the bowel and liver, eat more meat, fat and vegetables, eat fewer carbs, drink lots of quality water and exercise moderately daily. If you stop putting new layers of crap on top of the old layers, the body can start to deal with the old layers first *(see 'How We Can Heal Chronic Toxicity and Disease' later)*.

Every time you eat something unsupportive, the liver must deal with the recently ingested first, before it can begin to work on the chronic build-up of toxins and body fat. Save your money on buying expensive weight-loss programs and make the choice to take control of your own health today.

The average Australian consumes 700g of sugar per week. Simply eating an Australian Heart Foundation approved breakfast cereal and a glass of fruit juice each morning can provide you with just under half a kilogram of sugar per week. And that's without pastries, chocolate bars, soft drinks and shakes.

Artificial Sweeteners

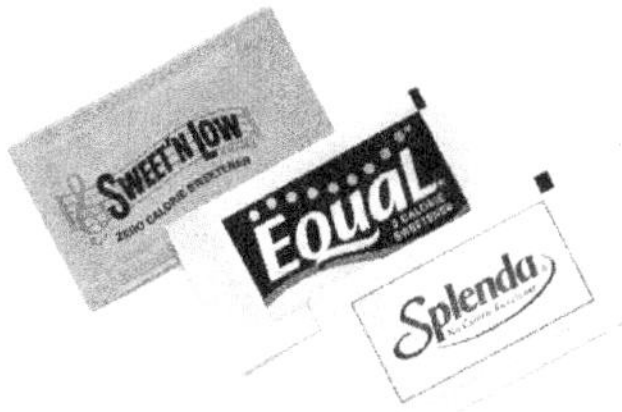

So, what about substituting sugar with artificial sweeteners? Aspartame and Saccharin are technical names for active ingredients used in brands like NutraSweet, Equal, Splenda, etc.

Aspartame is a chemical that was accidently discovered to be extremely sweet and has been marketed for the last few decades without adequate scientific human health studies being conducted. In fact, the few studies that have been conducted have basically shown that aspartame is detrimental to the health of rats, but because of the negative results, very few studies were conducted on humans. There have been no long-term studies on continuous use of aspartame in humans because there's no money to be made from such research. In fact, there is lots of money to be lost by chemical giants like Monsanto.

Science shows that when ingesting something sweet (without the equivalent energy — that is, a carbohydrate providing an actual boost of energy); the brain receives a signal saying, "I have received energy" and instigates insulin production which becomes imbalanced. Remember, insulin's basic function is to store fat, so the excess insulin races around the body to find sugars for storage. However, the body doesn't receive the expected energy boost, so, searching for balance, the brain then kicks in hormones to trigger hunger and cravings to justify the signal (perceived balance) — encouraging us to eat more.

Australian scientist, Dr Karl Kruszelnicki points out, "A study on rats at Purdue University in Indiana found artificial sweeteners break down the link between sweet tastes and calories, causing the rats to eat more and get fatter".

Artificial Sweeteners are Chemicals

Then there are the toxic chemical issues... too much aspartate, glutamate (from MSG (food additive 621 to 635) found in most spicy packet food) or both in the brain kills certain neurons by allowing the influx of too much calcium into each cell. This influx triggers excessive amounts of free radicals, which kill cells. This can lead to symptoms like memory loss, hypoglycaemia (low blood sugar), dementia, epilepsy, headaches, anxiety, sleep problems, depression, asthma or fatigue. You may not feel many of these symptoms immediately; it seems to take a few decades for symptoms to evolve.

There is a lot of concern lately about mental health issues, especially depression and aspartame may be a major contributor. The FDA approved Monsanto's aspartame application in 1974. At the time of approval, around 40 people employed by the FDA and involved in the approval process were later to receive highly-paid executive positions inside Monsanto, one of the world's largest chemical companies — hmmm... could there be a connection? *(reference: NEXUS Magazine)*

There is also a lot of conjecture about aspartame being carcinogenic — search it and have a look for yourself to see if you want to risk using aspartame.

Zero Coke and a Pizza Syndrome

I observe many people justifying eating pizzas, chips or burgers because they had a Zero Coke with it "to balance out the extra calories". Interestingly, I observe many diet-drinkers who are overweight. Watch out for labels promoting "No Sugar," "Sugar Free," "Low Calorie" or "Diet"; they will usually contain artificial sweeteners.

I know of several people where diabetics have changed their diet and taken herbal/fibre supplements to clean out their bowel and stabilise blood sugar. Now they have reduced weight, inflammation and have better circulation.

Some information on this topic has been gathered from
'Sweet Poison' *by David Gillespie, www.howmuchsugar.com.*
Also, information was obtained from www.mercola.com.

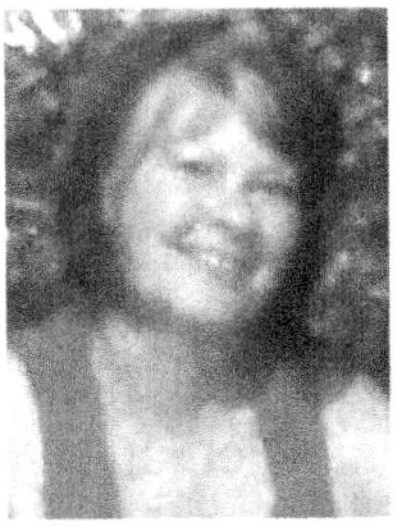

I'm 64 years old and have been diagnosed as a diabetic for 15 years now. Along with insulin for my diabetes, I have been on a number of medical drugs for hardening of my arteries, high blood pressure, high cholesterol and thyroid issues. At times, I have felt depressed and had no energy, especially in hot weather. Winter seemed okay, but summer got me down.

Just before Christmas, I was introduced to Herbal FiberBlend® and LeafGreens® and I have since reduced my insulin intake from ten to twelve units a day down to about four units (within six months).

We've been trying to sell our home, so over summer, I worked hard in the yard all day — something I couldn't do previously. Nothing seems a worry to me now and life seems less of a struggle, I feel clearer in the brain and look forward to more reductions in medication.

Janet — Cleveland Qld, Australia

Testimonials should not be construed as representing results everybody can achieve. Results may not be typical and may vary from person to person.

MSG the Hidden Additive

MSG (monosodium glutamate) is another food additive that has profound negative effects on the body's health, despite government administration approval. I believe the companies that put MSG in their packaged food don't really love you; they just want your money, again, again and again.

MSG is a flavour enhancer that can be created whilst cooking, but is also extensively added to spicy food, BBQ, vinegar or chilli-type flavours, noodles, soups, gravy, snacks, crackers, chicken salt, fast food and packaged food under the disguise of **Flavour Enhancer 621 to 635** (or similar). MSG can also be named hydrolysed vegetable protein (HVP), yeast extract, natural flavouring and numerous others.

MSG increases the amount of insulin created in the pancreas, can be addictive and encourages people to eat more. This can cause obesity, headaches, migraines, can trigger asthma and ADHD and increases the risk of heart attack, stroke, insomnia and diabetes. When dining out, especially at Asian restaurants, ask the proprietor if their food contains MSG?

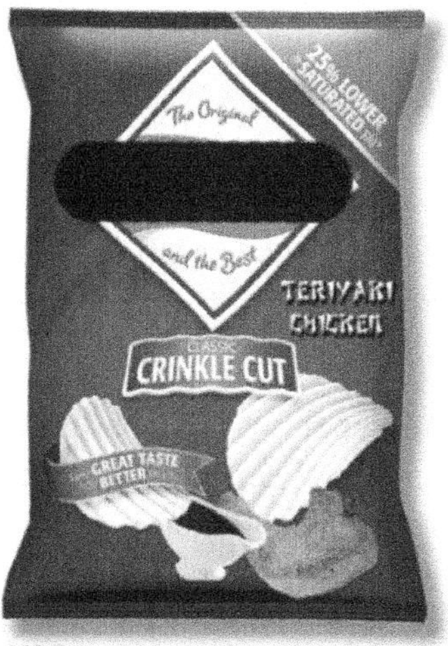

MSG is commonly found in most spicy snack food under the guise of 'Food Additive 621 to 635'

MSG is an 'excitotoxin', in that its chemical make-up is similar to serotonin (brain neurotransmitter), and the sudden oversupply over-excites and fatigues brain and nerve function leading to cravings, depression, chronic fatigue, mood swings, irritability, disorientation, learning difficulties, memory retention problems, Alzheimer's, Parkinson's and eye damage.

You won't hear much about the negative effects of MSG in lamestream media, as MSG is used everywhere in the fast food and packaged food industry and there is too much advertising revenue to be lost. So, you should do your own research☹.

For more evidence, search "MSG obese" or "MSG dangers".

Much of the information in this section came from Excitotoxins: The Taste that Kills *by Dr Russell Blaylock,* Slow Poisoning of America *by John Erb*, Chemical Maze *by Bill Statham*

Gall Bladder

As mentioned previously, the gall bladder is essentially a reservoir for bile (containing bicarbonate and salts) produced in the liver. The gall bladder also acts as a reservoir for waste released by the liver that is in turn released into the bowel for excretion from the body. The gall bladder bile reservoir sits ready for use should we ingest a highly acidic, fatty meal of dairy, sugar and refined flour (for example cappuccino and donuts).

When this type of meal is eaten, the gall bladder receives hormone signals in the blood (triggered from the intestines) which contracts and injects bile into the duodenum to aid in digestion and neutralise the stomach and food acid and start dissolving fat. The gall bladder holds around 50ml (1 ½ fl oz) of bile.

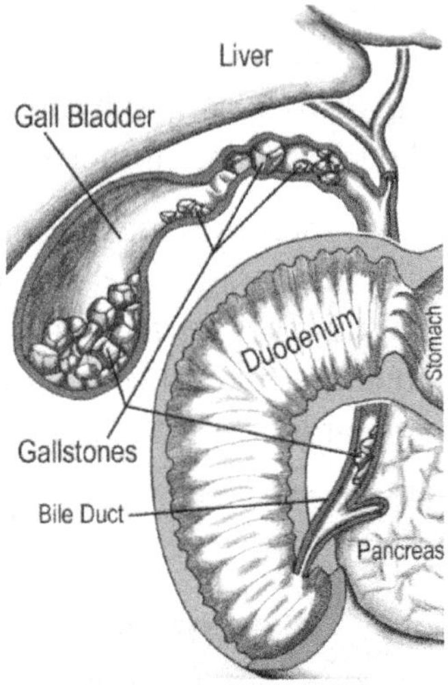

Gallstones

If we eat too many carbs and/or Omega-6 seed oils, the liver can have an oversupply of less supportive LDL cholesterol (fat), leading to clumps of cholesterol combining with unprocessed calcium accumulating in the liver, which then can be passed through to the gall bladder. These are called 'gallstones' and can be harmless until caught in the bile duct, which could then cause severe pain. A partially or fully blocked bile duct, can lead to inflammation and degeneration (rotting) of the gall bladder, sometimes necessitating removal of the gall bladder through surgery. Gallstones blocking the duct that is shared with the pancreas can lead to pancreatitis and pancreatic cancer *(see 'Pancreas' later)*.

Symptoms and Risk Factors

Symptoms of gall bladder problems include pain under the right ribs, fever, jaundice, nausea and vomiting. Overweight people, females, those with fair complexion and over 40 years old are the main risk groups. Gallstones don't cause cancer, but they are nearly always found in cancer patients, which can be an indication of a poor diet and lifestyle choices, therefore creating cancer.

Cholecystitis

Cholecystitis is the term used for an inflamed gall bladder. The gall bladder can be successfully removed through surgery with no apparent affects.

However, over the longer term, unless the diet is corrected to be significantly more alkaline with fewer carbs, the body could become more acidic — providing a nest-bed for disease. Also, something caused the initial inflammation, usually diet and lifestyle; so, unless changes are made, choices may continue to impact negatively on the liver. *(see 'Understanding Acid/Alkaline' previously)*.

My Experience

My stepfather-in-law had a gall bladder that turned gangrene through lack of circulation due to a blocked bile duct. Ultimately, because the decay infected the other organs around the gall bladder, he went through a very uncomfortable eight-week period of slowly dying, which caused a great deal of stress and discomfort to himself, my mother-in-law and our family.

Ever since I first met him in 1996, he always had strong breath (halitosis), which can be indicative of gut organ decline and dysfunction, though we didn't know this at the time.

Gall Bladder Flushes

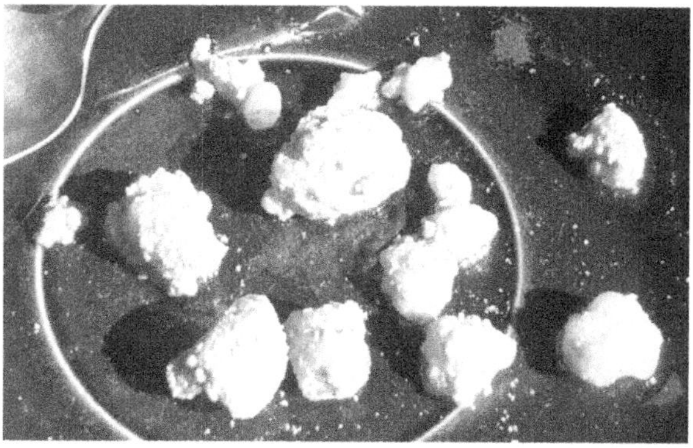

Gallstones removed from my gall bladder in 2006

The need for gall bladder surgery may be reduced by having regular gall bladder flushes. I have personally conducted many gall bladder flushes and removed thousands of gallstones. My wife and I perform an overnight gall bladder flush once or twice a year.

see instructions below

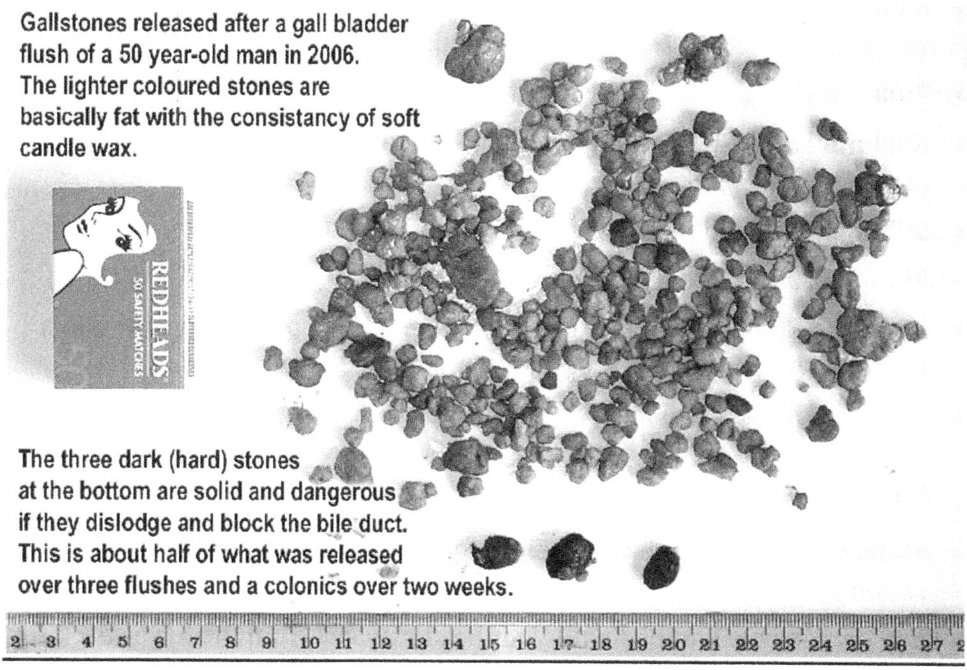
Gallstones released after a gall bladder flush of a 50 year-old man in 2006. The lighter coloured stones are basically fat with the consistancy of soft candle wax.
REDHEADS
50 SAFETY MATCHES
The three dark (hard) stones at the bottom are solid and dangerous if they dislodge and block the bile duct. This is about half of what was released over three flushes and a colonics over two weeks.

Gall Bladder Footnote

In January 2011, my wife was conducting one of her regular gall bladder flushes the same day our sister-in-law was having her gall bladder surgically removed. We all have choices.

12-Hour Gall Bladder and Liver Flush

Ingredients:

Epsom salts (magnesium sulphate)

Lemons (5–10 should be enough)

Olive oil (cold-pressed extra virgin)

Equipment:

Juicer (for lemons)

Glass or plastic jar with lid (to hold 700 ml (3 cups)) Colander (optional)

Water jug, metal spoon, saucer (optional)

Instructions:

Times are indicative only, but the **time spacing between** actions should be adhered to when possible.

- **2:00 pm** Don't eat after this time
- **6:00 pm** Dissolve 4 tablespoons of Epsom salts into 3 cups of warm water. Drink 200 ml (¾ cup) of the solution, leaving the rest aside
- **7:00 pm** Drink 200 ml (¾ cup) of Epsom salts solution
- **8:00 pm** Drink 200 ml (¾ cup) of Epsom salts solution. Feel free to pass motions as required.
- **9:00 pm** Drink 200 ml (¾ cup) of Epsom salts solution
- **9:45 pm** Juice 300 ml (1¼ cups) of lemon juice
- Pour the 300 ml of lemon juice and 400 ml (1½ cups) of olive oil into a jar with a lid and shake vigorously for a minute or two.
- Prepare your bed with pillows to elevate your body from the hips up (to minimize reflux).
- Place a bucket and towels beside the bed (just in case☺)
- **10:00 pm** Stand beside your bed and take five minutes only to drink the lemon juice and olive oil mix.
- Lay on your **back** in bed with your head elevated from the lower back for at least **20 mins**, then you may lay however is most comfortable.

- After 20 mins, you can lay in any position that is comfortable.
- **In the morning,** take 3 teaspoons of Epsom salts in water. This should move your bowel motion along within an hour — you can then follow with a coffee enema if you wish. Then follow with a probiotic and a good serve of fibre like psyllium husk, AIM Herbal FiberBlend® and/or Fit 'n Fiber®* along with plenty of quality water.

Notes:

If you want to measure how successful your gall bladder flush was, you can do the following:

1. To capture your stools, place a colander between the toilet bowl and lid.
2. After passing, use the water jug to pour water over the stools whilst running your spoon through the faeces to rinse the motion. Using the spoon, place your result on a saucer and photograph if you wish. Because gallstones are made of fat, they will not keep for long.

- The gallstones should appear with a green tinge and vary in size from 1–15 mm (1/16"– ½"+). There may be some brown gallstones too — these are mature, harder and may be more dangerous, being released from the bile duct, blocking flow and circulation.
- You may want to pass motions during the night, but mostly next morning.
- You may feel lethargic and slightly ill during the morning. This may be the toxins releasing from the liver. By lunch you should be feeling much better, then fantastic later. Avoid heavy work, dairy, carbs and sugar. Eat mostly vegetables and/or soup for a day (at least) if you can – to support your liver which has just had a huge shock.
- The Epsom salts relax and dilate the ducts of the liver and gall bladder so that gallstones can pass easier. Epsom salts also acts as a bowel stimulant.
- The lemon emulsifies the olive oil, making it easier to drink, and which causes the liver and gall bladder to constrict, squeezing out the gallstones and fat.
- The olive oil causes the liver to spasm, which helps release bile from the liver.
- Whitish to yellowish floating stools may be released during the afternoon and for a day or two after — this is mostly fat from your liver releasing, bile production catching up or both.
- Colonics experts recommended having colonics on the day of the treatment for safety and best results. (That is, colonics during the day, then gallbladder flush that evening, as well as, more importantly, colonics the

next day). Personally, I've never had colonics before or after; I find an enema sufficient. Your choice.

- If a large number of green and some brown gallstones appear, it is best to repeat this again weekly for three weeks, then twice a year. *"Bon Voyage Gallies!"*

Note: You should always consult your natural health practitioner prior to treatment. The supplier of this information is not responsible for any unexpected outcomes or consequences from this treatment. This is purely indicative of treatments I have given myself and result may vary from person to person.

Hulda Clark's book, *The Cure for all Diseases* offers a method that is similar to the above, but less dramatic and easier to handle. I have had the best results from the above method; however, some may find Hulda Clark's method more effective and easier. Search "Hulda Clark gallbladder cleanse".

Pancreas

The pancreas is a yellowish-coloured organ that sits behind the stomach and shares the entry point into the duodenum with the bile duct from the gall bladder/liver. Depending on your blood-sugar levels from food and activity taken around 15–60 minutes ago, the pancreas should release insulin, bicarbonate and enzymes to treat the chyme for digestion.

Insulin

Insulin acts like a key to access glucose for conversion to energy (ATP) in the liver. After this process, if there's too many carbs and sugars ingested, insulin's overriding message is to store sugar as fat. Insulin also acts as an appetite suppressant and once you have eaten enough food (to provide enough energy), the insulin should decrease your appetite, stopping you from eating. However, nowadays with the over-consumption of sugar and grains, the pancreas becomes overworked and with continual pumping of insulin into the blood, your body becomes insulin-resistant, which leads to diabetes. *(for more information, see 'Duodenum' and 'Fat and sugar' previously).*

Enzymes

The pancreas also makes digestive enzymes that are needed in combination with friendly gut bacteria to break down proteins into energy that the body can use. Often, because of our unsupportive diets, we can't make enough enzymes to digest food, especially gluten, lactose and casein (in the case of celiacs or food allergies or intolerances), so digestive enzyme supplements are recommended. Enzyme supplements won't diminish pancreatic enzyme production but will greatly enhance digestion and absorption.

Pancreatitis

The two main causes of pancreatitis are excessive alcohol consumption and gallstones blocking the common duct entry into the duodenum. Symptoms of pancreatitis are similar to gall bladder problems (plus itching under the left ribcage and weight loss) and can develop into pancreatic cancer which is the fourth most common cause of death from cancer in Australia.

Spleen

Though not really a digestive organ, I didn't want to leave the spleen out as it performs a vital role within the immune system: producing white blood cells (alkaline, oxygenated cells), returning iron to the blood, making disease-fighting components of the immune system (including antibodies and lymphocytes) along with destroying old red blood cells (acidic cells), releasing them as waste. The spleen also stores extra blood for emergencies, when short of breath (lack of oxygen), exercising or bleeding excessively.

The spleen can enlarge (often due to a struggling liver) if the body is under hypertension (high blood pressure), has a disease resulting in abnormal red blood cells, certain viral and bacterial infections, or in the case of some cancers and metabolic diseases.

Every 120 days the spleen systematically recycles and eventually removes hardened red blood cells by sending them to form part of the faeces and combined with green/yellow bile from the liver, gives the stool a darker-brown colour.

Chapter 4

Elimination System — Liquids

Kidneys

The first of the elimination organs are the kidneys. The kidneys filter most of the fluids in the body and regulate the mineral, salt, sugar, water and toxin levels, depending on the amount of water consumed and work performed.

Surprisingly, at any one time, the kidneys can hold almost 25% of the blood circulating around the body and filters about one litre (2.2 pints) every eight minutes.

Kidney Function

The kidneys' main function is to remove one to two litres (two to four pints) of waste daily from the blood and return the cleaned blood back into the body, excreting the waste through urine and in the process, also maintains correct mineral and body fluid levels.

The kidneys also produce red blood cells and balance the absorption, re-absorption and excretion of sodium salts, potassium salts, calcium, water and

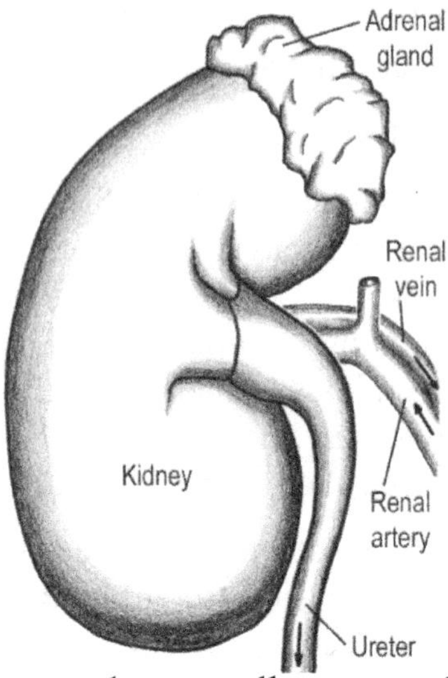

hormones regulating blood pressure. If we overeat, drink too much alcohol, or work excessively hard and perspire greatly causing dehydration, the kidneys over the next day (or so) should compensate and balance out the optimum fluid, salt and glucose levels. Often the kidneys will recirculate minerals to maintain body balance, and then excrete them when no longer needed.

Sugar and Kidneys

Overconsumption of sugar will have a detrimental effect on the kidneys. The fructose component of sugar stimulates the body to produce **uric acid** (an antioxidant, but when produced in excess, becomes a waste product usually removed through urine and faeces) which, if the kidneys fail to function optimally, can accumulate in the joints causing gout or arthritis. Uric acid also leads to chronic inflammation of the body's organs, which is the precursor to high blood pressure (hypertension), heart attacks and strokes. Uric acid clogs the small blood vessels inside the kidneys, leading to renal failure where the only solution is usually regular kidney dialysis or a kidney transplant. Kidney disease is **the major cause** of hospitalisation in Australia.

Vitamin 1,25D and the Kidneys

The best form of vitamin D is "activated 1,25D" (hormone 1,25-dihydroxy vitamin-D). Vitamin D3 is initially produced by sunlight hitting the skin (or from food or supplements containing vitamin D2 and D3), then transferred to the liver where it is converted into **calcitriol** (25-hydroxy-vitamin D) and is stored.

The sun's UVB rays convert a derivative of cholesterol – already prevalent in the skin – into Vitamin D3, which then travels to the liver.

Mushrooms are the only stable, natural vegan source of vitamin D2 with adequate potency. There are no vegetable sources of vitamin D3. Vitamin D3 supplements are derived from animals and the most prevalent being from lanolin on sheep's wool due to its availability and low cost.

When needed (triggered by the parathyroid glands behind the thyroid), 25-hydroxy vitamin D passes onto the kidneys, where enzymes convert it into vitamin 1,25D which only has a **life of just 6–8 hours**, but is **1000 times more active** than stored 25-hydroxy vitamin D which can be present in the body for 20 days or more.

Vitamin 1,25D has many effects throughout the body, including enabling calcium absorption in the intestines, therefore important for bone strength and healthy teeth.

The sun is the best source of Vitamin D. However due to seasons, weather and location, supplementation can help you build on the lack of vitamin D in the body. It's estimated that 59% of western society is vitamin D deficient, resulting in many diseases you are soon to read about.

Importance of Sunlight

Just 15–20 minutes of direct sunlight on the skin (not through glass or

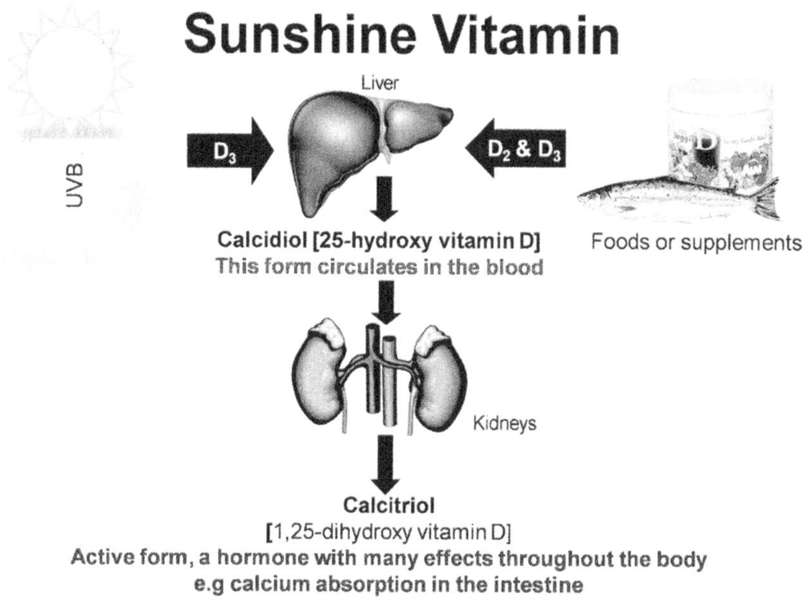

sunscreen) is enough to create sufficient vitamin D each day. If you are unable to obtain this, then food sources or supplementation is a good idea.

Too much sunlight in one sitting may cause your skin to burn and should be totally avoided. Applying 30+ sunscreen on children every time they venture outdoors for a short period is not supportive either as most sunscreens are made of chemicals the skin readily absorbs. Also, when the sun strikes the skin for a short period, it initiates the production of melanin in the skin which develops a protective tan, giving long-term protection to the skin. If the sun's rays are blocked every time, the skin doesn't develop any long-term protection and is more likely to burn under any amount of sun exposure.

I have noticed this phenomenon on my forearms which have received sunlight virtually every day, all my life. If I venture out in the harsh Australian sun without a shirt for over an hour, my shoulders and back will burn. However, I can stay out in the sun all day wearing a T-shirt and my forearms never burn,

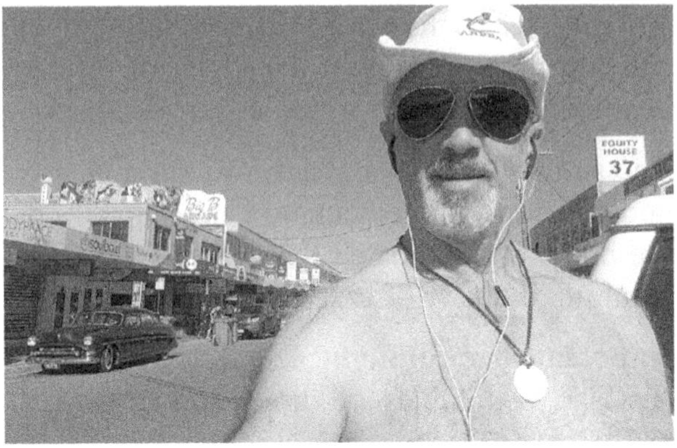

they just become darker. To try and improve my situation; when walking each morning and when weather permits, I take my shirt off which builds melanin on my chest, back and shoulders (the body's largest solar collection areas). I receive 'wolf-whistles' from 'chicki-babes' as I stroll around my neighbourhood and down the main street; however, I can handle the embarrassment.☺

Lack of sun exposure on the skin can also compromise the immune system and can encourage food allergies. Children need **education about sun protection**, not sun-fear, suppression and restriction.

According to *The China Study*, the impact of minimal sunlight is demonstrated in multiple sclerosis (MS), which is about **seven-fold** more prevalent in southern Tasmania (43ºS) than Townsville (19ºS) in Queensland, Australia.

Vitamin D's Function

Vitamin 1,25D is a vital hormone as indicated by its responsibilities for maintaining proper operation of the parathyroid glands, muscle, pancreas, bone, intestines (detoxing processes), heart, kidneys and brain.

Correct levels of 1,25D and vitamin D can prevent cells from becoming diseased. Diseases related to **vitamin D deficiency** are multiple sclerosis (MS), osteoporosis, rheumatoid arthritis, depression, schizophrenia, autism, prostate/breast/ovarian and colon cancer, asthma, heart disease, stroke, rickets, diabetes and obesity.

Vitamin 1,25D, Calcium and Dairy

Adequate amounts of vitamin **1,25D are needed to enable calcium to be absorbed.** Ingested animal protein (especially dairy) blocks the ability of the kidneys to produce the enzymes needed to convert vitamin D into 1,25D, therefore inhibits the production of vitamin 1,25D and consequently the absorption of calcium. Pasteurised milk inhibits calcium's own absorption and contains antibiotics (growth hormones) which inhibit gut flora production in the colon, compromising the immune system. *see 'Gut Flora and Bacteria'*

Overconsumption of dairy and animal products may cause 1,25D to reduce activation, and a build-up of unprocessed calcium can occur in the kidneys.

Unprocessed calcium, oxalate and uric acid can form kidney stones. These can be very painful when trying to pass through the urethra and sometimes requires hospitalisation and laser surgery. Vegans rarely get kidney stones.

This is where the dairy industry's claim of "milk being good for your bones" fails; in fact, they don't mention bones anymore. Vitamin D in milk is depleted during pasteurisation, negating calcium absorption down to about 8%. The dairy industry knows this and produces milk blends or drinks fortified with vitamin D and calcium (they no longer call it 'milk'). Look for the word 'milk' on the carton of milk-blends next time you're shopping.

Coupled with this is the fact that milk is inherently acidic and is inclined to draw calcium **from** bones.

The over-consumption of milk is considered to be as important a contributor to MS as insufficient sunlight exposure. Men who are chronic milk drinkers also have four times greater risk of prostate cancer than men who don't ingest dairy regularly. Some dairy products like cheese, cream and butter, are okay in moderation.

Bone Density

One of the main contributors to low-density bones is an acidic system produced through stress and an unsupportive diet consisting of excessive amounts of dairy, grains, sugar and alcohol. Calcium is alkaline in nature and is drawn from the bones to help balance acid levels in the body *(see 'Understanding Acid/Alkaline' previously).*

Whilst the glands, kidneys, liver and skin should do their best to balance the calcium and vitamin D content in the body, you can assist by ingesting the recommended daily intake (RDI) of calcium which is around 1200mg for an adult over 50 and less for younger people. It's not supportive to ingest more than your RDI of calcium.

After menopause, by the age of 65, some women have lost 50% of their skeletal mass. On average, 50% of women and 25% of men over the age of 50 will have an osteoporosis related fracture; however, **you** don't have to be average.

Be careful taking calcium supplements as this can lead to 'free calcium excess'. Initially when you take calcium you may feel better, however, over a couple of years, your energy declines because the excess calcium (that can't be dealt with by the kidneys) begins to block cell receptors, lowering your energy. You're better to eat more green leafy vegetables and apply magnesium to the skin daily, which will keep the calcium inside your bones.

Much of the information on this topic came from The China Study *by T. Colin Campbell.*

Essential Magnesium

As mentioned previously in the *'Salt'* section, minerals mostly exist within rocks and soil and are designed by nature to be integrated into plants as they grow. When animals such as cattle, sheep and poultry eat grass, they absorb and integrate minerals and Omega-3 EFAs into their flesh. In a perfect world, when we eat plants or meat, we should in turn integrate minerals and Omega-3s into our bodies too.

Today most animals raised for meat consumption are kept in feedlots where they are continually fed pellets containing mostly soy (high in oestrogen and inflammatory omega-6), low quality GMO grain and unwanted by-products from industry. Also, our farm soils are depleted through poor, large-scale farming practices, therefore we miss out on adequate mineral and Omega-3 intake from plants, resulting in the need for supplementation as discussed earlier.

Your body absorbs less magnesium when supplementing orally via tablets or powder (only about 10-20%) than simply applying magnesium to the skin. When supplementing magnesium orally, magnesium temporarily peaks in the blood and the kidneys pass excess magnesium out of the body through urine.

The only exception to ingesting magnesium is to ingest small amounts (3-6 flakes) of Magnesium Chloride in a glass of water when combined with medical grade Bicarbonate Soda to form Magnesium Bicarbonate. The Bicarb enables magnesium to pass through the cell wall into the mitochondria, energising and detoxing cells as discussed earlier in the acid/alkaline section.

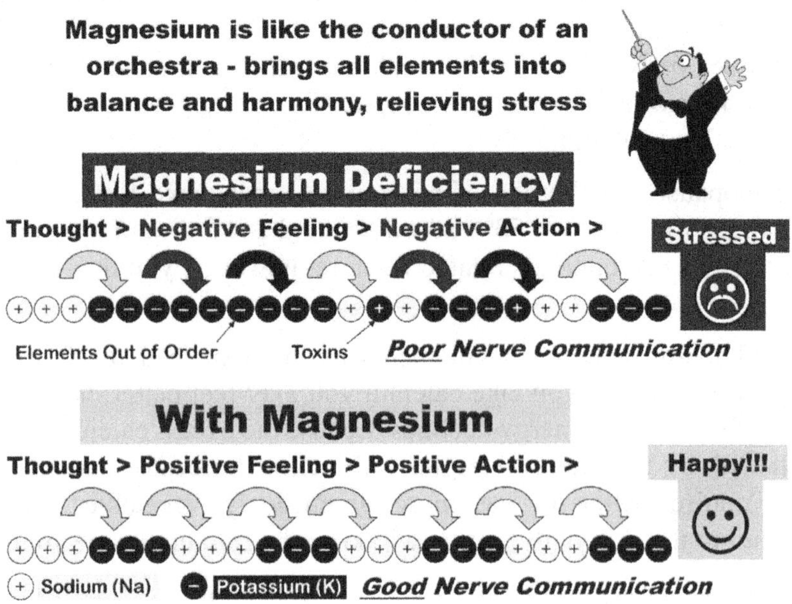

Our ancestors used to obtain their daily dose of magnesium by swimming in the ocean or bathing in hot mineral pools. We often hear how people 'love those negative ions' when visiting the sea and breathing in the salt air or they are around Himalayan salt lamps. When you breathe in the negative ions suspended in the air, they attach themselves to free radicals in your body and neutralise their harmful effect, making you feel better — less stressed. Magnesium is part of that process.

Magnesium absorbed through the skin (transdermally) is fully absorbed at a cellular level within 20 minutes of application. Skin applications include gels, sprays, lotions, creams and flakes that can be added to water for bathing or foot spas. When using transdermally, it's helpful to know that Magnesium Chloride is retained better by the kidneys and has more bioavailability than commonly used Epsom Salts (Magnesium Sulphate). *See resources section.*

Magnesium is the master mineral. Like the conductor of an orchestra, magnesium brings all vitamins and minerals into concert, correct balance, placement and harmony within the body.

Without magnesium, cell walls become weak and leach magnesium from inside the cells into the blood, so your kidneys register an excess of magnesium. Thus, the kidneys expel even more magnesium from the body (with the intention of creating balance) however; the body becomes accidentally more depleted. Blood test may show plenty of magnesium; however, you may actually be depleted in your bone, muscle and tissue cells.

Magnesium makes up 65% of bones and teeth, 35% of tissue, muscle and fluids with the highest concentrations in the heart and brain cells. Magnesium balances the electrical (nerve/brain) signals in the body and magnesium is involved in over 300 body processes and is essential for the utilisation of cell energy, detoxification and communication.

Magnesium relaxes muscles, converts protein for use, supports the heart, brain and nerves, enhances liver functions and helps balance the acid/alkaline balance in the body by allowing calcium to return to the bones in highly acid bodies. Magnesium also assists with detoxing, balances out hormones and enzymes like glutathione, melatonin (secreted by the pineal gland in your brain when night falls, encouraging sleep), adrenaline and EFAs. Without sufficient magnesium in your body, you may feel chronically stressed, fatigued, anxious, irritable and have poor quality sleep leading to unsupportive emotions and habits as detailed earlier.

The diagram above shows (simplistically) how magnesium supports nerve communication. This is not exactly how it works, but the result is the same and the actual process is amazingly complicated for simple minds like mine☺

Are You Magnesium Deficient?

As everything in this list depletes the body of magnesium, you can gauge your need to supplement personally: soft drinks (soda), fruit juice, dairy, coffee, tea, energy drinks, alcohol, ice cream, deserts, cakes, biscuits (basically all sugar), fluoride (drinking/shower water and toothpaste) and anyone on medication including the contraception pill and HRT.

Also, if you suffer from any of the following symptoms: Headaches, muscle pain, chronic fatigue, depression, insomnia, emotional and physical stress, anxiety disorders, anger, mood swings, muscle cramps and twitches, cognitive difficulties or you are over 55 years of age when magnesium levels are depleted even further.

As you can see from this comprehensive list, most of the population are probably magnesium deficient.

I used to supplement with a sweet-tasting magnesium powder for many years without noticing significant improvements. Since I began supplementing with transdermal magnesium, I have noticed an incredible improvement in my stress levels, muscle twitching (happened regularly after my seizures), mental focus and clarity. I sleep much deeper and awake refreshed every morning.

Like most men, I like to shower daily, dress and get on with my day with a cursory swipe of deodorant under my armpits. However, nowadays I always take an extra few minutes to apply magnesium to my skin before getting on with my day. I never miss out — it's so important and makes such a difference to my quality of life.

My Magnesium Deficiency

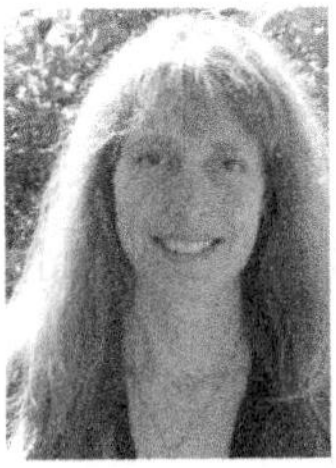

The past six years have been quite challenging with many periods of stress (at times quite chronic), anxiety and grief. This coupled with a diet no doubt deficient in essential minerals led to what I now believe was a spiralling magnesium deficiency.

Looking back, particularly at the last 12-18 months, I can now identify a steadily (and until recently, alarmingly) increasing number of symptoms which at times had me feeling I was losing my grip on my health, my life and reality.

Some early symptoms were pricking sensations all over my body (but especially my hands/arms and feet/legs) as though I was being stabbed by pins and tingling, especially in my fingers and hands and later my feet. Also numbness in my hands and fingers mainly at night. As time passed these sensations began to creep into my daytime hours as well.

I also began to experience disturbing lapses of memory, of conversations, actions (as in where I had placed something or things I had done) and had difficulty retrieving information. I simply could not remember things. This was commented on by my husband and was genuinely worrying to us both.

Once a sound sleeper, over time I had become restless and frequently wakeful throughout the night often waking totally exhausted in the morning.

I was sensitive to noise, irritable and not at all relaxed.

Then, a few months ago I began experiencing episodes of breathlessness and rapid heartbeat even with very minimal exertion. At times my heart felt it would skip out of my chest with sudden fluttering and palpitations. My "resting" pulse was at times at least 100 beats per minute. I would experience tightness in my chest and have trouble taking a deep breath. One day I even ended up at the doctor's having an ECG in case I was having a heart attack. Nothing showed up as being wrong.

In fact, I had many tests throughout the year; just about every organ in my body scanned, blood tests, nothing was revealed. But I was gradually feeling worse and it was starting to scare me.

My hands began to tingle and "buzz" constantly, though the sensations moved around. I began to experience muscle weakness in my legs and hands (it was hard to make a strong fist and my legs felt really wobbly and like they might fold under me). I had the most disturbing sensation that I can only describe as feeling like I was "not properly in my body", it was as though I couldn't look at things properly through my eyes.

I started experiencing anxiety and panic and all these later symptoms arrived and escalated within a couple of months. I was waiting for an appointment with a neurologist at this time and felt like I was really in trouble.

I was wracking my brains for possible answers for what I was experiencing and in an inspired moment I wondered if I could possibly have a mineral deficiency. Basic research quickly showed it was indeed possible that all my symptoms could be a sign of magnesium deficiency (though admittedly, also a number of other things). So, I began taking an oral supplement just to see if it would help me. Then, in a series of wonderful synchronicities I learned about transdermal magnesium therapy and that it is a much more effective way of getting magnesium into our cells than oral supplementation. I had nothing to lose, I gave it a try.

I am being completely truthful when I say that within 24-48 hours of starting to use AIM's magnesium products (I started with the gel and spray and recently added the crystals) I started to feel different. I simply started to feel "better" within myself. Within a few days my pins and needles were improving. In less than 2 weeks the tingling, muscle weakness, spacey light-headedness, anxiety/panic and fluttery heart were all but gone.

Now, after about 8 weeks I feel more relaxed, sleep better and I am symptom free. I have also had an amazing improvement in the arthritis in my neck, much less pain and inflammation. I know it can take several months to get magnesium levels back into the normal range so I still view

myself as journeying back to health. However, the improvement I have experienced has been nothing short of dramatic and has felt miraculous.

At 44 years of age I feel I was potentially headed for an unpleasant disease diagnosis in the future if things had continued on their original path and life was becoming scary and difficult. I believe I am heading in the direction of regaining good health because of AIM's

magnesium products and I will be using them life-long. For me, they have literally changed my life. They may have even saved it.

(Incidentally, my results from the neurologist recently where normal and I honestly don't know if that would have been the case a few months ago.)

Angela Macpherson — Eagle Heights Qld, Australia

Testimonials should not be construed as representing results everybody can achieve. Results may not be typical and may vary from person to person.

Iodine and the Thyroid

Iodine deficiency is linked to numerous ailments, especially those associated with the endocrine and lymphatic systems (chiefly the thyroid, parathyroid, thymus, pituitary and adrenal glands, and the hypothalamus, pancreas and gonads) of which each is an important hormone signal trigger for other functions in the body, from hormone signalling, cognitive function, immunity and sleep quality.

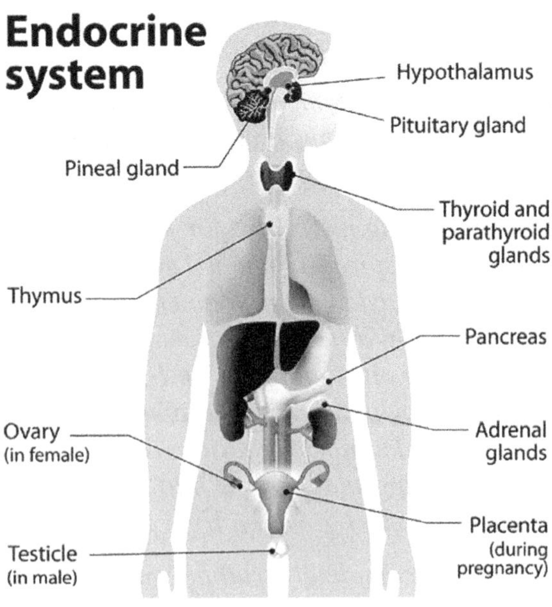

The key organ of the endocrine system is the

thyroid gland which is controlled by the pituitary gland through thyroid stimulating hormone (TSH). The thyroid gland combines Iodine and the amino acid 'tyrosine' to make the thyroid hormone thyroxine (T4 – inactive). The liver and kidneys then convert T4 into triiodothyronine (T3 – active). **Thyroid cells are the only cells in the body that can absorb Iodine.** If the thyroid doesn't obtain enough Iodine, hormone signals to the rest of the body will be weak and out-of-whack, and you may feel confused, irritable and an unreasonable 'misery-guts' to everyone around you.

Soy, fluoride, mercury, lead and radiation will displace Iodine from the thyroid, so if you've fallen for the sickness industry's mantra of drinking soy milk, brushing your amalgam-filled teeth with fluoride toothpaste, drinking tap water and having regular mammograms, your Iodine levels are likely to be through the floor and you will feel chronically fatigued.

In fact, if must have X-rays; drinking half a glass of water with 4-8 drops of Iodine one hour before should protect you from most thyroid radiation damage. Potassium Iodide is approved by the US FDA as a non-prescription drug for use as a 'blocking agent' to prevent the human thyroid gland from absorbing radioactive iodine.

Stress, smoking and other negative lifestyle habits like alcohol, sugar and carb intake, pesticides, dioxins, high estrogen levels, some medications and HRT are implicated with low Iodine levels too.

Eating a low carb diet will increase metabolism and reduce the need for T3 by around 40% by making T3 and insulin more sensitive, which is a good thing. Conversely, eating a high carb diet will place pressure on the thyroid, liver and pancreas, by increasing the need for more T3 and insulin.

Together with Iodine, selenium and tyrosine (an amino acid found in dairy, meat, eggs, coconut and nuts (fat)) help Iodine to be absorbed into the thyroid.

Iodine Level Test:
You can easily test if you have sufficient levels of Iodine in your body...

Place one drop of Lugol's Iodine on the inside of your wrist, smudge it on your skin with a finger, then take note of the time. The rate of absorption will indicate Iodine levels in your body. If the brown/yellow stain disappears within 3-4 hours, you are probably Iodine deficient. If the stain is still showing 6-8 hours later, you probably have enough Iodine in your body. Once your test stain remains visible for 8 hours, then take 1-4 drops in half a glass of quality water, twice a week then test monthly and adjust accordingly.

Lugol's Iodine?
Lugol's Iodine is a type of Iodine mixture (not a brand) and was developed in

the 1800s by French doctor, Jean Lugol. Lugol's Iodine is a 2:1 ratio of 10% Potassium Iodide (KI) with 5% elemental Iodine (I_2) in distilled water which provides what is commonly known as **full-strength 15% Lugol's Iodine**, which has been found to be the most effective Iodine supplement for daily use. *See resources later.*

Iodine Uses

Externally: Iodine can be used to help heal cuts, wounds, warts, polyps, cysts, sunspots or skin blemishes. Apply Iodine directly the area and re-apply if needed. It may take a few weeks areas to dry-out and peel-off, so be patient.

Iodine will kill bacterial, viral and fungal infections externally and internally.

Internally: If you are Iodine deficient, slowly introduce Iodine into your body, gradually increasing relative to your body's Iodine levels according to the test above.

Start with 1-6 drops in half a glass of quality water, three times a day with meals. Do this for one month, then test again. Iodine is best taken with meals, especially fats like butter, coconut oil or cream and animal fat. Because the thyroid regulates metabolism and protein synthesis, having plenty of Iodine with fat should assist your body to change its body mass composition over time to build more muscle and store less body fat.

People with **Hyperthyroidism** (overactive thyroid) may not need as much Iodine. Taking Iodine orally can also stain your teeth, so drink it without touching your teeth or use a straw. **Hashimoto's Disease** is where the body's immune system becomes unbalanced and attacks the thyroid, leading to an underactive thyroid for which correct Iodine levels should assist.

If you are using Lugol's Iodine with a dropper that has a rubber teat, please note that Iodine will degrade rubber within a few months. You are best to use soft plastic pipettes.

Stress and Adrenal Fatigue

*Also see **Step 1** of '14 Principles for Health, Wealth and Happiness' previously.*

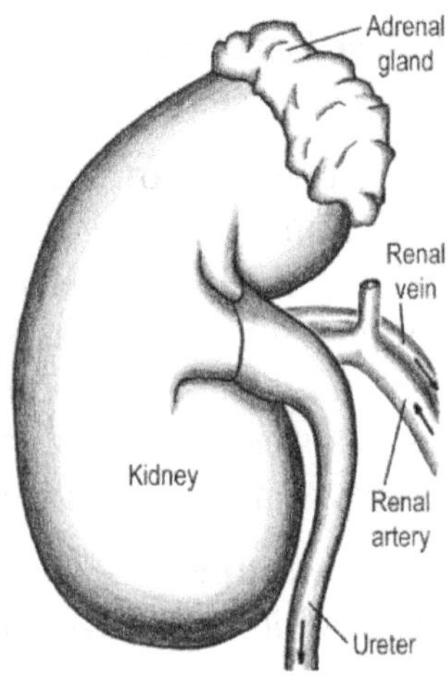

About 75% of people believe they experience stress at least once every two weeks and half of them describe their stress as high to extreme. Recent surveys show that 90% of people believe stress is a major cause of illness in their lives, and about 80% of the population suffer from adrenal fatigue.

Ongoing stress can cause the adrenal glands to

continually create adrenalin (short-term stress hormone) and cortisol (long-term stress hormone which is highly acidic), however, these tiny glands that sit on top of the kidneys can't keep up hormone production and so trigger carb, sugar and salt cravings as they struggle to balance the blood sugar and salt levels. This often results in frequent ingestion of addictive fast food, coffee and sweets, because the carbs, sugar, caffeine and salt stimulates energy in the short term (relief/escape), which has a deleterious effect on the body over the long-term.

Stress Impacts

Stress fatigues the adrenal glands, tenses muscles causing joint pain, headaches and insomnia, and can cause constipation through a highly-strung, twisting bowel that restricts flow, leading to a dysfunctional colon and liver, impacting your blood pressure, immune system and heart.

Stress can also be the catalyst for unsupportive (escape) **addictions** like alcohol, cigarettes, gambling, sugar, caffeine and drugs which have a negative impact on obesity, health, relationships, work, productivity and income — causing more stress, and which can ultimately lead to depression and suicide. *(see 'How we Create Our Own Reality' previously)*

Stress is your body's internal response to external events based on how you've perceived similar events in the past. Events trigger emotions, judgement based on beliefs and attitude, and ultimately reactions. Stress reactions can become habitual (for example food cravings), even something as simple as an odour, a song, a few words spoken or a judgemental glance or wink from another can cause reactions. The foundations of what cause people to become depressed or overweight are based around habitual reactions to their emotions. *(see 'Emotional Memory' in Chapter 2)*

As chronic stress continues, thoughts consistently turn towards worry, dwelling on issues outside one's control. Worry focuses on potential negative outcomes which, because of focus, usually eventuate. Worry can lead to powerlessness, a victim mentality, blame and choosing to not take responsibility, which increases stress.

In 1988, Bobby McFerrin released the first a-cappella song to reach number one in Australia and the US called *Don't Worry, Be Happy*. At the 1989 Grammy Awards, the song won Record of the Year, Song of the Year, Best Male Pop Vocal Performance and ranked number 31 in the Greatest One Hit Wonders of the 1980s. The merits of this rather simplistic song possibly lie in the reflection of how much stress and worry there is in society. People have an urge to feel happy, but don't know how to achieve it.

Stress can also impact on the body from physical internal and external situations and substances from tooth infections, joint or muscle injury, chronic pain, caffeine, sugar, cigarettes, alcohol and prescribed drugs (with this particular stress commonly called 'side-effects').

Incidentally, side-effects are not really on-the-side – they are real effects impacting the body, caused by the drug or treatment. They should really be termed 'other-effects' to not negate the importance and impact prescribed chemicals may have on the body.

Hormones

It's commonly known that adrenals produce adrenalin and cortisol for fight or flight responses but nowadays these same hormones are regularly triggered by sugar and caffeine. What's less commonly known is that adrenals also produce about 40% the body's sex hormones such as oestrogen, testosterone and progesterone, along with about 50 other hormones necessary to sustain health.

Menopausal women may feel the impact as their ovaries begin to shut down and the adrenals react to take up the slack and produce more oestrogen and progesterone. Some women are prescribed hormone replacement therapy (HRT) using synthetic progestin hormones, which have numerous side-effects. Often women feel 'out-of-sorts', irritable and can't explain why.

According to Dr John Gray (author of 'Men are from Mars, Women are from Venus'), men over 55 years probably have more oestrogen than their wives which causes 'man-boobs', belly fat and prostate issues. Eating more cruciferous vegetables, less alcohol, more water and exercise should help.

Women naturally process oestrogen, whereas men don't have that capability and with the mammoth amounts of oestrogens in our environment from processed foods, Omega-6 overload, toxins, spays and plastics, men become less able to make testosterone, leaving an abundance of oestrogen.

Adrenal Fatigue Symptoms

Symptoms of adrenal fatigue are feeling tired or run down for no apparent reason, morning fatigue, needing caffeine or sugar (e.g. chocolate) for energy, feeling better after lunch followed by an afternoon low, a 6pm energy pick-up, feeling continually stressed, slow recovery from illness, depression (feeling of a lack of fun in life) and decreased sex drive.

Pharmaceutical drugs like anti-depressants or relaxants might help in the short-term by relieving symptoms but often have side-effects, and over the long-term (I believe) can exacerbate stress.

AIM Composure® is a combination of natural herbs that work harmoniously to provide a gentle relaxant, without impinging on thought processes or making you drowsy. Feeling more relaxed can provide more opportunities for better-quality sleep which in turn supports better choices to help you lead a more relaxed life.

Reduce Stress — Increase Happiness:

- Firstly, stress is more a perception of events than reality. Sometimes things just happen and don't need to be judged — they simply are...
- Only work on things you have control over and that involve you directly.
- Take responsibility and wear any consequences as a lesson. Nothing is really negative about learning from something that didn't work last time.
- Avoid overwhelm. Make a list of what you need to achieve today, prioritise and do the next thing on the list with focus.
- Make your next thought happier than your last. Have a positive attitude, change your mind-set.
- Find your passion and work your passion. Make plans and take action to make income from what you enjoy doing.
- Still the mind, meditate and stop thinking. Stop judging everyone around you; it's their problem, not yours. Let go and be happy!
- It's none of your business what others think about you. Detach from unsupportive people and family. Move on and attract a more supportive crowd that align with where you want to be.
- Adjust your lifestyle — it's okay to have time off to do nothing. Assess whether your actions are simply laziness or your need for some time-out.
- Be happy more often; see the funny side of life and people, rather than giving them control by reacting negatively. Instead of swearing at something that goes 'wrong', try exclaiming to your work colleagues, "I'd prefer that didn't happen" (whilst smiling). Make a joke of it!
- Avoid TV shows like soap operas and reality shows that frame negative judgemental, emotional, ego-driven responses. Only watch educational documentaries, comedy, quality drama and the occasional trusted news item (once or twice a week, just a little to keep informed).
- Add positive music to your playlist. Listen to quality, happy, positive music throughout your day and during exercise. Use 'commute time' to learn from positive audiobooks.
- Reduce unsupportive food and drink like alcohol, caffeine, sugar, MSG, packet food, pastry, and so on.
- Get plenty of quality sleep and rest. Immune system cells in the brain are

activated by cytokines created in the bowel through proper delta-brainwave sleep and food. Try to have a 'siesta' after lunch if your lifestyle allows.

- Exercise regularly. Exercise produces positive hormones that assist your happiness *(see 'Exercise' later).*
- Drink plenty of quality water and electrolytes.

Glutathione

Glutathione is a molecule that has many supportive attributes when abundant in the body, but when depleted, has serious ramifications for your health and longevity.

Glutathione is the master antioxidant, the key to detoxing, the secret to balancing your hormones and reducing inflammation. Glutathione supports mitochondria (cell's power station or engine room) improving energy levels and your immune system. Thus, you have more energy, a clearer mind, feel more positive, vibrant and happier.

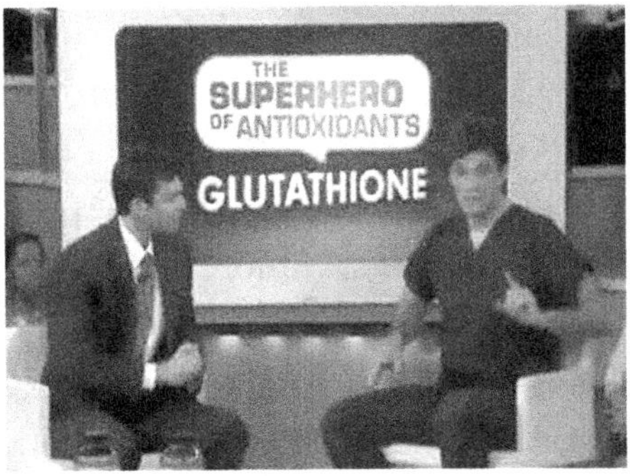

Dr Mehmet Oz calls Glutathione the *"Superhero of Antioxidants - It's the most important antioxidant you've* ***Never*** *heard of. It's the key to fighting-off diseases you fear the most..."*

Glutathione is **made by every cell of your body** and is the most important antioxidant used to protect every cell and which the body naturally relies upon to clean up toxins, supply energy, support the immune system and reduce inflammation.

However, glutathione's production declines around 1% every year after 21 years. Therefore, a person 50-60 years of age may be operating on just 50% of their optimum energy – how I used to feel before I **cleaned up my act**.

Glutathione can't be effectively ingested as a supplement because your body's own digestive system will destroy any externally introduced glutathione in the stomach.

The secret to glutathione's power is the sulphur-rich chemicals it contains which are sticky, smelly molecules that stick to toxins and heavy metals and escorts them out of the body via the bile and eventually through the bladder and bowel (if you eat enough fibre and drink plenty of quality water).

In a perfect world, glutathione should normally be recycled, but in our toxic world, glutathione is so busy dealing with everyday toxins, attacks from free radicals and body waste that it becomes even more depleted.

One of the reason glutathione is known as the master antioxidant is that it has numerous spare receptors that attract free radicals. Not only does it recycle itself, but also allows other antioxidants like vitamin A, C, & E to be recycled and do more good work too, especially detoxing.

Lifestyle factors such as an acid diet, stress, lack of sleep, disease, injury, infections, heavy metals, toxins, pollution, household chemicals, vehicle exhaust, tyre rubber dust, medication, smoking, sugar, flour products, coffee, alcohol, electromagnetic radiation from electronics and phones, excessive exercise and aging all add to the depletion of glutathione levels. Panadol and other acetaminophens destroy glutathione production in the liver.

Are you beginning to see the pattern? Similar, unsupportive lifestyle choices impacting on numerous vitamins, minerals, enzymes and processes that should be abundant in the body but aren't, therefore depleting energy, health and happiness whilst building toxins, blockages and disease.

The key to cell energy is the mitochondria, which is like the engines of your cells. Mitochondrion (plural) are made essentially of three molecules; **glutamic acid, glycine and cysteine**. The first two are in plentiful supply; however, **cysteine is often depleted**, causing mitochondrion to run on just two cylinders instead of three.

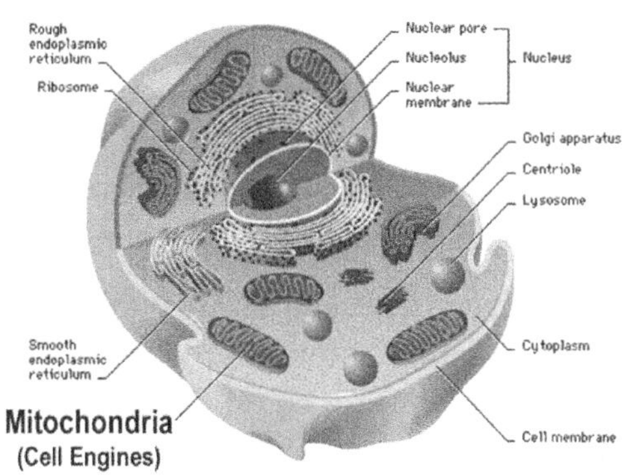

Your body's glutathione levels may be supported through regularly eating selenium and sulphur-rich foods like cruciferous vegetables – broccoli, cabbage, Brussels sprouts, cauliflower, garlic, onions, kale and asparagus. Eggs, grass-fed beef, animal organ meats, poultry, cottage cheese, Brazil nuts (soaked overnight), turmeric and seafood also assist. Milk Thistle, N-Acetyl Cysteine, Lipoic acid, vitamins B12 & B6 and magnesium all add to the production of glutathione along with sound sleep and regular, moderate exercise. Avoiding alcohol helps too. Essentially the basis of a Ketone diet mentioned in the "Losing It" section of this book.

Water Quality and Intake

Adult human bodies are made up of around 70% water. Enough quality water is vital to balance the salt/mineral/sugar/waste levels in the blood (via the kidneys) and in the faeces (via the colon). Enough water is also required to hydrate the brain allowing nerves to communicate through the utilisation of minerals. Dehydration can lead to memory loss, depression, Alzheimer's and dementia. *see 'Serotonin, Zinc, Depression and Dementia' later*

If your entire water intake of fluid is mixed with food, sugar, tea and coffee or soft drinks (sodas), your kidneys may find it difficult to flush and create the desired balance, ultimately leading to the kidneys withholding body fluid to balance the concentrations of sugars (osmosis). Stagnant food particles can rot over time, becoming toxic leading to kidney, liver and bowel disease.

Urine Colour and Frequency

Urine should be a very pale-yellow colour (straw). If urine is dark yellow (and you haven't been taking vitamin B supplements or you're significantly detoxing), you need to drink a lot more water. The average person should pass about two glasses of urine every two hours. Generally, the water you drink should pass as urine over the next few hours, after the water has been used by the body to expel waste and balance blood sugars — depending on work, perspiration, temperature and humidity.

To exercise your bladder, hold onto your urine for as long as you comfortably can. When you first feel the urge to urinate, see if you can hold on for another 10-20 minutes. This will stretch and exercise your bladder muscles, which over decades, will increase your holding capacity and strengthen your bladder and prostate (for men). Also when urinating, take your time and fully empty.

I've had many situations in public toilets at shopping centres; where I've started urinating, another guy has walked in next to me, started urinating and walked out before I've finished. The other guy may eventually have a small holding capacity and weaker bladder muscles over time.

Fat to Water Ratio

The interesting implication which easily explains body fat's role in creating diabetes is a simple observation of how fat and water don't mix when you are cooking. Fat separates from water and floats on top.

Similarly, in your body fat and water don't mix. The greater the percentage of fat, the smaller the percentage of water, therefore the less viscose the blood, the slower the circulation and the more toxic deposits left behind to clog up the smallest capillaries around the feet, ankles and eyes. Eventually after 10-20 years, circulation stops, limbs die – requiring amputation and vision is impaired (diabetes).

Conversely the more muscle, the more hydration (water), therefore less percentage of body fat. Muscle burns more Calories, and because there is more water present, the blood is more viscose, circulating more readily and removing body waste and toxins to the kidneys and bowel for release.

Thirst Responses

Every time you urinate, it's supportive to measure your thirst and drink the desired amount of quality water.

If you're feeling continually, unjustifiably thirsty, then this may be a symptom of diabetes, so visit your healthcare practitioner for a check-up.

Kidney problems can also impact negatively on the body's natural thirst response by not giving the body a clear signal to drink water when needed, leading to dehydration, toxin build-up and constipation. People with such conditions should make a special effort to drink quality water often.

Work Habits

Often in our society, habits, routine, work commitments and situations can cut in and override the body's thirst.

For example, you may work in an air-conditioned office on the tenth floor, (air conditioning can dehydrate the body) and enjoy a coffee for morning tea each day at 9:30am. Your body might normally signal thirst at, say, 10am, but before your thirst is signalled, it's quenched with a dehydrating or diuretic beverage like coffee, tea, energy drink, soft drink, juice, sports drinks or milk which further concentrates acids and dehydrates the body.

Try drinking a glass of water ten minutes prior to your morning tea break at work or take two litres of water with you to sip during the day.

People driving busses, taxis etc. or working in mines or similar and can't access a toilet easily will purposely drink less water which solves the immediate problem but is injurious to their long-term health. There is a consequence for every choice you make.

Water Intake and Constipation

Water is needed to form chyme for digestion. If you are not drinking enough water, you can hamper digestion and elimination, leading to constipation and all its complications *(see 'Constipation' later)*.

Water is drawn from the colon to help form a solid stool for elimination. Constipation has a compounding effect on the stool; the longer the stool sits in the descending colon, the more water is drawn from the stool and the harder (and dryer) it becomes, making it more difficult to pass a motion. You may have experienced this when finally being able to pass a stubborn motion, where the first part is hard and dry and the remainder of the motion passes easily after the 'plug' has been released.

Water Replacement

As adults, our bodies are made of around 70% water, so the idea is to replace the liquid expelled during the day. Simply walking can produce 250–500ml (two cups) per hour of perspiration and up to 1.5 litres (three pints) per hour during strenuous activity. On top of this, the body uses water to urinate and excrete waste from the colon along with lubricating blood and joints and aiding cell nutrient transfers and reproduction. The body also uses water to create stomach acid and to balance the salts, sugar and food we eat.

I've found drinking about one litre per 25kg (2 pints per 55 lbs) of body weight per day is a good guide. This quantity may vary depending on season, temperature, humidity and activity. Personally, I drink around two to four litres a day, which is about right for this formula. Therefore, a typical person 70–80kg (180 lbs) should drink up to three litres a day.

A good start for the day is to drink two to three glasses of quality water first thing in the morning to flush out toxins collected in the liver and gall bladder overnight. This amount of water should also hydrate the body when most needed from fasting overnight.

Tap Water

Avoid drinking unfiltered tap water. **Chlorine** is added to tap water to kill bacteria; therefore, chlorine kills and disrupts gut flora (good bacteria) production and processes too, leading to numerous problems mentioned later. Most common tap water filters can't filter out **fluoride** which is a government-registered **S6 poison** and is noted in official Materials Handling Data Sheets (MHDS) as "toxic if swallowed". I think our governments and dentists are lying to us☹

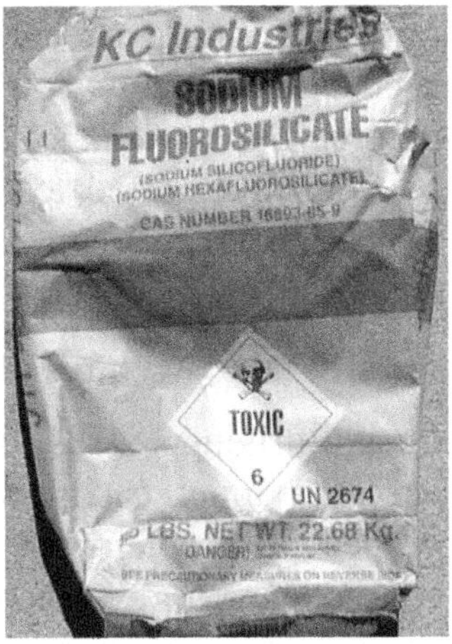

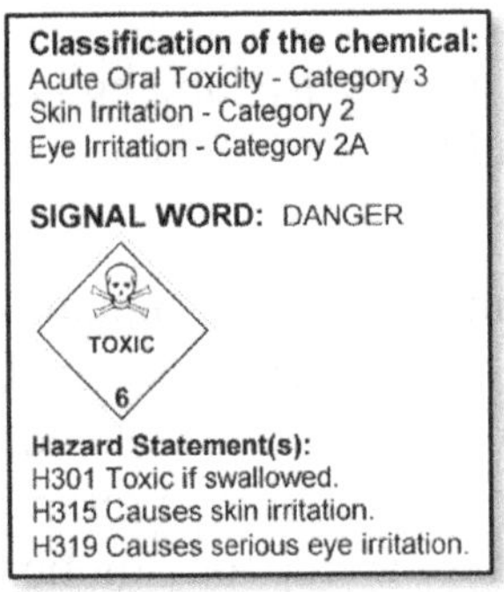

Fluoride dissolves Iodine from the thyroid with all the negative implications mentioned previously. Fluoride is also a neurotoxin and over 300 studies have revealed reduced intelligence and impaired learning in children, www.fluoridealert.org Fluoride also combines with aluminium and oxygen in the body which has found to be a contributing factor to Alzheimer's Disease.

Distilled Water

Distilled (and reverse osmosis) water is surprisingly acidic due to a lack of minerals, therefore can draw minerals from your body (especially bones) to bring the ingested distilled water back into balance. Though toxin-free, distilled water is not recommended unless you are gaining sufficient amounts of minerals from your food or supplements or re-mineralising by adding liquid trace minerals.

Tank Water

Rainwater is essentially distilled water with pollutants gathered from the environment as it falls and should therefore always be filtered before drinking. Bird poop on roofs, decaying leaf debris, worms, grubs, bugs and algae/mould growth further necessitates the need for filtering.

Storing rainwater in concrete tanks is best as the water will draw minerals from the rock and concrete that makes up the tank, making the water more alkaline.

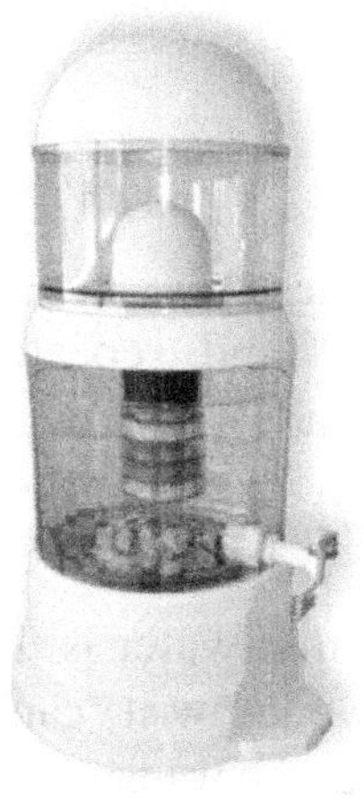

However, today more affordable plastic and metal tanks are becoming more popular. Metal tanks mostly have a plastic coating for protection against rust and therefore essentially have plastic characteristics.

We've previously used plastic tanks and I've measured filtered rainwater to have a pH of 1.5 – highly acid. To bring our pH back into balance, we store and filter our drinking water utilising a water purification system as seen in this photo. Using tank water; this system brings our water as near as possible to be perfect for consumption. There is a fluoride reduction option if you are using city supplied tap water.

What's Best?

Filtered water from a concrete tank is best, for the reasons mentioned.

When we lived in a unit on the Gold Coast and couldn't capture our own rainwater, I filter our tap water utilising the water purifier above with the fluoride reduction cartridge. This set up was economical because I gained a return on my investment in just 14 weeks, compared to buying bottled water. *See resources later for details or www.quantumk88.com*

When away from home, I use BPA-free plastic, glass or stainless-steel bottles to carry water with me. Commercial plastic water bottles are designed to break down in the environment and therefore can leach toxins into the water; however, polycarbonate and BPA-free bottles don't have this issue.

On our water journey, we invested in an expensive $3000 water ioniser that produced various grades of alkaline or acid water. This unit needed to be connected to plumbing, used electricity and waisted a lot of water during the flushing processes. It also needed maintenance to descale the plates every six weeks and replacement filters were very expensive. So, we sold it on eBay and now use the water purifier above which is much cheaper and far easier to maintain.

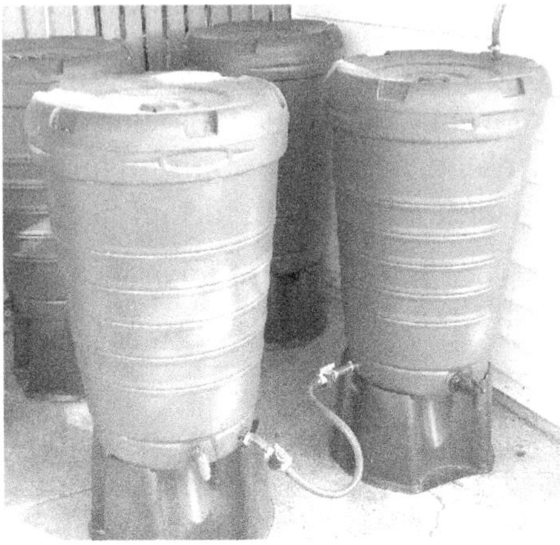

If you're renting, you can simply divert one downpipe into smaller, portable 100-200L plastic tanks. The set up photographed, provided our family of four, enough drinking and cooking water for more than two months during dry spells.

The best water ultimately is uncontaminated, fresh spring water straight from the ground, but it's a little hard to find in the city.

Water and What You Think

In his bestselling book *The Hidden Messages in Water*, Japanese scientist Dr Masaru Emoto documented evidence through controlled and repeated experiments that simple thought-form, pictures, text, labels, signage, chemicals, toxins and music can change the molecular structure of water, either positively or negatively.

After a lifetime of studying water, Dr Emoto hypothesises that water is the universal communicator and makes the point that life (as we know it) can't exist without water and that water retains a memory which can be transmitted to the next life it supports, even if pure and distilled.

At a lecture presented by Dr Emoto at Bond University on the Gold Coast several years ago before his passing, Masaru pointed out that every year, around ten million tonnes of ice meteors from other parts of our universe vaporise into clouds when entering the earth's atmosphere — the giver of earth's life and intelligence from a universal source.

So, what's the ultimate thought-message to energise your next glass of water with? "Love, appreciation and happiness!" Remember our bodies and the food we eat both contain water, so what you think about your food and yourself actually matters.

Appreciate what you have,
rather than struggle with what you've got!

Chapter 5

Elimination System — Solids

The 'Poo' Word

Most of the remainder of this book talks a lot about poo. Poo is known by many names... The official scientific, medical term is 'faeces' also spelt 'feces' by our American friends. Faeces is formed once chyme has passed into the cecum (first part of the colon) from the small intestine, and once most of the water has been extracted, forms a brown paste called faeces.

For the more colloquial minded, faeces can also be known as a stool, a motion, turd, dump, excrement, number two (really bad ones are called number threes), defecation, dung, a job, doo-doo, crap, poop or just plain old poo.

I've even heard the term "a brown dog sleeping in the kennel" or "a brown dog barking at the back door". Some people find the word 'shit' offensive, so I won't use it here... oops!

Crapper

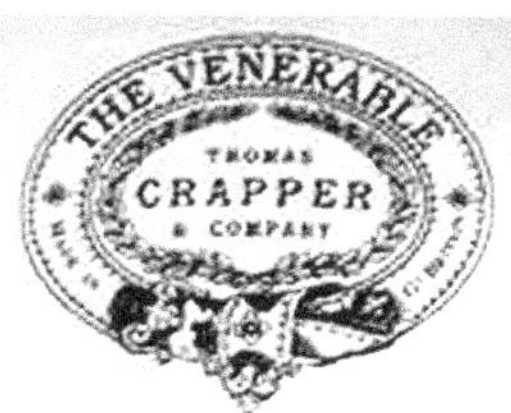

The word 'crap' is derived from Thomas Crapper in the 1800s in England — a plumber and installer of (the then new) flushing toilets. Crapper didn't invent the flushing toilet (as legend might lead you to believe) but having Crapper's name on most of the cisterns installed at the time, the term "I'm going to the Crapper" evolved. However, Crapper was an inventor and patented several plumbing devices. Just think, this morning you didn't know any of this!

Speaking of number twos, two children were holidaying in London and were about to visit Downing Street with their parents when one said, "If 'number one' is a wee, and 'number two' is a poo, I don't want to be anywhere near Nº10".☺

Now to push the boundaries of toilet humour...

A woman was trying to convince her husband to pay for her breast enlargements, when her husband came up with a brilliant idea. She asked, "Why do you think rubbing toilet paper on my breasts will make them grow larger?"

Her husband replied, "Well, it worked on your bum".☺

Now for Foxtrot, Alpha, Romeo, Tango

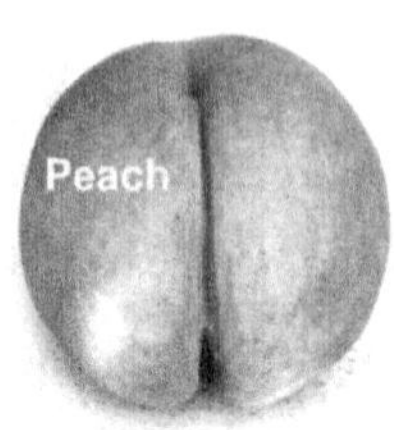
Peach

Polite words for farting are pop-offs, fluffs, pass wind, broken wind, gas, bottom burp, etc.

Farting is officially called 'flatulence' – which sounds like a romantic name for French perfume. "Flat-u-laance – It's me; it's you, no wait... (sniff- sniff), it's me."☺

Farting is a natural part of life, especially if you have not been eating supportively and your gut is internally fermenting food, rather than digesting it. It's the undigested carbs and sugar that create the smell. Apparently even the Queen does it – so I've been told.

One of the better comments I've invented after I have farted is, "Put that on Facebook and like it!"☺ ...one of my only claims to fame.

Another trick when you free a 'SBD' (silent, but deadly), is to ask your nearby friends, "Can you smell petrol?"☺

Alternatively, when working on a computer, ask someone from a desk nearby to, "Come and have a look at this". It's nice to share and pointless wasting the event☺.

If you're the driver of a car with passengers and have electric windows, and you are successfully able to negotiate a SBD, quietly lock the windows, wait and smile☺.

Back in the 1970's, when CB radios were new and connected to most cars, our group of friends used to call "Foxtrot, Alpha, Romeo, Tango" to announce to the world about their latest expulsion☺.

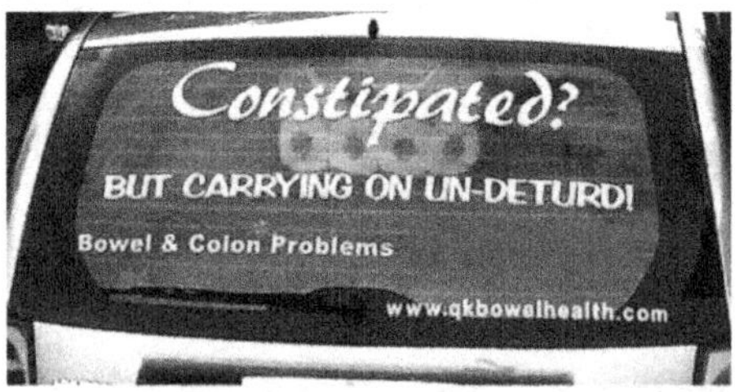

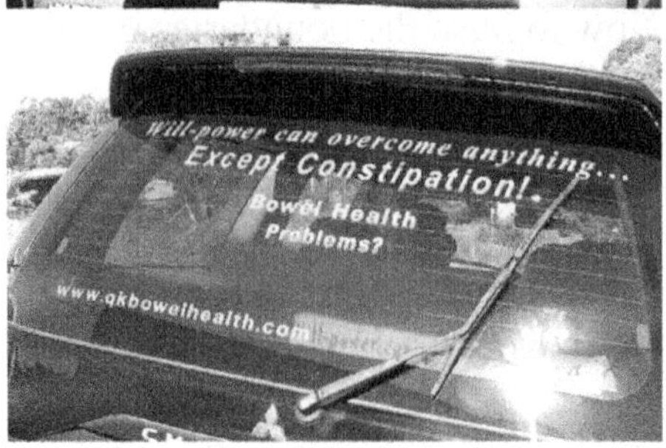
Will-power can overcome anything...
Except Constipation!
Bowel Health Problems?
www.qkbowelhealth.com

We provide a lot of laughs through the signage on our vehicle windows, especially when we carry toilet paper on the back shelf

This one takes a lot of front, but when in a queue, and you let go a 'thunder from down-under', turn and loudly blame your friend behind you. It's even funnier if you don't know anyone in the queue – you can simply turn around and look inquisitively at the person behind you☺.

I try to encourage humour around bottoms and poo. Everybody has one and does it, but because of our 'anally-retentive' upbringing, most are too embarrassed to talk about it.

When people ask me what I do for a

living, I tell them: "I talk crap for a living and I'm not even a politician" It certainly initiates a conversation.

I am setting up a YouTube Channel soon – search for "Quantum Knowledge" or "Ramiah Selwood" and keep up with the latest information from my research.

Now I have the humour out of my system, let's get serious and carry on 'un-deturd'...☺

Groom of the Stool

In the 1500s, King Henry VII and VIII had a servant dedicated to wiping the king's bottom after each motion. Though it sounds disgusting, this was a much sort-after position as the servant would live in-chambers and share the luxury and travel of the king. The position was abolished later when Queen Elizabeth I came to the throne (literally).

These days, surprisingly, a similar position still exists for the US President (and presumably other important world leaders). When the US President travels, all his or her excretions are contained and disposed of (back in the USA) by a secret service member. Whitehouse toilet paper is also brought with the President.

The reason for this is to stop samples of urine or faeces being collected by foreign intelligence agencies and analysed for signs of an illness or disease — information which might compromise the President. The CIA would know of such a threat — they reportedly did just that to Soviet President Mikhail Gorbachev during his visit to Washington in 1987, towards the end of the cold war.

Colon — Large Intestine

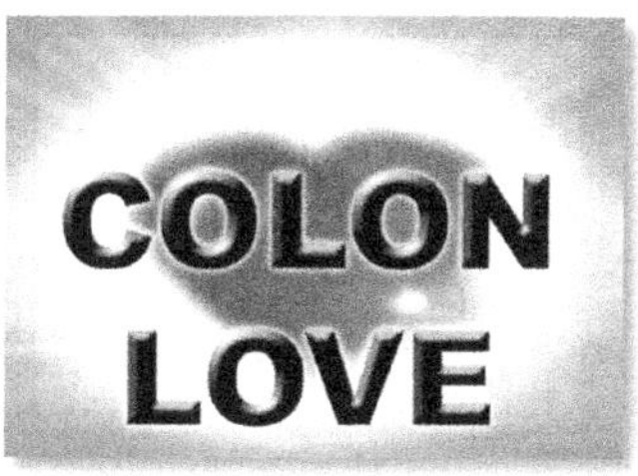

The colon is also referred to as the large intestine, large bowel or sometimes more simply as "the bowel" (which can also refer to the gut in general). To avoid confusion, I will refer to it as the colon. When I mention 'the bowel' I will be referring to the small and large intestines together.

Also, note that if the colon, kidneys or both are overwhelmed, dysfunctional or diseased and cannot handle the load of waste and toxins to be eliminated, the body can use mucus, lungs, the skin, eyes, mouth, hair and any external body orifice to eliminate as well.

The colon is about 1.5 meters (5 ft) long and 6.5 cm (2½ in) in diameter. Of the 11 litres (2.5 gal) of food and liquid ingested every day by the average Australian or American, only about 350 ml (12 oz or 1½ cups) reaches the colon. The rest is absorbed and used for energy and body functions or stored as fat or toxins.

Unlike the small intestine where the internal surface is lined with villi, the colon has a smooth internal surface lubricated by mucus.

Water and water-soluble vitamins B6, B12 and C are absorbed into the liver from the colon for use in the body and are **not** stored. Therefore, they require ingestion regularly.

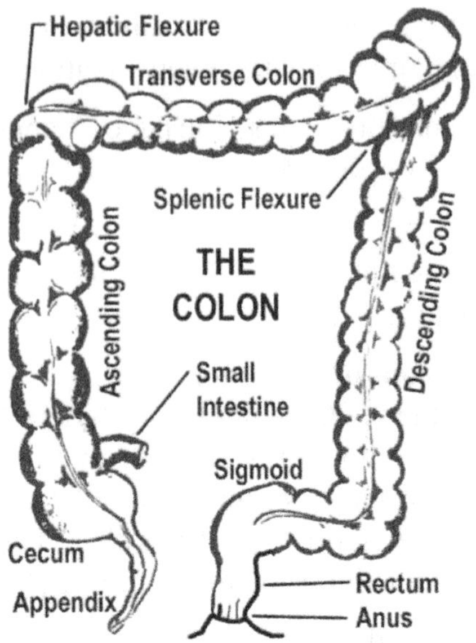

Cecum
The first part of the colon is the cecum which is a 'blind area' just below the entry point of the small intestine into the colon. Because this area is 'blind' (not in the flow of chyme/faeces), often parasites can live quite nicely there. Tapeworms are known to anchor in the cecum and reach into the transverse colon for nutrition. Colonoscopies sometimes don't find parasites in the colon as the scope does not turn down into the ascending colon as far as the cecum.

The time chyme or faeces sits in the cecum depends on its consistency (water content) and the amount of roughage (fibre) contained within. The more fibre, the quicker the faeces should be moved up the ascending colon; relieving constipation.

Appendix
Attached to the cecum is the appendix, which on occasion can become infected (appendicitis) due to lack of fibre and good bacteria and can require removal by surgery. For most of medical history, it was believed the appendix has no use; however, research by Duke University Medical Centre in North Carolina USA has shown that after a bout of diarrhoea and the expulsion of the offending bacteria, the reserves of good bacteria stored in the appendix are used to repopulate the colon.

Peristalsis
The cecum extracts most the water from the chyme, turning it into faeces, which is a thicker, pastier material; allowing the faeces to be manoeuvred up the colon using a series of muscle contractions and stretches called peristalsis

(snake-like movement).

The more fibre in the faeces, the easier it is for the colon wall to push against the faeces and move the stool up the ascending colon, thus negating one of the causes of constipation.

Ascending Colon
From the cecum, the faeces is pushed up the ascending colon where gut flora is mixed with water and fibre, and the remainder of the nutrients are mostly extracted. It then travels around the first bend (right hepatic flexure), which is attached near the back of the ribcage. At this point fibre begins to ferment and encourages the friendly gut bacteria needed for digestion.

Transverse Colon
Faeces then travels along the transverse colon and at about the halfway point, the faeces becomes more solid and is readied for elimination. Also, at the halfway point, gut flora begins to outlive its usefulness, dissipates and is excreted with the faeces. In a healthy colon with enough stem cells available, new gut flora should then be reproduced in the small intestine and ascending colon to treat the next meal.

Descending and Sigmoid Colon
Beyond the halfway point in the transverse colon, the faeces should be a solid stool and move towards the second bend (left splenic flexure, again attached near the ribcage), then down the descending colon towards the sigmoid which is slightly 'S' shaped, but narrower than the descending colon. However, the sigmoid expands to hold faeces which is about to be released when the time and place is right. There is very little gut bacterium in this area of the colon and water is continually being extracted from any stagnant faeces, which can exacerbate constipation.

If the bowel is constipated, the descending colon and sigmoid area can expand to house the extra faeces waiting to be released, this can cause diverticulitis and segmentation as you will read later.

Rectum and Anus
To release faeces, the internal sphincter muscle known as the rectum opens, and the stool is released through the anus. The anus is the external opening that you would see if we had a long-enough neck or a strategically placed mirror☺. I will spare you from listing the colloquial terms for anus for obvious reasons.

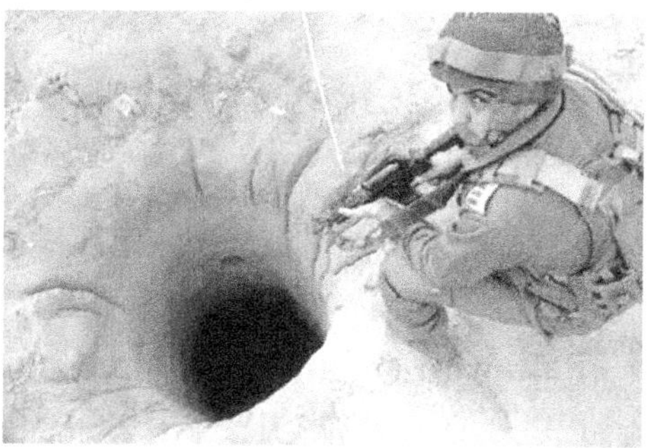

No Blood

There is no blood within the digestive and eliminations system (from mouth to anus), which is about 9 metres (10 yards) long. So, if blood shows in your stool, you should take special note! Most often, blood in the stool can indicate haemorrhoids, which is quite common, but may also indicate something more sinister (like polyps or colitis which can turn cancerous) and you should seek advice from your healthcare professional.

Mucus Lining

The internal lining of the colon wall has a smooth mucus coating, which is continually replenished and binds and lubricates the faeces to slide along the colon wall. Consuming insufficient water can cause this mucus to become thicker, stickier and more viscid, which can form mucoid plaque and compound constipation.

The Shape of Poo...

Your morning stool is the best stool to assess your internal bowel situation.

- The **optimum stool** should be easily released each morning (or one to three times a day) and should be about 2 cm–2.5 cm in diameter (3/4"– 1") or greater; soft, moist, mostly continuous and dark amber/caramel in colour with little or no odour and should float most of the time. The colour can vary depending on the colour of food eaten the day before (for example, eating lots of beetroot can make the stool much darker). The odour should be more of an earthy, compost type of smell, rather than a sulphurous rotten egg smell. Stools released later in the day (after the first stool) are often floating, less dense, broken with sharper edges, but are still healthy. The reason they are lighter and less dense is because the colon has had less time to extract liquid from the stool.

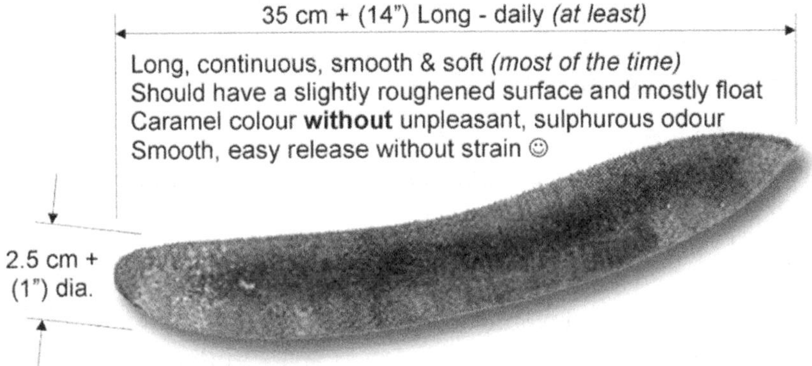

- **Pale-whitish**, light coloured stools may indicate a lack of bile being produced by the liver, which could indicate a struggling, fatty liver or possibly gall bladder duct blockages.

- An abundance of easily identified, **whole pieces of food** (peas, carrots, capsicum) can indicate that you need to chew your food better or that nutrition from your food is not being properly absorbed in the small intestine. This can be indicative of too much sugar and processed food being consumed, which tends to ferment food rather than digesting.
- Indicators of a poor diet based on carbs, sugar, animal products and too-little plant fibre are **short, smelly stools** which are **hard, dry, dark brown, separated, lumpy** segments or nut-like balls.
- Ongoing **offensive odour** can be indicative of sugars and carbs causing fermentation of food (rather than digestion, as previously discussed) or an imbalance of unfriendly bacteria in the colon (from similar causes), or both. Short-term offensive odours can relate to recently eaten food with strong odours like onions, garlic or coffee, or (if you have started to eat well or take supplements) can be a temporary release of toxins from the liver or colon (detoxification).
- **Thin, continuously streaming stools** or **ongoing runny diarrhoea** can be an indication of faecal build up on the colon wall or blockages. This is often accompanied by constipation and diarrhoea cycles.
- **Light, fluffy, floating, semi-liquid/gel-like and broken** faeces can be an indication that you are over-stimulating your bowel with too much fibre and/or water and your transit time (that is, the time taken from eating food to passing the same food through the anus) may be too short. When you make changes like adding extra fibre, often it needs to be introduced progressively. Sudden changes can overstimulate and overwhelm your digestion and elimination system, so it's helpful to 'sneak up' when you make changes.

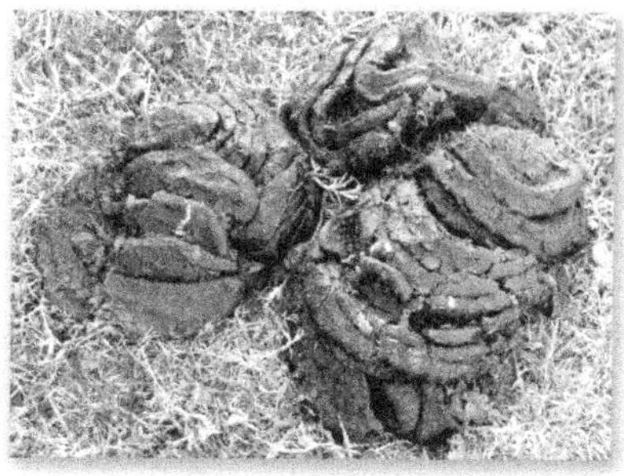

If your poo looks like this, then you're probably an old cow

Of all the above shapes and situations, one-off events are usually nothing to worry about, however, if you are regularly experiencing any of the above situations, you might like to consider changes like eating less carbs and more water, animal protein, vegetables and fibre or supplementation.

The primary indicators of an unhealthy bowel are blood in the stool, regularly having difficulties passing motions (constipation) or regularly have runny stools (diarrhoea), or cycles of both.

Syndromes, Symposiums and Terminology

A syndrome is the association of several clinically recognisable features whereby other symptoms may be expected. Therefore, **irritable bowel syndrome** (IBS — also known as a spastic colon or gut flora imbalance), **leaky gut syndrome** and **inflammatory bowel disease** (IBD — also known as colitis or Crohn's disease), are examples of what is actually a combination of many of the issues discussed in this book. Syndromes are often diagnosed and treated with drugs, diminishing specific symptoms. Most drugs are simply designed to relieve symptoms, rather than rectifying the cause.

It's interesting to note that the symptoms of a dysfunctional digestion and elimination system are similar for most bowel disorders because they are all ailments of some part of the bowel, liver, kidneys, and other digestive organs.

Big Pharma spends around $30 million annually on five-star hotels and restaurants for dining, symposiums and conferences held to 'educate' doctors, gather consensus and officially name each particular degree of a disorder.

I have found medical terminology describing the "build-up of pressure and lack of movement or stagnation of material waste in the sigmoid colon" used instead of simply saying "constipation". Such spin terminology keeps mere mortals like us confused, out of the system and in need of doctors who study how to interpret such names, much like the legal profession does.

In my view, all diagnosed diseases and syndromes in the digestive and elimination system mostly boil down to a couple of causes: there are toxins present in the bowel, liver or both due to introduced chemical intoxication, or food either not being digested correctly or becoming stagnant (constipation) and contaminating other organs. And that's it!

Constipation has an impact as a knock-on effect causing stress on the liver through hormone imbalance, toxicity, bacterial infection and inflammation, which stresses the entire body. All the names the sickness industry wants to give to the symptoms that affect impacted organs are somewhat irrelevant.

Simply clean out the bowel, eat supportive food and water, exercise daily, have happy thoughts and regular bowel motions. Life can be easy... really. We're designed to be happy and well.

Serotonin, Zinc, Depression and Dementia

According to Dr Hugo Rodier *(see www.hugorodier.com)*, 95% of the body's serotonin is created in the bowel. Nerves use mostly water, zinc, magnesium, manganese, potassium and sodium to transmit signals. Dehydration can slow the signal rate of the brain, hampering transfer of information and building concentrations of toxins and minerals, which in the short-term can cause the brain to signal a headache, tiredness and vagueness. In the long-term, prolonged dehydration, toxins and lack of minerals can lead to memory loss, depression, Alzheimer's and dementia.

Originally, serotonin was thought to be only a brain chemical (a neurotransmitter which sends messages from one synapse to another in the brain), but now recent research has turned that idea on its head — figuratively speaking!

Serotonin, along with vitamins K2, B6 and B12, is produced in the colon, therefore it stands to reason that if the bowel is clogged with toxic faecal matter, the chemicals and vitamins transmitted to the brain are more likely to be toxic too, or at least be reduced in their production or functionality.

Dr Rodier suggests poor diet and impaired gut function will cause cognitive and mental problems, along with neuro-degeneration in addition to bone-thinning and inflammation.

The brain becomes clouded, foggy and confused. Do this decade after decade and **depression, anxiety, senility and dementia** can set in.

US research also found walking for 40 minutes a few times a week boosts the hippocampus, an area of the bran that makes memories. Exercise helps preserve memory and reduces the risk of developing dementia.

Zinc

Researchers from the Massachusetts Institute of Technology and Duke University have also discovered that **zinc** plays a vital role in brain activity, relieving anxiety, depression, dementia and possibly epilepsy.

Zinc is highly-concentrated in areas of nerve cells called 'vesicles' which are pockets that contain neurotransmitters (serotonin) that are released for cell communication with other nerve cells.

The greatest concentration of zinc is in the hippocampus, which is involved in short and long-term memory and spatial navigation, and is often involved in epileptic attacks.

Prozac

The sickness industry will often prescribe anti-depressant drugs like Prozac, typically to preserve the remaining serotonin, rather than cleaning up the toxic area of serotonin production — the bowel. Prozac has side-effects like insomnia, weakness and loss of appetite.

Flamboyant Australian stockbroker Rene Rivkin, who was diagnosed with depression and prescribed Prozac, said in May 2003 (two years before his death), *"I take Prozac. Nothing worries me. I'm serious. That's the effect that Prozac has had on my life. Nothing worries me anymore."*

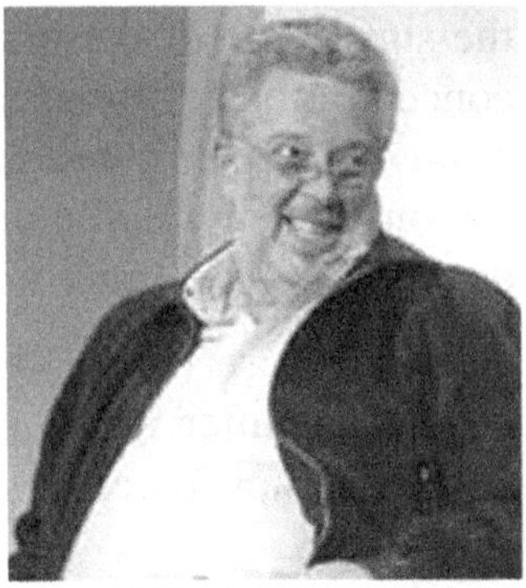

Rene Rivkin died at just 61 years. Perhaps diet and medication contributed to his situation?

Rivkin also took sleeping tablets to override his insomnia, a side-effect of Prozac.

Gut Flora and Bacteria

We are continually bombarded with advertising telling us that bacteria (commonly known as germs) are bad for us. Regular contact with unfriendly bacteria can be a good thing, as these builds, exercises and strengthens the immune system, creating antibodies to fight future infections.

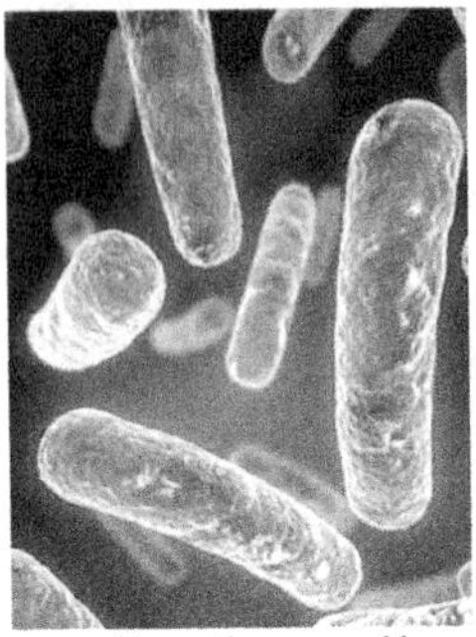

Overall, society tends to believe advertising and purchase disinfectants, antibacterial sprays and soaps that kill both friendly and unfriendly bacteria. Over time, this can compromise the body's immune system making us more susceptible to disease and allergies.

Bacteria outnumber cells in the body by ten to one. The body contains around 10 trillion cells and 100 trillion bacteria weighing around 1.8kg (4lbs). Bacteria are much smaller than cells and the majority are mostly housed in the bowel (especially the colon). You could say we are actually made of bacterium.

Immune System

The digestive system is responsible for the functioning of about 80% of the immune system. Immune system cells in the brain are activated by cytokines created in the bowel through proper delta-brainwave sleep and food. Stress levels may also impact on the quality and quantity of cytokines. Therefore, the lack of quality sleep (for example as a consequence of snoring) and a compromised digestion system may have a significant effect on the body's overall health and susceptibility to infectious diseases.

Bacteria Names

Bacteria in the colon can be called different names: good or bad bacteria, acidophilus, micro flora, **gut flora,** and **friendly** and **unfriendly bacteria.** I mostly use the highlighted terms.

Probiotics are often incorrectly called gut bacteria. Probiotics can be ingested to promote bacterial growth by providing supportive bacteria that encourages certain gut flora to flourish. It's like adding compost to a garden.

Prebiotics is a fibre that passes through the small intestine undigested and becomes fermented when it reaches the large colon.

Faecal Make-Up

Around one third of the faecal matter that the body should pass every day is made up of the body's own gut flora (friendly and unfriendly bacteria), designed to assist with digestion and steer the body towards better health. Another third consists of undigested food we've eaten (fibre), but if our diet is acidic and high in sugar, the fibre could be replaced with food that your body has not been able to digest due to the fermentation process that sugar introduces. The remaining third is waste removed from the body via the blood and bile (dead cells and toxins).

Under normal conditions, the ascending colon produces its own gut flora assisted by the appendix. This friendly lactobacillus, acidophilus bifida bacterium (amongst others) produces vitamin K2, B6, B12, folic acid and supportive amino acids. However, because of today's unsupportive (acidic) western diet and lifestyle, much of the friendly bacteria are destroyed by antibiotics (usually in dairy products and medicines), alcohol, stress, sugar, food and so on.

***Un*friendly Bacteria**

Counter-intuitively, unfriendly bacteria thrive in an alkaline colon of 7.1 pH and higher but also loves acid food like carbs and sugar. Unfriendly bacteria produce acidic bodies, hazardous chemicals and toxins as well as gas, providing the most offensive flatulence.

If the body does not produce enough of its own friendly bacteria, symptoms like flatulence, bloating, diarrhoea, constipation, lowered immune system and depression can evolve. This can be known as **irritable bowel syndrome (IBS).** Chemical laxatives, medications and eating food such as sugar, fruit juice, dairy and most processed food support unfriendly bacteria like candida yeast and fungi. Drinking chlorinated tap water may also kill friendly bacteria.

Anytime you eat refined carbohydrates (carbs – like sugar, cakes, biscuits, bread, etc.), you automatically **within minutes**, support the proliferation of **unfriendly gut bacteria**. In turn, unfriendly gut bacteria will send signals for carb-cravings to support their survival, then you tend to eat too many Calories and become overweight and provide the foundations of chronic disease. *Search YouTube for 'Catalyst Gut Reaction (Parts 1 & 2)'*

Bacteria Support

You can help support the bacteria in the bowel by eating vegetables that encourage friendly bacteria. Vegetables contain fibre and friendly bacteria and enzymes that actually feeds on fibre. The metabolic process of properly digesting vegetables produces chemicals that act like weedkillers towards unfriendly yeast and fungi. You can also eat fermented food like sauerkraut, olives, miso soup, vinegars, pickles, raw natural yoghurt and properly fermented soy sauce, which contain and encourages friendly bacteria. Contrary to advertising and popular belief, most commercially produced yoghurt does not support gut bacteria greatly due to the pasteurisation process and added sugar and flavourings. *(See also 'Celiac Disease' previously)*

Try eating as organically as possible. Sprays and pesticides used on normal supermarket vegetables are designed to kill bacteria and are not conducive to a healthy bowel. If you choose to eat fruit and vegetables that have been sprayed, either wash them in a mixture of water and vinegar prior or peel off the skin. Generally, fruit and vegetables won't absorb sprays past the skin because they know toxic sprays are unsupportive for growth.

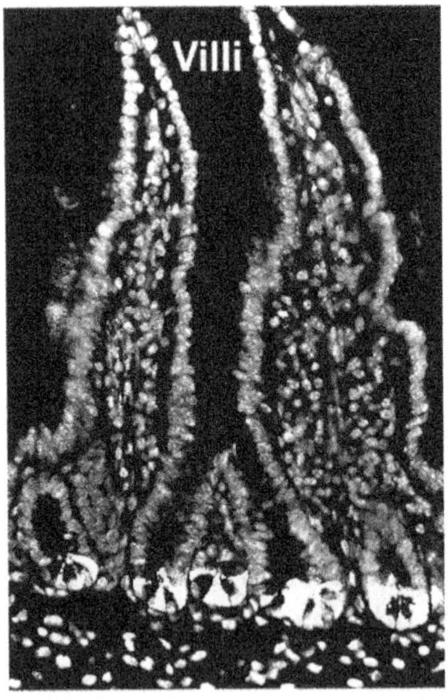

Stem cell activity highlighted at the base of villi, initiating friendly gut bacteria renewal

You can further support the regrowth and proliferation of friendly gut bacteria by ensuring you have a high number of adult stem cells circulating in your body. Stem cells are involved in the initiation of renewal of every cell in the body, and intestinal bacterial regrowth has one of the shortest renewal cycles. Stem cells can be increased by either intermittently fasting or taking supplements that encourage adult stem cell release from bone marrow.

You can also introduce friendly bacteria daily through supplementation. Of the more than 100 species of friendly bacteria, only around 12-15 (including the commonly known **lactobacillus, acidophilus and bifida** bacterium) can be implanted into the colon through ingestion.

These are commonly known as probiotics (as opposed to 'kill everything' antibiotics). Again, counter-intuitively, as the name acidophilus would suggest, these friendly bacteria thrive in an acidic colon environment, between 5.5–6.5 pH, but support the body by aiding in the establishment of a more-alkaline body.

The Best Probiotics

Probiotics have been used for decades, but there are a few things to look for...

1. Animal bacterium strains should be of human origin rather than dairy.
2. Should not contain anti-caking agents like magnesium stearate.
3. Should be stomach-acid resistant and bile-resistant. To dissipate the impact of stomach acid on the friendly bacteria, it's helpful to take your probiotic either with meals or 10–20 mins before a meal.

There are only a couple of supplements on the market that adequately supply 12 or more strains of probiotics produced from fermented vegetables.

One last tip... it's supportive if you double your dose of probiotics when travelling overseas to help counteract the new and different bacteria you may encounter during your journey.

Child Autism and Gut Flora

Dr. Natasha Campbell-McBride MD, *(www.doctor-natasha.com)*, states that autism in children is directly related to the imbalance of gut flora in the bowel of the child's mother prior to birth. Non-vaginal births and bottle- feeding impact a child's potential mental state too.

Natasha has found that 100% of the autistic childrens' mothers she has treated have abnormal gut flora which is passed onto the child as they pass through the birth canal. If a child is born from a caesarean section, then the child does not receive the correct amount of gut flora from the mother. Natasha believes autism and other child behavioural disorders (ADHD, dyslexia, dyspraxia, depression and schizophrenia) have similar origins. Natasha calls this 'gut and psychology syndrome' (GAPS) and such children are particularly vulnerable to normal vaccine regimes.

Flour Preservatives and Behavioural Problems

There is significant research to show that food preservatives E280-283 (propionic acid and propionates) used in flour products like bread, cake, biscuits, crackers, snacks, cereal and pasta are linked to behavioural problems such as hyperactivity, anti-social behaviour and autism.

Supporting Research

Natasha's research is supported by Professor Patricia Conway, of the School of Biotechnology and Biomolecular Sciences at the University of NSW in Sydney Australia, where she has found that babies born through non-vaginal methods are more prone to gut flora imbalances, asthma, allergic infections and viruses.

Recent research in Finland shows that providing mothers with good gut bacteria during pregnancy reduces the chances of their baby having allergies.

Building Strong Gut Flora Foundations

Natasha believes GAPS can be treated through correctly cleansing and conditioning the child's bowel and establishing the correct balance of gut flora through diet and supplementation.

Pregnant mothers can also assist a child's potential health by ensuring their bowel is clean prior to and during pregnancy and breastfeeding, ensuring the correct balance of gut flora is present and avoiding constipation which can happen easily due to the foetus placing pressure on the colon.

Breast-feeding also naturally introduces colostrum from the mother's milk, initiating the first peristaltic action in the child's bowel, instigating the elimination system for solids. Within hours of birth, the foundations of the child's digestive and elimination tract are laid down for life.

If the first bacteria come from the mother's milk, then supportive acidophilus bacteria will begin to breed in the gut. If the first bacteria are unfriendly, then unfriendly bacteria will breed and the child may be heading towards a potentially unhealthy future with allergies, intolerances and potentially autism. Whatever the foundations laid down, ongoing nutrition can change and determine the bacteria balance in the bowel and therefore the child's long-term health and mental faculties. The condition of the baby's bowel matters.

After breast feeding, commercial baby food from the supermarket may not be your best option. Perhaps mashed vegetables are a good alternative and skip the dairy and sugar. If they don't have it early in life, they won't want it later.

Parents need to be aware and give their child the best opportunities for health and learning, but unfortunately, most parents are ignorant and provide unsupportive food in the early years of development, then pay the price with extra tutoring, drugs, and doctors' and lawyers' bills later in life.

Genetically Modified Food (GMOs)

According to Dr Donald Huber *(search for "Don Huber interview" on www.mercola.com),* we have a huge negative impact evolving from genetically modified organisms (GMOs), as the body is not designed to digest artificially-modified cells which **impacts on supportive gut flora production** and suppresses the uptake of minerals and vitamins in the liver, which in turn effects the immune system negatively.

I believe that GMO food is the primary reason for the growing trend of food allergies and intolerances. It's too late, GMOs are already substantially in our environment and the best we can do is support our bodies to digest these mutated food-cells by consistently ingesting probiotic and enzyme supplements.

The following represent the percentages of total crops grown in the US in 2019 that are genetically modified (mostly through Monsanto GMO products)

- 94% of **soy**
- 90% of **corn**
- 90% of **canola**
- 98% of **cottonseed oil**
- 95% of some crops are **Roundup Ready** (seeds), meaning the crops can be sprayed with Monsanto's chemical weed killer, Roundup, which will only kill the weeds and not the cash crop.

In 2018, Monsanto was purchased by the German company Bayer and soon after faced several US lawsuits claiming that Roundup caused cancer. Three lawsuits have been found against Monsanto with one awarding a staggering US$2+ billion in damages. There are a further 18,400 lawsuits on file waiting to be heard. Meanwhile in Australia, our government departments ignorantly continue to support Monsanto's claims of safety.

The above figures are part of the reason why I don't recommend eating soy, especially when considering soy's digestive problems and its ability to negate the uptake of minerals like zinc, manganese and magnesium. Pigs are mostly fed corn and the GMO content of corn has created problems with pig reproduction.

Grain-fed beef is often promoted as a high-end cut; however industrial style feedlots feed cattle pellets made of soy, corn and other grains. Cows are designed by nature to eat grass! Grass fed beef is much better for you.

Remember, in the 1990s when mad cow disease was rife throughout the United Kingdom? It was originally triggered by feeding cattle pellets which contained contaminated animal matter. Why work against nature? Cattle aren't carnivorous!

Try to eat organic or grass-fed meat and encourage our governments to label food properly, so we have a choice. As a free person, you can also boycott purchasing products from companies that supply GMO chemicals and food or companies who choose not to label correctly.

Enzymes

For many years, I'd heard about enzymes but didn't give them any attention, until one of my acquaintances sent me a link to a 90-minute webinar that provided so much fantastic information and I've since given enzymes a priority in my life.

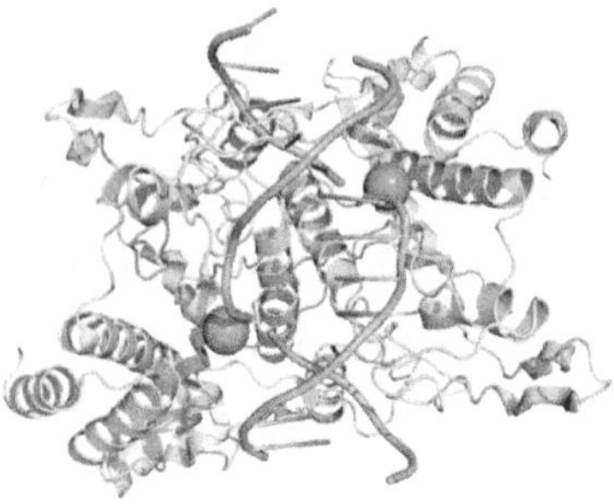

Generally, enzymes are created in the pancreas to assist with digestion later in the small intestine. Enzymes are incredibly complicated in structure and are so small; they couldn't be seen with a microscope until recent technology advancements made it possible. Scientist knew they were there, saw their positive impact, but couldn't find them. Their complicate 'squiggled' structure is necessary for their protein-conversion processes and when de-natured or contaminated (by toxins, chemicals, stress, etc.), enzymes become elongated and don't work effectively causing dysfunction in the body.

Friendly gut bacteria also create and engage enzymes to process food proteins that pass through the digestive tract. Once processed, these enzymes are transported to the liver and converted into energy (ATP, etc.). Without enzymes, we have minimal energy, and therefore poor quality of life and a shortened health span.

Enzymes also form part of raw food, to assist with its own digestion. Cooked food is depleted of enzymes.

It's estimated that around 80% of the body's energy is diverted to process a meal that the bowel finds difficult to digest, such as eating a large, sugar and carb-based lunch at Christmas. By 2-3 pm, we are so tired that we must sleep to empower the body to continue into the evening.

The same happens if we eat junk food day-after-day. That's why we feel tired and disempowered after eating and eventually create disease and depression.

Enzymes also support people with allergies and food intolerances (like Celiacs and gluten, lactose and casein intolerances), autism, Asperger's Syndrome and other chronic cognitive issues. Studies have shown significant improvement in each of these areas due to the addition of enzyme and probiotic supplementation.

Because the pancreas is usually over-burdened by production of insulin from unsupportive food choices and we generally don't eat enough raw food, it's desirable to supplement with enzymes – take a capsule (or two) **with** each meal. This takes the load off enzyme-producing organs and organisms in the body and can only aid the digestion and energy process.

Chapter 6

Constipation

Elvis' Constipation

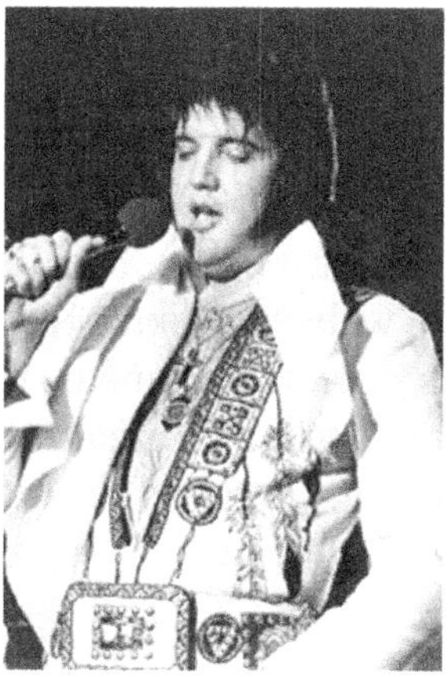

Elvis Presley's doctor has claimed the legendary singer did not die from an irregular heartbeat as first thought, but of an embarrassing case of chronic constipation.

Some myths also say that Elvis died from an over prescription of medical drugs by his doctor. Naively prescribing excessive medical drugs to Elvis may have however, also contributed to Elvis' constipation as his doctor laments...

Dr George Nick Nichopoulos, who was by Presley's side for the last 12 years of his life and tried to resuscitate him the day he died, has released a book titled *The King and Dr Nick*. It reveals his belief that it was chronic constipation that actually killed the King of Rock and Roll in 1977.

Presley, who was found dead in the bathroom after going to the toilet, was thought to have died from cardiac arrhythmia, possibly brought on by drug dependency, obesity and a weak heart.

"After he died, we weren't sure [of the exact cause of death], so I continued to do some research and I had some doctors call me from different places and different med schools that were doing research on constipation," the now-retired Memphis MD told FOX News.

According to Nichopoulos, an autopsy revealed that Presley's colon was 12–15 cm (5–6 inches) in diameter (normal width is 5–7cm (2–3 inches)) and instead of being the standard 1.2–1.5 meters (4–5ft) long, his colon was 2.7 metres (9ft) in length (indicating severe prolapse of the colon).

"We didn't realise until the autopsy that his constipation was as bad," the doctor said. "We found stool in his colon which had been there for four or five months because of the poor motility of the bowel."

In 1975, treatment involved removing part of the colon, known as a colostomy, and at the time Dr Nichopoulos was in talks with a surgeon at the University of Memphis to perform the procedure.

However, Presley's ego got in the way.

"He would get embarrassed; he'd have accidents onstage. He'd have to change clothes and come back because of the way we were trying to treat his constipation," Dr Nichopoulos said.

He also believed that Presley's prominent weight gain in the years prior to his death was not a result of overeating or eating the wrong foods, as they initially assumed. The doctor says that Presley's bloated appearance was due to his severe constipation.

Constipation — the Primary Cause

Don't believe everything you read, especially on the internet. I do my best to cross-check all information from several sources: books, websites, textbooks, documentaries, practitioners, etc. I've found numerous doctors and medical websites quoting that just "one motion per week is okay if that is normal for you". It might be normal (or heading towards average), but logic tells us it can't be healthy, especially over the long term.

One of the primary reasons I believe this is due to my personal experience and the fact that seeing, thinking about or chewing food instigates digestive-acid creation in the stomach, and that peristalsis action in the colon is triggered by food entering the stomach. The occurrence of these natural reactions indicates that as we eat, we are meant to release (daily at least).

Along with this, the longer food and toxic waste sits in the colon, the more toxic material is absorbed back into the blood. The body unwittingly utilises these toxins as a foundation to build the body's cells, and the cells are acidic, depleted of oxygen, creating the foundations of disease through autointoxication.

I have read in several places (and personally believe) that transit time through the digestive and elimination system should be 12–24 hours. Any longer and the food ferments, then putrefies and starts leaching toxins into the blood – the foundation of most diseases. We should have 1-3 relaxed bowel movements every day (I'll explain why in the next topic).

Prominent gastroenterologist Dr Wesley Jones found that virtually all digestive problems have one single underlying cause — **constipation**. "Our modern diets and stressful lifestyles can make poor digestion a common experience that sometimes people don't even recognise as a problem."

Fibre and Water

If faeces doesn't have enough fibrous material, water or both, the faeces may move slowly through the colon because the mucus lining and muscles on the colon wall have little to push against or is too dry and hard. The slow movement of the faeces allows extra water to be extracted, causing the faeces to become more dehydrated, harder and more compacted than intended.

Hard, solid faeces makes it difficult for the colon wall to work its peristalsis action and move the faeces towards the anus. It's a bit like trying to move a long, smooth piece of wood using a wet, silk pillow. A chronically constipated bowel won't pass a motion until enough pressure (waste) has built up behind the stool to force it out the anus.

As mentioned previously, the internal lining of the colon wall has a smooth mucus coating, which is continually replenished and binds and lubricates the faeces to slide along the colon wall. Inadequate water consumption and the resulting constipation can cause a build-up of sticky, dehydrated mucus on the colon wall which combines with other old, stagnant faeces to make a type of glue which adheres to the colon wall forming mucoid plaque, slowing the movement of faeces. The plaque can slowly build from a snake-skin-type of material, to leather-like and finally like tyre rubber with an adhesive inner surface. At the same time, water and nutrients are extracted by a series of veins connected to the colon that lead to the portal vein, which feeds to the liver for processing or storage. The longer faeces sits in the colon, the more toxins are extracted leading to autointoxication of all organs via the liver and blood.

Fibre acts as a prebiotic that passes through the small intestine undigested and becomes fermented when it reaches the large colon producing friendly gut bacteria. One of the best sources of natural fibre supplements is psyllium husk combined with ground flaxseed (20-30%). Take 20 minutes before meals with 2-glasses of quality water.

Autointoxication

Autointoxication is the term used when the digestive and elimination system is not working properly (constipation) and the accumulation of putrefied waste in the colon leads to toxins being continually absorbed and which essentially chronically poisons all other organs in the body.

The fact that you're having regular motions daily is not a true indication that you're not constipated either. Thick encrusted build-up (mucoid plaque) on the colon wall can sometimes only allow a thin, narrow stream of faeces to move through, whilst continually building up the solid faecal matter on the colon wall. Often such people may have up to 3-5 thin (often runny) bowel movements per day *(see 'Blockages' and 'Shape of Poo').*

One Excellent Solution to Constipation

If your colon is in poor condition (which may be indicated by a combination of the following disorders), then you might need to consider supporting your colon through taking supplements like AIM Herbal FiberBlend® which has soluble and insoluble fibre combined with 19 active herbs. Through our family's experience, I can certainly vouch for this product.

AIM Herbal FiberBlend® was formulated by Teresa Schumacher in 1988 and is patented by AIM, so no one else can copy Teresa's unique and proven formula. AIM Herbal FiberBlend® was the first blend of herbs and fibre in the world and nothing else comes close. Being on the market for 30+ years speaks for itself.

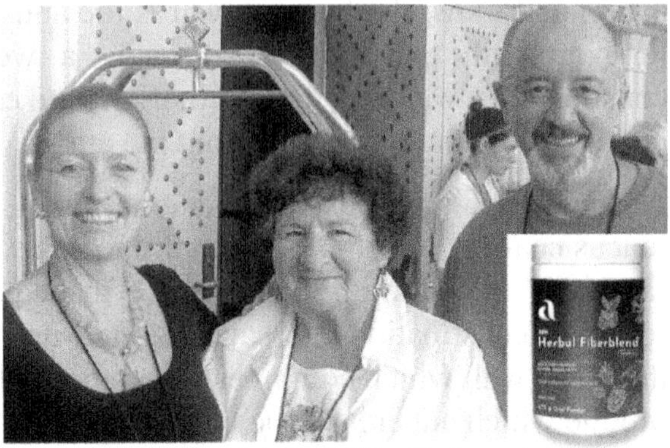

Shakti & Ramiah in 2009 with formulator of AIM Herbal FiberBlend, Teresa Schumacher

Conditions that May be Caused through Constipation

This next section discusses the complications and 'diseases' arising from constipation. They include: Diverticulitis, Colitis, Crohn's Disease, Segmentation, Blockages, Prolapsed Colon, Ballooned Colon, Diarrhoea, Bloating and Flatulence, Parasites, Chronic Fatigue and Lethargy, Allergies, Candida, Haemorrhoids, Varicose Veins, Skin Rashes, Fertility Problems, Prostate Issues, Inflammation, Toxic Build Up, Muscle and Joint Pain, Weight Gain and Cravings, Halitosis, Irritable Bowel Syndrome (IBS), Leaky Gut Syndrome, Inflammatory Bowel Disease (IBD), Insomnia and Snoring, Depression, Anxiety, Senility and Dementia

Though **heart disease and cancer** are not specifically colon problems, they are related to problems of the colon because they too can result from a low-fibre diet. A recent medical study concluded that, "If we could increase the daily per capita consumption of fibre by 13 grams, the risk of colorectal cancer in the US would decrease by 31%." **That translates to two lives saved every hour!** Various forms of cancer, including breast cancer, have also been shown to be related to a low intake of dietary fibre.

How Constipation Can Easily Happen

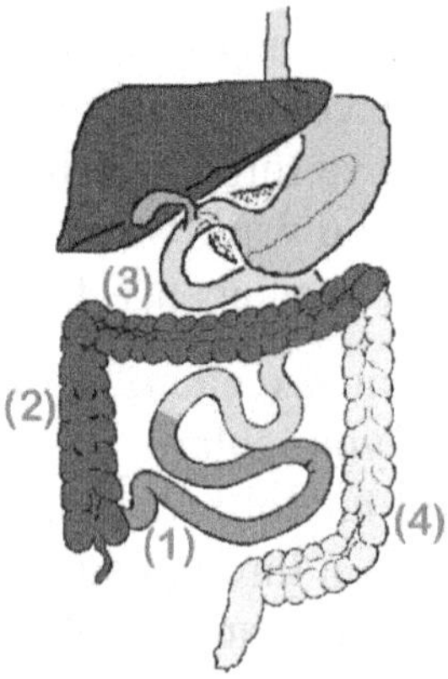

If you eat breakfast at **8 am**, then four hours later (at 12 noon), breakfast should have reached the end of the small intestine *(see picture, (1))* by which time most of the soluble oil and mineral nutrients should have been absorbed and the remains are ready to be passed into the colon.

At **12 noon**, lunch is ingested, which by 5 pm has reached the end of the small intestine *(1)* and breakfast has fully entered the ascending *(2)* and transverse *(3)* colon.

At **5 pm**, dinner is eaten and by 9 pm has reached the end of the small intestine *(1)*, lunch has reached the ascending *(2)* and transverse *(3)* colon and breakfast is sitting in the descending *(4)* colon, ready for elimination.

If the waiting stool is **not** released at this time (approx 12–16 hours after ingestion), four hours later lunch backs up in the descending colon *(4)*, then if still not released, dinner backs up on top of breakfast and lunch. Thankfully the colon has a built-in mechanism called the sigmoid (near the rectum), which expands to hold extra faeces if not released.

At the very least, a full bowel motion next morning should relieve the previous day's ingestion. Failing this, breakfast is ingested again, then lunch, then dinner. By day two, if you have not passed a motion you have six meals backing up — you are CONSTIPATED, and feeling bloated, irritable and uncomfortable as the colon distorts to house the excess faeces and toxins start leaching into your body.

The average time for regular bowel motions in western society is once every 96 hours (four days – about twice per week).

If you Think Constipation Isn't a Problem...
Now if you think passing a movement every 3-4 days is okay, just imagine...

<u>Mix a blend of the following food:</u>

Minced beef, milk, flour and sugar – leave **on the kitchen bench** for 4 days at 38°C (100°F) – body temperature. What would happen?

The meat mix would decay, turn toxic, grow bacteria and smell disgusting, attracting flies, maggots and other parasites. If you ate the meat mix you would most likely become ill from the bacteria and toxins.

<u>Now EAT a blend of the following food:</u>

Minced beef, milk, flour and sugar – leave **in your colon** for 4 days at 38°C (100°F) – body temperature. What would happen?

The same happens in the bowel — meat combined with sugar, dairy white flour and left in the gut for four days will create a putrid, toxic stool that smells strongly, as will the gas produced during its fermentation.

You'll also provide a perfect nest-bed to attract parasites like roundworms, pinworms, tapeworms and intestinal fluke, some of which only need 36 hours to reproduce. The toxins produced may leach into the body through the colon wall. In the short-term, you'll probably feel fatigued and grumpy at the very least. In the longer term, you're promoting an acidic environment that supports disease, cancer and a low quality of life.

Transit Time Test

You can easily test how long your transit time is for meals by doing a simple test. Eat normally, but during your evening meal, include corn kernels. Over the next day or so, observe your stools and see if they contain yellow corn kernels.

If your first motion is next morning and yellow corn kernels are visible, then your transit time can be regarded as excellent (around 12 hours). If your first motion is around lunch or dinner time, and corn is visible, then it can be considered reasonably acceptable too. If no corn is visible in your first motion after consuming corn, then you are probably releasing a previous motion, so wait for a corn-ladened motion to pass.

The sickness industry also has a method that involves swallowing a solution containing twenty or so small plastic chips. The following day the abdomen is x-rayed to view their progress and check for blockages.

In my view this is expensive, intrusive and potentially unhealthy as you ingest artificial products and expose your body to unnecessary radiation. But that's how Big Pharma makes their profit. *see chapter 10*

Causes of Constipation

Constipation is usually caused by five major factors:

1. Stress, anxiety, fear and emotions
2. Lack of fibre
3. Acidic food (high consumption of carbs – sugar/dairy/flour)
4. Poor quantity and quality of water
5. Lack of exercise (sedentary lifestyle)

However, anxiety, tension, tobacco, medications, steroids, chemicals, toxins, pregnancy, occupational sedentary vibration (for example driving trucks, buses, taxi) and 'holding on too long' can all contribute as well.

Conversely, many diseases like acidosis, colitis, Crohn's disease, IBD and IBS can encourage constipation. Constipation may not be the original cause of the disease, but once constipation is encouraged by a disease or prescribed medication, and subsequently stress increases, it can be exacerbated and contribute to disease. The notorious 'vicious circle' leads the body towards your Sickness Cycle, but the good news is that it can be stopped and reversed.

Changes in Pipe Diameter

A natural phenomenon surrounding constipation (but not the cause), is the fact that the colon is about 65mm (2½ in) diameter and the faeces is trying to fit through the anus, which (as you know) should be water tight — if it wasn't, life could get messy.

This is one of nature's little quirks; with the correct diet, enough water and exercise it's usually not a problem. However, should you choose a sedentary lifestyle and eat unsupportive refined food and drink little water, the faeces may become more dehydrated and compacted, making it more difficult to release through the small opening of the anus.

Spastic Colon

Stress and anxiety can cause parts of the colon to become either twisted or inactive, often referred to as a spastic colon and can be diagnosed as IBS. This inactive or twisted state can cause constipation and, assuming there is no nerve damage, magnesium and AIM Composure® may assist with relaxation of the colon muscles, allowing a gentle passing of faeces and regaining colon strength.

Prolapsed Colon

A prolapsed colon lengthens and stretches the colon significantly and can disengage nerves and muscles, leaving parts of the colon thin and dysfunctional *(see 'Prolapsed Colon' later).*

Cancer Risks

Constipation can be an indicative condition that can lay a foundation for cancer, reflecting unsupportive lifestyle choices that, overtime can develop diseases and encourage or exacerbate cancer.

Statistics

In 1908 the five leading causes of death were influenza and pneumonia, tuberculosis (TB), diarrhoea, heart disease and stroke. Cancer didn't gain a mention 100+ years ago.

Statistics show that one in two Australians will be diagnosed with cancer before the age of 85, making cancer Australia's leading killer which wasn't the case even 50 years ago. According to the National Bowel Cancer Screening Program, 80 Australians die each week from bowel cancer (most common in people over 50) which is Australia's second highest cancer killer behind lung cancer (due mostly to smoking). Third is prostate cancer in men. Many in the sickness industry believe that most cancers start in the bowel, and then spread to other organs via the liver and blood.

An 11-year study of 1,300 people by the University of Western Australia showed that men between 55 and 84 with type 2 diabetes had double the chance of developing bowel cancer.

The World Cancer Research Fund mentioned in a recent report involving ten studies that eating (acid-forming) red meat, sugar, dairy and alcohol, along with a sedentary lifestyle increased the risk of developing cancer. The stats surrounding red meat have since been found dubious and unreliable.

The Western Australia Institute for Medical Research showed in a study of over 2,000 men that sedentary office work increased the risk of bowel cancer by 44%.

Men who have been heavy consumers of milk for most of their lives have a four times greater chance of developing prostate cancer.

Causes and Risk Factors

Diseases caused by diet and lifestyle choices can cause constipation, which can impact on your chances of developing cancer.

The causes of constipation are similar to the causes of cancer — get the picture? Can you see why constipation can lay a foundation for future illness?

Remember that **cancer is often the end result** of diseased organs which degenerate due to lifestyle choices. Generally, cancer doesn't happen first, something else has gone wrong prior to the cancer diagnosis, whether it's found by the doctor or not. If a doctor diagnoses cancer, they are not going to check for lesser ailments. Cancer can be developing unnoticed in the body for ten years or so prior to diagnosis.

I believe in most cases; cancer isn't just bad luck and doesn't just happen! I believe it's caused by choices of food, work, exercise, water quality and level of happiness.

Stress has a considerable impact on cancer. Emotional stress is acidic to the body through triggering the release of cortisol (2.4 pH) from the adrenal glands; happiness is alkalising, as you will read later.

Traditional medicine believes that all illness is caused by unresolved negative emotional conflict, which causes stress on the body by clouding choices which in turn results in relief and escape. Stress begins in the brain and transfers to actions which become habits. Habits become comfortable. If your habits are not supportive for optimum health, you will chronically impact the body's health which, over time, can lead to cancer.

That's why I focus so much on being as positive and happy as I can in every thought, elevating my happiness level little by little, whilst considering my impact on my health and others around me.

Genes have little to do with it

Latest research is showing that genes don't cause disease or cancer but react and mutate according to what is fed to the cells (food, water, stress, emotions and the resulting hormones and enzymes).

There have been many experiments where cancerous cells (genes) can be switched on or off, depending on the type of food ingested.

There have been countless studies showing that people who leave their European homeland and immigrate to Australia or the US and then take up the local high dairy, carb and sugar-ladened (low fibre) diet tend to increase in weight and develop common diseases typical of their new country. It's not the genes; it's the food and lifestyle you provide to your genes.

Cancer and gene research institutions don't want you to know this; they would like you to continue contributing to keeping their staff employed and maintaining profits through cancer research charities - thank you very much.

There is Plenty of Opportunity
Cancer can only thrive in a de-oxygenated, acidic body which is primarily caused by the fermentation of sugar. Reduce your sugar intake, supply your cells with plenty of alkaline vegetables which oxygenate the cells, exercise regularly, drink plenty of quality water and you should starve cancer growth.

This has been known and scientifically proven since 1931 by Nobel Prize winner Otto Warburg who said: *"The prime cause of cancer is the replacement of the respiration of oxygen in normal body cells by a fermentation of sugar (glucose)... all* ***cancer cells*** *without exception must ferment".* —

Dr Johanna Budwig went on to develop Warburg's work and created an effective cancer treatment based around essential fatty acids (EFAs), namely omega-3 and 6 combined with cottage cheese and blended in a specific way. The flaxseed oil is activated by the sulphur-based proteins found in cottage cheese. Budwig claims a 90% success rate.

Dr Burzynski's 'antineoplaston' treatment has a success rate of around 50–60% but has been hindered in its development and availability by Big Pharma and government bureaucracy *(see 'Big Pharma and Your Health' later)*.

Don't believe everything the cancer industry tells you and don't take my word for it either; please do your own research...

Documentaries:
Search the internet and watch...

- *Cancer is Curable Now*
- *Burzynski Movie*
- *One Answer to Cancer*

- *Forks Over Knives*
- *Cancer Conquest*
- *Fat, Sick and Nearly Dead*
- *Healing Cancer from the Inside Out*

Websites:

- www.budwigcenter.com
- www.gerson.org
- www.dr-gonzalez.com
- www.oasisofhope.com
- www.drconnealy.com
- www.anoasisofhealing.com
- www.naturopath4you.com
- www.healthranger.org

In March 2012, the Brisbane Sunday Mail championed the headline "Colon cancer drug hope". Upon reading the story it turns out that the drug simply blocks the actions of enzymes involved in digesting food, therefore relieving the symptoms IBD, one of the causes (or precursors) of colon cancer. Symptoms are simply warning lights that something is out of balance.

However, because the enzymes are blocked, the food goes through the bowel undigested. What impact is that going to have on the rest of the digestion and elimination process? The results of the expensive ten-year study into relieving symptoms (not resolving the problem) have been published in the Journal of Pharmacology and Experimental Therapeutics *(see Chapter 10 for the reasons behind this article).*

Before you hand over responsibility for your life to the methodology and dogma of orthodox medicine, do yourself a favour and conduct your own research (as I've done). Your life (or the life of someone you love) might just depend on it.

Start by cleaning out the colon and detoxing the liver through supplementation, diet, water and exercising.

Important Question: Which One Will Win?

- Cancer

☹ *Sugar, excess dairy, refined packaged food, fast food, tap-water, stress, sedentary lifestyle, fear, negative emotions and reactions*

- Wellbeing
  ☺ *Meat, fat, vegetables, wholefood, quality water, detoxing, supplementation, exercise, intermittent fasting, fulfillment, inner peace, happiness, giving and love*

Answer: ***"The one You Feed!"*** *It can't be any other way.*

The fuel you provide must result in an outcome for your health, positive or negative. You can't beat natural laws. You create your reality – full stop!

I've Bet my Life on It!
After a significant family history of cancer, diabetes and heart disease, I've bet my life on natural preventions and treatments. I've decided not to take out health insurance or have a colonoscopy after my father passed with colon cancer; instead I've changed my lifestyle to produce better outcomes.

I have seen first-hand orthodox medicine's attempts to deal with cancer and have personally found it ineffective, toxic, expensive and degrading. I choose not to go the same way. My current health indicates that I'm on the right path.

How to Relieve Constipation

Old Ways
The original way to relieve constipation was to become a mathematician and 'work it out with a pencil'☺. (That's an old one from high school.)

For decades, the sickness industry has used chemical-based laxatives to resolve constipation, but laxatives work by essentially 'inducing diarrhoea' which can become problematic, habit-forming, can lead to dependency and can irritate the colon.

As a child, I remember listening to radio ads that I didn't really understand at the time: *"Keeps you looking slim and healthy; keeps you really regular. Buy Ford Pills"*. Laxatives don't stimulate or exercise the colon muscles by utilising the peristalsis action, rendering the colon wall-muscles unfit, inactive and disempowered over time. With such chemical laxatives, the colon wall is not exercised and becomes lazy.

Practical, Natural Solutions
There are several things you can easily do to relieve constipation, assuming your colon is in reasonable condition. Please don't dismiss this information as unimportant and fanciful! Making these changes can make a significant difference — however, you must give it time.

1. **Walking** naturally massages the bowel, stimulating movement of blood, bile, toxins and bowel motions. Exercise increases oxygen content to the cells, which alkalises the body. If you've ever walked a dog, you'll notice

that usually within the first 15 minutes, the dog will pass a motion because the walking action has stimulated (massaged) its bowel. The same happens to humans — once you get home of course.

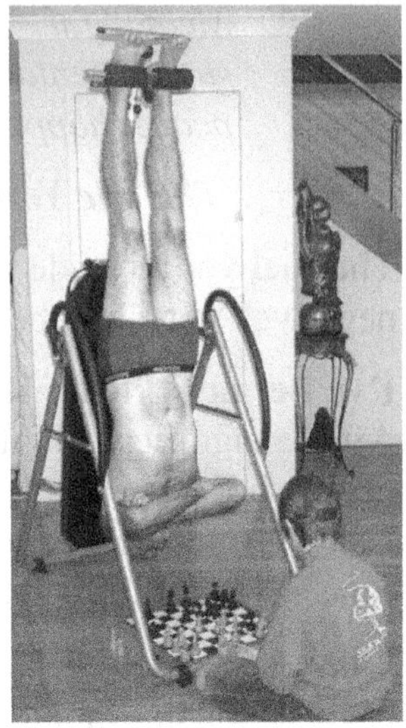

Inversion bed — just hanging around playing chess with my son

2. **Invert daily**. Using an **Inversion bed** daily drains and flushes the gut organs of blood and stimulates movement in the intestines and liver. When inverting back to a vertical position, the rush of blood through gut organs flushes toxins and debris out into the bloodstream where the waste can go through the excretion process. Yoga has been using this principle for thousands of years. The inversion bed has the added advantage of stretching the spine and balancing the hips too.
3. Rub **magnesium** into your skin daily. Magnesium is not only necessary for nerve communication, but also bowel contractions and is a bowel relaxant.
4. Reduce **stress and anxiety** and increase sleep.
5. Drink plenty of <u>quality</u> **water** as discussed earlier.

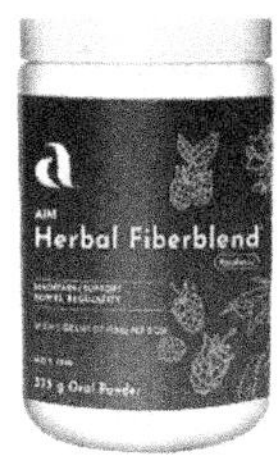

6. Supplement with **fibre,** like psyllium husk, AIM Herbal FiberBlend® or AIM Fit 'n Fiber®* *see resources later*
7. Improve your **diet** by eating less refined food and eating more animal protein and fibrous vegetables (especially) and fruit.
8. Include in your diet natural support like:

   Prunes, rhubarb, broccoli sprouts, beetroot, beans, peas, apples, legumes, Senna (herb), Cascara Sagrada (herb), cayenne pepper, capsicum (peppers), ginger, Oatstraw, rice fibre, turmeric (curcumin), avocado, barley grass, flaxseed, fennel, parsley, slippery elm, liquorice, alfalfa, coconut oil, nuts, apple cider vinegar, psyllium husk, bran, rye, oats, wholemeal bread (but minimal grain is best) and diatomaceous earth. Avoid white bread and processed cereal.

Relax and Set --it Free

The body also needs to be relaxed to pass a motion. Tension, busy-ness, young children, interruptions, fear, phone calls, laptops, tablets, smart phones, anxiety, worry, aggressive music or conversation at home or work can 'make it go back up' (so to speak). Allow yourself time and space to relax.

Remember, "Will power can overcome anything, except constipation" ☺

Supermarket Solutions

Be cautious of advertising and promotion of mainstream, supermarket high-fibre products and detox programs that come in sweet tasting drinks, cereals, wafers, shakes and biscuits. Most contain significant amounts of sugar, or if labelled "Sugar Free" or "Low Calorie" are likely to contain artificial sweeteners and colouring. Sugar compounds constipation, and whilst these products supply a sweet-tasting portion of fibre for the gut, they also create a highly acidic environment which constipation and cancer loves *(see 'Sugar' previously).*

Go ASAP

The greatest support you can give your colon is to pass a motion as soon as possible when your rectum signals 'there's a brown dog in the kennel'. This will stop the faeces backing-up, dehydrating and becoming harder and more difficult to release.

Natural Supplements

Sometimes the colon can become dysfunctional *(see 'Symptoms of Constipation' below)* and may need support to regain its former capacity or ability. There are plenty of natural herbs and fibre you can use.

Fibre and Water

Fibre has long been recognised as one of the best food ingredients for maintaining bowel regularity and preventing constipation, and because it normalises bowel movements, it can also be used to treat and manage chronic diarrhoea. Fibre requires enough water to function properly in the body.

Professor Denis Burkitt

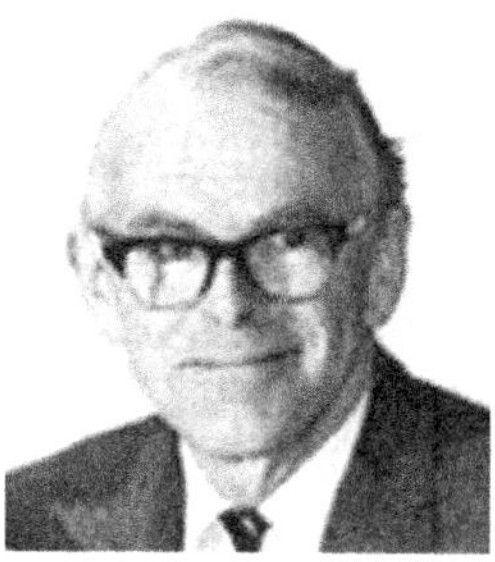

Prof. Denis Burkitt

Professor Denis Burkitt of Dublin University is considered the grandfather of dietary fibre research. After driving through Africa for many years studying native diets, he emphasised in his 1979 book, '*Don't Forget Fibre in your Diet*', that low fibre in the diet was an indication of future bowel cancer, heart disease and diabetes. Burkitt's studies showed that primitive diets (the diet our body is designed to eat) protected native Africans from most diseases and he also found that natives passed 2–4½ times more faeces than the typical western diet in the 1970s. Today's typical western diet contains much less fibre than 40 years ago.

Fibre's Benefits

Consuming fibre reduces transit time by giving the faeces substance to push against during peristalsis and results in a more thorough evacuation of waste materials. It's known to improve all aspects of colon function. Fibre is found only in plants and not in animal products. Fibre is an indigestible complex carbohydrate, therefore adds few calories to the diet. There are two main types of fibre — insoluble and water-soluble (also known as 'soluble'). Both types of fibre are required in the daily diet, in the recommended ratio of 3:1 insoluble fibre to water-soluble fibre. At the very least, should be equal parts.

Insoluble Fibre

Insoluble fibre resists being dissolved in water, meaning that our bodies cannot digest it. This type of fibre includes the un-dissolvable parts of plant walls and is found in its greatest amounts in cereals, bran and vegetables. The primary function of insoluble fibre is to collect water that increases stool bulk in the colon. This promotes bowel movement, and when the bulk faeces works through the intestine, it scours the intestinal walls of waste matter, reducing the risk of colon-related problems.

Water-Soluble Fibre

Water-soluble fibre readily dissolves in water and is found in oat bran, legumes, psyllium, nuts, beans, pectin, and various fruits and vegetables. It forms a bulky gel in the intestine that regulates the flow of waste materials through the digestive tract. Water-soluble fibre may lower cholesterol by preventing the re-absorption of bile acids. Bile acids are made from cholesterol, and after they aid fat digestion, fibre binds with them and escorts them out of the body through the anus. The liver then must pull more cholesterol from the blood.

Water-soluble fibre may also stabilise blood sugar by slowing down the absorption of carbohydrates into the blood. Plus, it can lower blood sugar levels. Researchers have found that increasing fibre intake results in a decrease in the body's need for insulin, therefore less fat is stored. Psyllium supplementation in particular, has been shown to improve blood sugar levels in diabetics.

How Much Fibre?

For adults who are 50 years and younger, the recommendation for total fibre intake is 38 grams per day for men and 25 grams for women. Adults over 50, the recommendation is 30 grams per day for men and 21 grams for women.

Personally, I take more than the recommended servings. Because my bowel was in poor condition originally, this amount seems to work for me. I have a relaxed, unforced motion every day after my walk. Test your own situation and take the amount that works for you.

It's important that you don't rely totally on fibre to do all the heavy lifting and detox work for the body and allow the proper processes of bile (produced in the liver) to do most of the work for the body – as nature intended. Fibre and water will assist in escorting toxins and waste out of the body, but bile and water do most of the organ and blood cleansing. Bile is best produced by eating more animal protein earlier in the day (especially) and eating minimal refined carbohydrates as discussed in *"Importance of Animal Protein"*.

Studies have found that in populations with high fibre diets, the incidences of colon cancer, appendicitis, and diverticulitis are very low. Industrialised countries, which largely have diets high in carbs and sugar and low in fibre, have high incidences of these diseases. Because fibre is low in calories, it can be added to your diet, providing a greater feeling of satiety (feeling satisfied, full) without significantly increasing your caloric intake.

The fibre found in plants serves as a source of complex carbohydrate, which most nutritionists consider to be a healthier choice.

In addition, fibre's ability to stabilise blood sugar, fibre may also curb the desire to snack. Fibre eaten about 20 minutes before a meal will trigger a hormone called CCK (Cholecystokinin) which sends messages to the stomach, "I am satisfied — don't eat much more." In other words, you should find yourself eating less, if you listen to the messages and not your habits. This is beneficial in weight-loss programs.

Kellogg Trivia

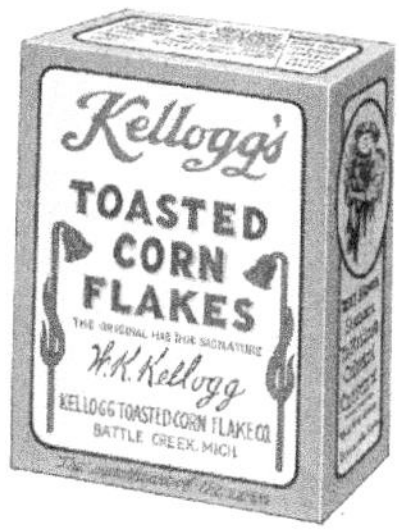

Dr Harvey Kellogg MD once said, *"Of the 22,000 operations I personally performed, I never found a single normal colon and of the 100,000 performed under my jurisdiction, not over 6% were normal."*

Dr Kellogg went on to invent Corn Flakes and form the Kellogg's cereal company to encourage people to eat more fibre.

Unfortunately, Kellogg's today serves as a means of delivering sugar to children with some cereals containing up to 32% sugar and not much fibre. It's also not desirable for health and weight control to have refined carbs for breakfast

Diatomaceous Earth (DE)

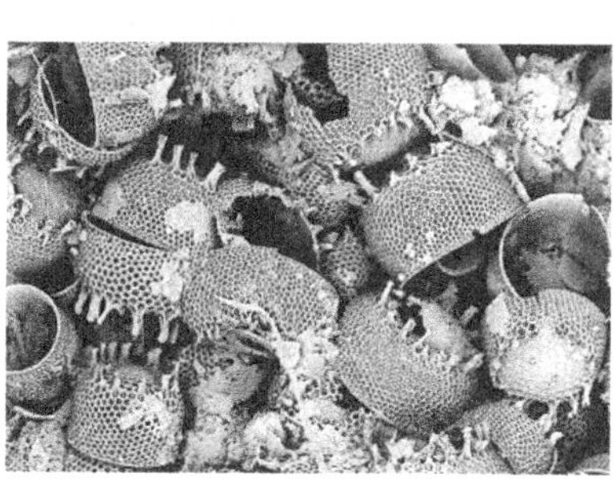

Diatomaceous Earth (pronounced *'diamacious'*) is a white powder of fossilized remains made from microscopic shells of freshwater plankton called diatoms. Made from about 90% amorphous silica with 28 trace minerals and shaped in the form of microscopic hexagonal tubes with a strong negative charge, DE provides an excellent vehicle to trap toxins, heavy metals, fungi, etc and escort them out the bowel.

Having a significant hardness and a microscopic structure, DE helps to clean the small intestine and colon walls as it passes through, keeping fresh bacteria and mucosa in place.

Freshwater DE has (and maintains) its hexagonal tubular shape, whereas saltwater DE is softer and has more irregular shapes, making it less effective.

DE helps normalise bowel function and assists with detoxing. It assists with keeping cholesterol in check and helps normalise blood pressure. Being made from silica, DE also supports skin, hair, nails, teeth, bones and connective tissue.

DE can be purchased from most health food stores or online. Personally, I take 1-2 heaped teaspoon daily which seem to work well for me.

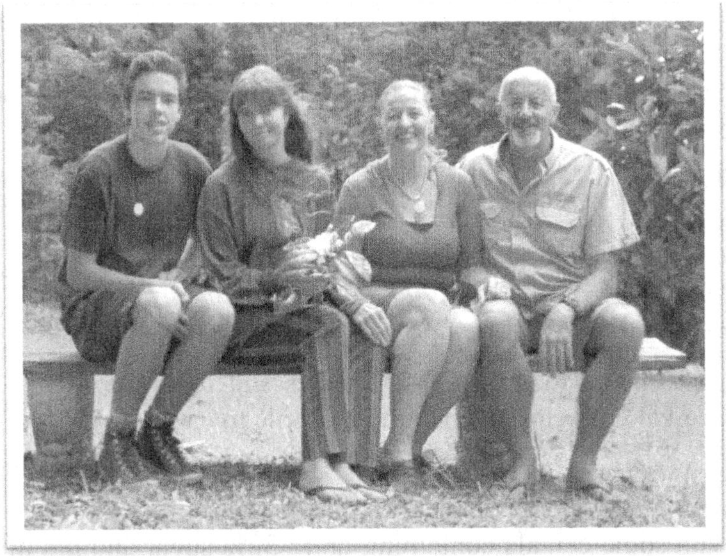

My family are living happy, healthy, adventurous lives following the guidelines in this book. Each of us are pursuing our income through our individual passions and taking responsibility for our actions. My son (21) is currently growing in the film industry. My daughter (22), is pursuing her art career. My wife (Shakti) helps people improve their lives through therapies and her intuition. I love researching and connecting information; painting a big picture through my written and spoken word. Shakti and I learn something new every day and grow that little bit more. Together, we market this book, along with products that saved our lives whilst educating and inspiring people to take responsibility and control of their health and wealth whilst caring for our planet.

Chapter 7

Conditions that Can be Caused Through Constipation

Common Features of Diagnosis

Study the table below and observe similar symptoms between common bowel diseases and mental problems (in UPPER CASE). Medicine tends to treat disease separately, rather than look at the whole body.

Disease Symptom Summary

Many BODY and MENTAL issues appear to derive their origins from a clogged BOWEL (colon) as a result of constipation, resulting in an overwhelmed and stressed liver, which is unable to filter the blood properly and therefore impacts negatively on every other organ in the body.	BODY						BOWEL							MENTAL ILLNESS			
	Acidosis	Adrenal fatigue	Diabetes	Gallstones	Liver cirrhosis	Toxin overload	Celiac disease	Colitis (colon)	Crohn's disease	Diverticulitis	Inflam. bowel disease (IBD)	IBS and gut flora imbalance	Leaky gut syndrome	Anxiety	Bipolar (nanic depressive)	Chronic fatigue syndrome	Depression
Abdominal pain				*	*		*	*	*	*	*	*	*	*		*	
ANGER and IRRITABILITY	*	*	*		*	*	*	*	*		*	*	*	*	*	*	*
ANXIETY and STRESS	*	*	*		*	*	*	*	*		*	*	*			*	*
Allergies and asthma	*		*		*	*	*	*	*		*	*	*				
Bleeding — anal or internal	*				*			*	*	*	*						
Bloating and gas	*			*			*	*	*	*	*	*	*			*	
Blockages / strictures in colon								*	*	*	*						
Bone density — low	*	*	*			*	*	*	*		*	*					
Cancer (can progress into)	*		*		*	*	*	*	*		*	*	*				
Circulation — poor			*		*	*	*									*	
Constipation (or cycles of)	*					*	*	*	*	*	*	*	*				
CONCENTRATION PROBLEMS	*	*	*		*	*	*	*	*		*	*	*	*	*	*	*
DEPRESSION / MOOD SWINGS	*	*	*		*	*	*	*	*		*	*	*	*	*	*	
Diarrhoea (or cycles of)	*					*	*	*	*	*	*	*	*			*	
Eye irritation or deterioration			*		*	*		*	*		*					*	
Fatigue and lethargy	*	*	*		*	*	*	*	*				*	*	*		*
Fever				*				*	*	*	*	*	*				
Headache	*		*			*							*			*	*
Immune system — low	*	*	*		*	*	*	*	*		*	*	*				
Inflammation	*		*	*	*	*		*	*	*	*						*
Insomnia						*							*	*	*		*
Kidney complications	*	*	*		*	*											
Liver complications	*		*	*		*	*	*	*		*	*	*				
Pain — joint and / or muscle	*		*			*	*	*	*		*	*	*	*	*	*	*
Siezures					*	*	*										
Skin rashes or discolouration	*		*	*	*	*	*	*	*		*	*	*			*	
Vomiting or nausea				*			*		*	*	*	*		*		*	
Weight gain	*	*	*									*			*		*
Weight (or appetite) loss	*		*		*		*	*	*		*	*	*		*	*	*

This table is not meant to diagnose any particular disease and is **not** comprehensive. The table has been compiled to display the similarities between symptoms of diagnosed diseases, and (also) the relationship between bowel disease and mental illness. Constipation may be a cause, or symptom, of the above diseases. One disease may also evolve into another. You should consult your healthcare practitioner for diagnosis.

Examples of distorted, diseased colons caused by unsupportive lifestyle choices

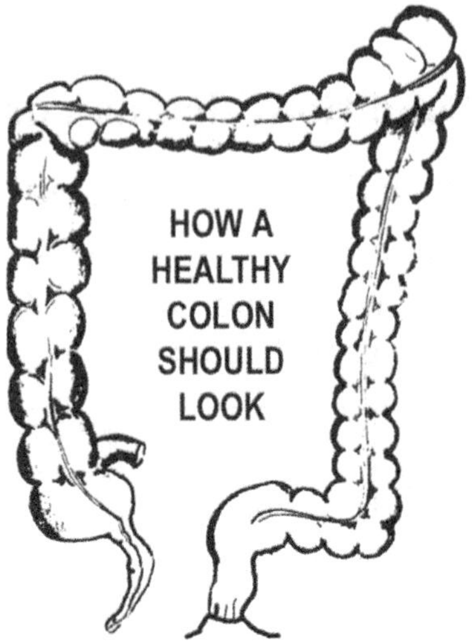

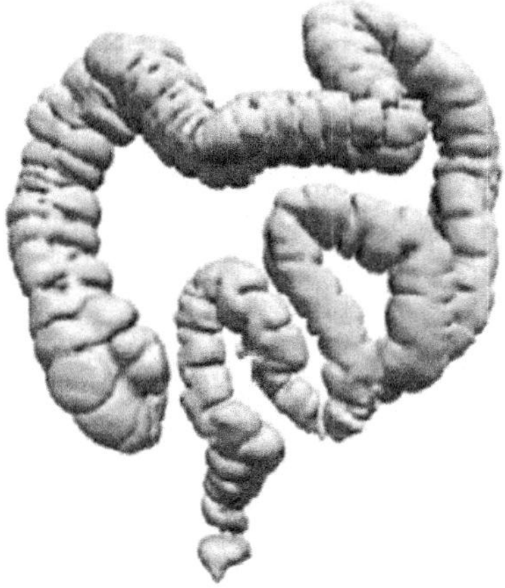

1

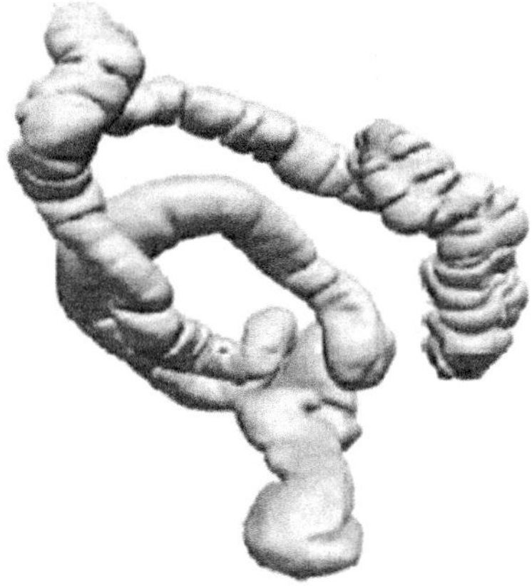

2

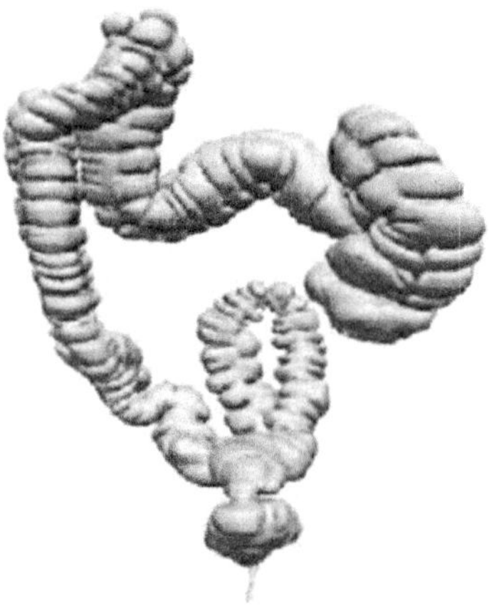

3

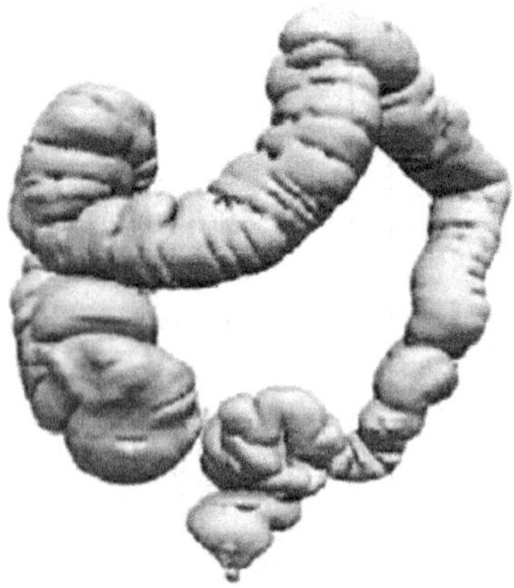

4

Diverticulitis

As faeces gathers at the rectum and the sigmoid is stretched to its limits, more faeces can back-up along the descending colon, then around the second bend towards the transverse colon. Accumulation of compacted faeces tends to stretch the wall of the descending colon and sigmoid making them thin. Under the strain of passing a dry, stubborn stool, the colon wall can 'pop out' in numerous balloon-like extrusions called diverticula. If diverticula become inflamed (infected), the disease is called **diverticulitis**. They can become infected from the intense focus of stagnant toxins within the faeces and often antibiotics may be prescribed to treat the infection, which further exacerbates constipation, rather than working towards fixing the problem — constipation.

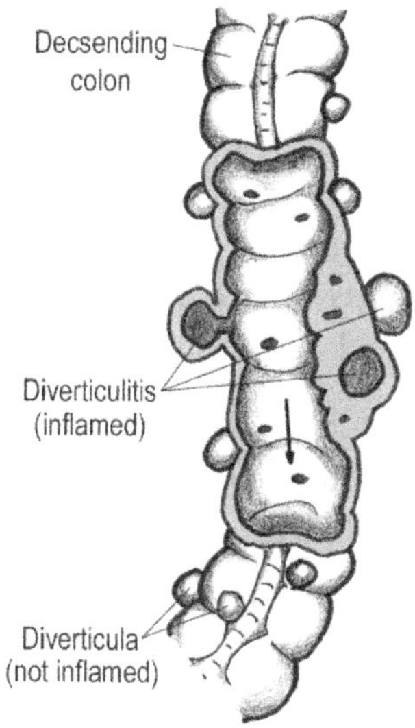

Colonic therapists note that people who eat a lot of bread have the most problems with diverticulitis.

Segmentation (Strictures)

Chronic constipation, diverticulitis, strictures and scar tissue can lead to segmentation (especially in the sigmoid and descending colon), where numerous pockets of diverticula become the norm and stretch to join together to form larger segments, leaving the 'between' sections of the bowel thin, narrow and weak, unable to move faeces forward through peristalsis, therefore exacerbating constipation.

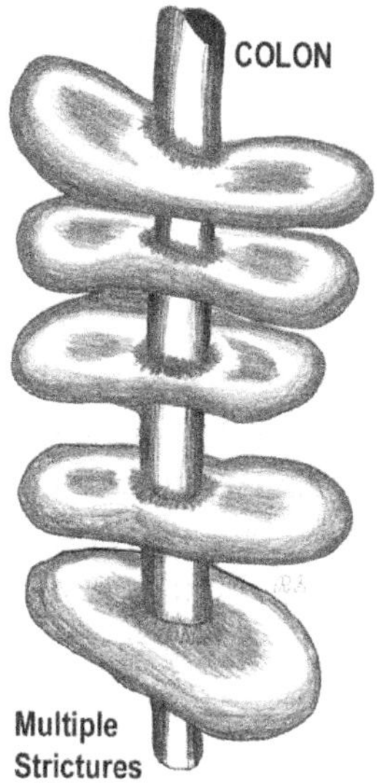

Though I was never clinically diagnosed with segmentation, I did remove a plaque lining from my colon wall that looked similar to this segmented shape I sketched.

Blockages

As faeces backs up from the rectum, around the second bend, a stricture (blockage) can form at the bend and the transverse colon can balloon to the size of a football, holding up to 5kg (11 lb) of toxic waste material. The material on the outer edge of the colon (near the colon wall) can harden and become immovable due to lack of peristalsis and continual dehydration through the colon wall. This hardened material can become like tyre rubber and adheres to the colon wall, blocking the production of lubricating mucus.

However, the faeces must get through, so paradoxically, the caked faeces can allow a narrow channel for liquid faeces to move through giving the appearance of diarrhoea or thin, soft poo. Sometimes this channel can be as narrow as a pencil. Ultimately though, this channel is likely to become blocked (as happened with Elvis Presley).

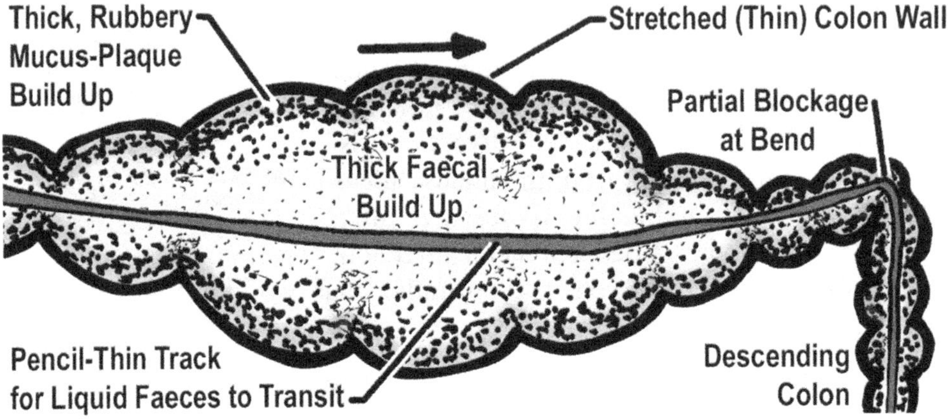

Nurses have related numerous unpleasant experiences of patients admitted to emergency wards with faeces backing up to their mouth. Faeces must be released one way or another.

Why Blockages Occur

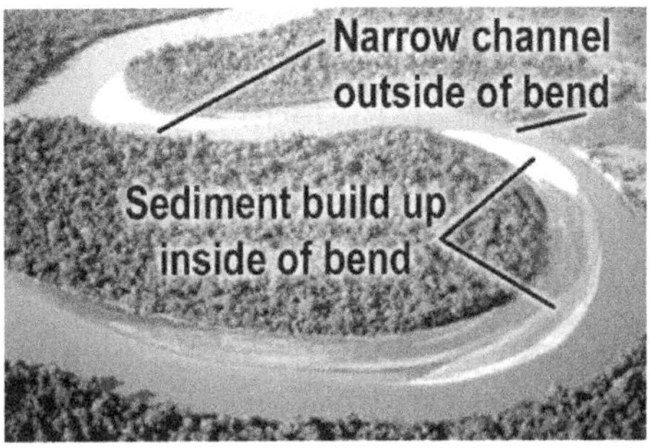

Besides the previously mentioned build-up of faecal matter, one of the main reasons blockages often occur on bends can be easily explained through a natural phenomenon in nature. If you look at a bend in a river, you'll find that the water travelling on the inside edge of the bend travels much slower than the water travelling on the outside of the bend. As the inside water travels slower, it drops sediment on the inside bank. Whereas the fast-moving water on the outer edge tends to carve a deep, narrow channel.

Likewise, in the colon, as faeces travels around a bend, it can often leave deposits on the inside of the bend. If the colon is not regularly cleaned out or emptied, over years, these deposits can lead to a blockage and a lazy colon wall.

Similarly, this effect can be seen in blood vessels, as suspended fat, sugar and toxins in the blood deposit on the inside of vessel connections and bends, causing arterial blockages that can lead to stroke and heart attack.

Blockages can also occur due to a large accumulation of parasites (such as roundworms) in one part of the intestine. Hundreds of roundworms can gather in a nest, blocking flow.

Also, through colon and visceral prolapse, the weight and extra downward drag of the colon can crease or fold each bend, causing blockages *(see 'Prolapsed Colon' later).*

The afore-mentioned bends of the colon are connected near the back of the ribcage. If the colon has a blockage (often around the second bend because the faeces is dryer at this bend), the colon can balloon out to the size of a football. Coupled with extra belly fat, this puts significant strain on the connections of the colon to the ribcage and tends to pull the ribcage forward, giving chronic lower back pain.

Diarrhoea and Constipation Cycles

Usually, faeces that is running through a narrow channel ultimately blocks and backs up to a point that the pressure finally forces the solid faeces out the anus. Much of the faeces removed comes from the softer, inner built-up area and is generally not the harder faeces caked nearer the colon wall. When this 'plug' is removed, the body may eliminate as much liquid faeces as possible over the next few days or weeks as diarrhoea begins to set in. Eventually, the faeces becomes more solid and compacts again, leading to the next cycle of constipation, as the faeces forms another pencil thin channel to release liquid faeces. This cycle is often diagnosed as irritable bowel syndrome (IBS), and depending on the condition of the colon, can repeat every 3-8 weeks, unless the colon is cleaned out.

Colitis

Colitis (and Crohn's disease) is mostly diagnosed as inflammatory bowel disease (IBD), but sometimes falsely diagnosed as irritable bowel syndrome (IBS) and should not be confused with a spastic colon which is usually caused by emotional tension. Generally, people with IBS don't lose weight.

As mentioned previously (when discussing the small intestine), colitis is a disease of the colon and can be exhibited especially in the ascending colon if the regular diet is too acidic. Constipation can back up faeces to a point where the water-reduced, pasty faeces wallows in the ascending colon allowing acid to irritate the superficial mucosa lining of the colon wall, causing colitis (like continual, internal nappy (diaper) rash). Sometimes colitis will combine with a ballooned colon making the walls thin and even more irritated giving pain feedback and leading to leaky gut syndrome.

Ulcerative Colitis

Ulcerative colitis occurs when the general irritation noted for colitis intensifies in a smaller, specific area, most often in the transverse colon. Because the faeces is more stagnant at this point, the irritation can evolve into an internal sore or ulcer on the colon wall which can bleed and become infected or inflamed. Because there is an open sore constantly exposed to toxic faecal bacteria, ulcerative colitis can progress into bowel cancer if left unchecked.

Most medical journals may tell you the cause of colitis is unknown, however, it's logical to construe that acidic food, stress and constipation are three main causes. There's not a lot of profit to be made by conducting studies that are likely to find that patients should reduce medication and be encouraged to change their lifestyle. Changing to a high fibre, alkaline diet including plenty of water (thus relieving constipation) should help relieve this condition.

Symptoms of colitis include bloody diarrhoea, a false urge to pass a stool, reduced appetite, weight loss, fever and skin rashes during flare-up cycles. Symptoms can vary depending on how severely and which part of the colon is impacted.

Crohn's Disease

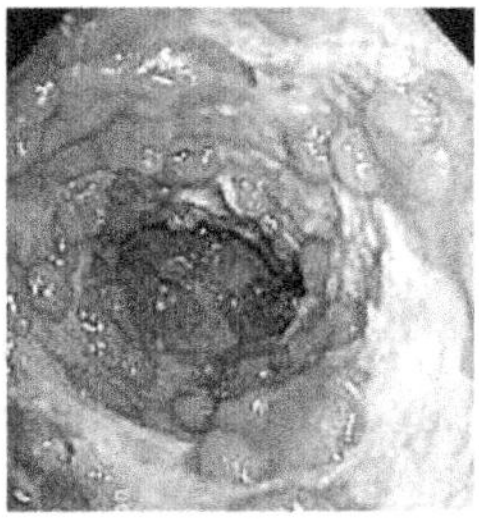

Crohn's disease inside the small intestine

As mentioned above, Crohn's disease is mostly diagnosed as inflammatory bowel disease (IBD). Many medical experts consider colitis and Crohn's disease to simply be two degrees of the same disease having the same cause, hence the IBD diagnosis.

Crohn's disease has similar origins to colitis, and though mainly found in the small intestines (especially at the end of the ileum), it can be present in the wall of the colon too and be diagnosed as colitis. Patches of Crohn's disease can be found in the stomach, oesophagus and mouth too, but are often simply called ulcers.

Colitis irritation tends to be diffused and uniform over a general area, mostly involving only superficial layers of the colon, whereas Crohn's disease is more inclined to be patchy and concentrated in areas, involving deeper layers of tissue.

Again, medical journals may tell you the cause of Crohn's disease is unknown, though again it's easy to surmise the same three causes are involved: acidic food (and therefore blood), stress and constipation.

Symptoms of Crohn's disease include abdominal pain associated with eating, diarrhoea, fatigue, poor appetite, weight loss and skin rashes. Symptoms can vary depending on how severely and which part of the small intestine or colon is impacted.

Both Crohn's disease and colitis may be relieved through effective diet and lifestyle changes that alkalise the body *(see 'Acid and Alkaline Foods' previously).* I've known several people who have combined ingesting AIM Herbal FiberBlend® (to relieve constipation), AIM Composure® (to relax the bowel), AIM BarleyLife® (to alkalise the body) and a probiotic with enzymes (to restore gut flora balance and absorption), which together can relieve colitis and Crohn's disease, though results may not be typical for every person.

Ballooned Colon

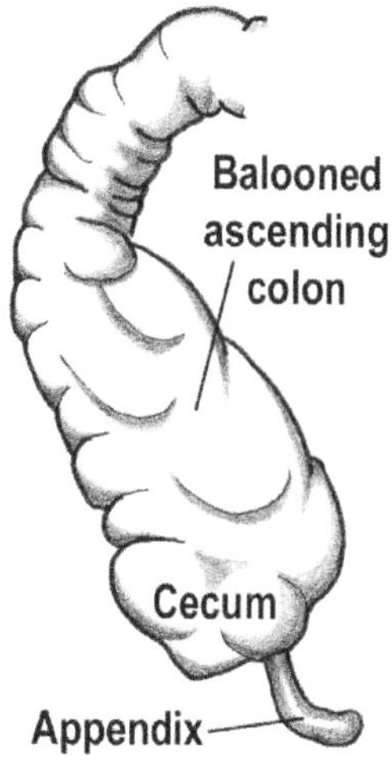

Chronic constipation can cause faeces to back up to the ascending colon, causing the colon wall to stretch and balloon to store the trapped faeces. When trying to release a motion, faecal and muscular pressure can cause the colon to expand and stretch in both the transverse and ascending colon. This can occasionally happen in the descending colon too.

When the colon prolapses *(see 'Prolapsed Colon' later),* partial blockages can form at the first bend, encouraging ballooning.

Ballooning is so called because it's similar to filling a rubber balloon with air — as the balloon increases in size, the walls become thinner. Similarly, the ballooning of the colon stretches the colon wall making the wall much thinner, leading to 'leaky gut', which (in essence) leaks toxins directly into body tissue, rather than via the blood where the liver should filter out toxins. This can make body organs quite toxic, leading to disease.

Leaky Gut

According to Dr Hugh Rodier *(www.hugorodier.com)*, in 1984 the Journal of the American Medical Assn (JAMA) published a report that said any yeast infection in the body (for example vaginal, ears, sinuses) is a spill-over of the yeast (candida) infection (or imbalance) in the gut flora within the colon. Other causes are stress, medication and diet, but don't necessarily lead to candida.

Some yeast is normal, but with the drinking of chlorinated water, excessive antibiotics (medical and dairy), eating too much sugar, preservatives, coffee, milk, processed food, and having a lack of B-complex vitamins, the flora in the bowel becomes imbalanced. *(see 'Gut Flora and Bacteria' previously)* Sugar is an excellent host for yeast to feed upon.

Medical journals also tell that the imbalanced bacteria in the colon can begin to produce antigens or proteins that are toxic *(see zeonulin next)* due to the above situations. These are so irritating to the colon that they cause the colon wall to be permeable (or cause the cells that make up the gut wall to become separated) and toxins leak through the space created in the colon wall into circulation throughout the body and bypass the filtering/enzyme producing processes of the liver.

Any metabolic depletion of gut flora, electrolytes, ATP, cytokines, or similar, can increase the permeability of the colon wall.

Zeonulin

The European magazine *Gut* released a report saying that they have isolated the very chemical that bacteria produce to separate the cells and allow the toxins to circulate into the body. They call these chemicals zeonulin. Leaky gut syndrome is at the heart of many diseases that cause spill over from the colon to the body and circulated back into the colon, where the liver then becomes loaded with toxins.

An alternative cause (as mentioned previously) is ballooning of the colon which stretches the colon wall making it much thinner, and coupled with increased internal pressure from constipated faeces in the colon, causes inflammation which can force toxins to leak through the colon wall into the body, again avoiding the filtering process of the liver.

Leaky gut (also can be falsely diagnosed as Crohn's Disease) stresses the endocrine system (immune system) and is involved in many mental diseases, autism, arthritis, inflammation, heart disease, asthma and allergies. A major part of the body's immune system is in the colon.

The first line of defence in the body is the good gut bacteria, second is the liver where whatever is passed 'legally' from the colon onto the rest of the body travels via the blood to the liver for processing and is then distributed around the body.

When the liver is bypassed and overwhelmed by toxins from the colon, it can become somewhat confused as it begins to try to attack these toxins — but it does this imperfectly and produces its own immune complexes, which are worse than the original toxifying substances and they start to attack the rest of the body producing autoimmune diseases with the thyroid, the adrenals, inflammation of the heart, arthritis, and the like. This is what I believe happened in my situation.

When the heart, liver or brain falters, it's often because there was a problem in the colon years before. The colon is the foundation of our well-being.

Prolapsed Colon

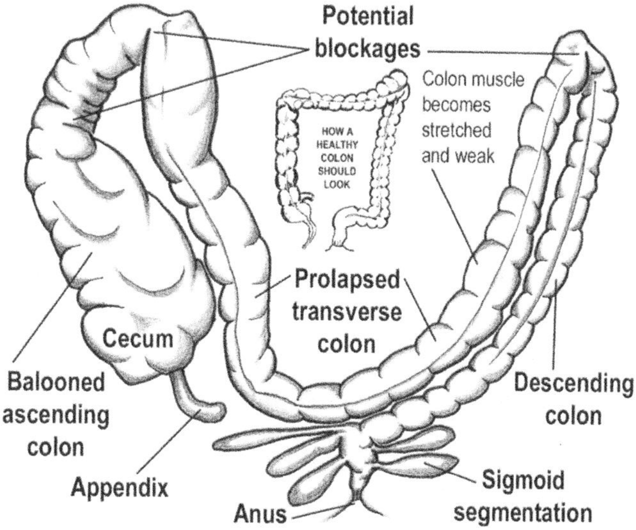

A prolapsed colon is a condition when the transverse colon drops and sags towards the groin. When all, or most, of the abdominal organs join the trip south (that is, drops and sags) the sickness industry calls this 'visceroptosis' which is the most common type of prolapse.

Prolapse is usually caused by being overweight or unfit with weak pelvic and abdominal muscles, and is overwhelmingly caused by a clogged, degenerated colon that can hold up to 5kg (11lbs) of waste in the transverse colon alone. That's equivalent to the size and weight of a large bag of potatoes!

When the transverse colon drops, it mostly remains anchored at the hepatic and splenic flexures (first and second bends) near the back of rib cage. Over time, the colon can form a deep 'V' shape and elongates (stretches in length), weakening the colon muscles and causing folds or strictures (blockages) at each bend. This can lead to ballooning of the ascending and transverse colon and constipation, which provides a perfect nest-bed for parasites to breed.

Prolapse and Women's Problems

In women, the weight of the prolapsed colon can place pressure on the uterus (disrupting blood flow during menstruation), which can cause infertility and irregular menstruation periods. I have a friend who was chronically constipated; therefore, her liver became diseased and she had part of her liver surgically removed. After taking AIM Herbal FiberBlend® and cleaning out her colon, the weight lifted off her uterus and she became pregnant, something she and her husband had been trying to do for many years.

Women who have had a hysterectomy can sometimes find themselves with a prolapsed colon as the abdominal organs drop to fill the vacant space.

Prolapse and Men's Problems

In men, the extra weight of the colon bearing down on the bladder and prostate can cause distortion and partial blockage of the urethra, making urination difficult and problematic. *(see 'Prostate' later)*

Bladder and Back Pain

When suffering from a prolapsed colon, both sexes share two common problems: bladder issues like incontinence and chronic lower back pain as the prolapsed colon continually pulls on the back of the ribcage, throwing the hips forward causing lower back pain.

Symptoms

The main symptoms of a prolapsed colon are indigestion (especially after eating), constipation, vomiting, abdominal tenderness, occasionally high body temperature, but there can also be no symptoms at all.

Support

The sickness industry often prescribes a corset or girdle to physically support and push the sagging gut upwards, but they don't recommend any change in diet — only improving appearance.

Logically however, I feel if you clean out the colon and reduce the waste products built up in the gut and eat more plant and animal-based wholefoods, the body has a better chance of correcting the situation. Combine this with supplementing with fibre, probiotics and enzymes with plenty of quality water and moderate exercise, then you are providing the best environment for your distorted colon to function as best as it can.

Stress and anxiety can cause parts of the colon to become inactive, often referred to as a spastic colon and can be diagnosed as IBS. Just a theory; perhaps the collapse of the transverse colon also detaches nerve connections to parts of the colon causing muscle inactivity, therefore sagging or becoming spastic?

Diarrhoea

Occasionally the body might contract a 'bug' (bacteria or virus) causing diarrhoea, especially when travelling in different countries. If the symptoms dissipate in a day or two, there are usually no ongoing problems, but it would be supportive to treat for parasites when you return home.

Taking good gut flora, fibre and drinking bottled water whilst travelling would be supportive in this situation.

Watch out for ice in drinks when travelling too. Mostly, ice is made from tap water and is generally not filtered, therefore can contain bugs and parasites.

Relax... Being a very considerate person, I have spared you from having to view images of diarrhoea ☺

Some people may boast they don't have a problem 'going'; in fact, they have the opposite problem of going too often with thin, runny stools. *See 'blockages' diagram previously.* These are often thinner people who are essentially undernourished; they might be eating plenty but are not able to absorb nutrients from their food. However, depending on their emotional state and habits, they can also be overweight, as they need to eat a lot of food to gain any nourishment.

This situation can be a derivation of the issues mentioned in 'Blockages' above, only that the constipated faeces is compacted all the way through to the anus from the transverse colon leaving a pencil-thin, narrow track through to the anus. The only way faeces can be eliminated is by semi-liquid faeces from the ascending colon being continually passed through the narrow channel, and because there is little 'storage space' left at the sigmoid. This can happen six or more times a day, often without much notice or control, and can go on for years with the ignorant owner thinking they are okay because it's normal for them, but ultimately time may catch up with them. People in this situation can often have haemorrhoids too.

Just think about it for a moment. Stale, stagnant, putrefied faeces continually lining the colon wall does not allow the uptake of nutrients through the colon wall. Instead, what is taken up by the body? Toxins leaching from the stale, putrefied faeces. The toxins are transported to the liver, which is already overloaded and can only pass this toxic mess onto other organs in the body (autointoxication). Is there any wonder why cancer rates are increasing?!

Bloating and Flatulence

Our American friends call flatulence 'gas' or 'wind'. We in Australia are a little more descriptive, commonly using the word 'fart' which is derived from the medical term to describe gas in the colon; 'flatus'. You learn something new every day, don't you?

Constipation can cause an ongoing, uncomfortable feeling in the bowel, always feeling over-full and finding it difficult to bend over or move around, with lots of embarrassing gas (flatulence). This is generally a result of hydrogen sulphide, methane, nitrogen and carbon dioxide (which, when combined, produce a flammable gas) being produced and trapped in the bowel, which is released under pressure through the rectum/anus. *see the 'Poo Word' previously*

Unfriendly Bacteria Imbalance

Ongoing offensive-smelling gas is an indication of **unfriendly** gut bacteria, incorrect diet (too many carbs and sugar) or toxin release from the liver or colon (from detoxing). *(see 'Gut Flora and Bacteria' previously)*

Creating Alcohol and Gas Within

In industry, sugar is used to ferment products like potatoes (vodka), wheat or barley (whisky), rice (sake), sugar (rum and ethanol fuel) which turns the produce into alcohol, creating gas as a by-product. The same thing happens when we eat sugar with our meals — we ferment food rather than digesting it, creating alcohol and gas.

The alcohol produced might go towards explaining how so many people are foggy brained during the day and want to sleep after a meal as their memory lapses with age.

Avoid eating sugar or fruit with meals. Also, avoid eating things that turn into sugar once eaten, such as grain-based products like bread, biscuits, cake, pasta and potatoes. If you're going to eat fruit, eat just one type of fruit at a time so that they don't ferment each other. Avoid adding sugar, honey, maple syrup, fruit or dried fruit to your cereal in the morning — you are only going to ferment that already unsupportive carb-based breakfast.

Parasites

Parasites are organisms that derive their nutrients from another organism known as the host, and constipation provides a perfect nest-bed for parasites to thrive.

The breeding cycle for some parasites is as little as 36 hours (1½ days). So, if you're not having at least one complete bowel movement daily, you are increasing your chances of harbouring parasites.

Because of the sedentary lifestyle and poor eating habits of western society, the average cycle of bowel movements is once in around 96 hours (four days). This provides a perfect space for parasites to proliferate.

Parasites use the body's food and blood as nutrition to grow and breed, all the while defecating into the host's body, creating a toxic mix for the body, which encourages degeneration of cells.

As mentioned previously, my wife removed a tapeworm that had been in her colon for years, despite numerous visits to doctors and

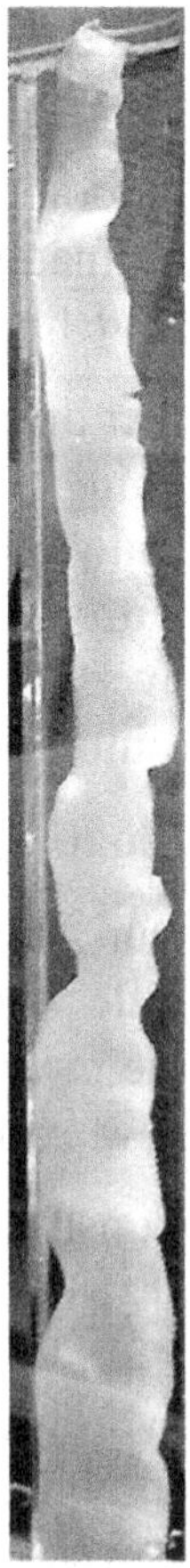

Part of a tapeworm

a colonoscopy. I personally removed hundreds of intestinal flukes. I've had several friends who have removed some pretty horrific critters from their colon; one a white crayfish-like parasite (without claws). Another 12-year-old girl released a bug that looked like a scarab beetle.

Common Parasites

There are over 300 different species of parasite that utilise the human body as hosts; here are a few of the most common:

- **Cryptosporidium** — microscopic parasite found in faeces, causing diarrhoea and abdominal cramping
- **Giardia** — microscopic parasite that thrives in the small intestines, causing diarrhoea, abdominal cramps, upset stomach and nausea. Most infection occurs in tropical areas through drinking unfiltered tank water. Fat absorption is decreased, and nutritional deficiency is also decreased through the lack of fat-soluble vitamins A, D, E and K1.
- **Toxoplasma** — another microscopic parasite. Has mild flu-like symptoms that can exacerbated when the immune system is low. Most infection is caused through cats and handling raw meat, especially pork. It's estimated around one third of the world's population is infected with toxoplasma. Recent research has linked toxoplasma with brain cancer.
- **Pinworms** *(enterobius)* — resilient parasites whose entire cycle takes place inside the human gastrointestinal tract and can be seen exiting the anus of infected people (especially at night). Pinworms are spread mostly by human-to-human contact and therefore are commonly found amongst children in schools with the most common symptom of an itchy anus. Pinworm infection in humans is called enterobiasis and it's estimated that 209 million people worldwide are infected.

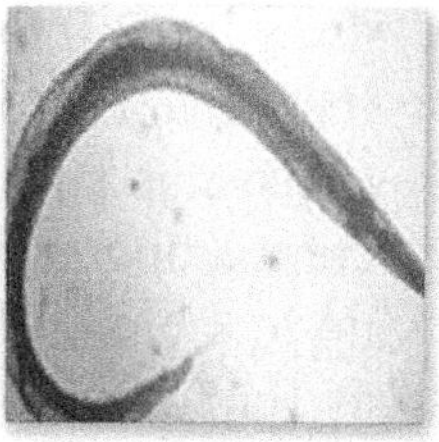

Pinworm

- **Roundworms** *(nematodes)* — there are thousands of species of roundworms varying from microscopic to 20cm long (8 in). Their fertilised eggs can be found in most places including soil, food and water. The larvae hatch and invade the intestinal mucosa, then move to the lungs via the circulation system. Once mature, they ascend the bronchial tubes to the throat where they are swallowed and develop further in the intestines, repeating their breeding cycle. They can live for one to two years and when clumped in the intestines, can cause blockages.

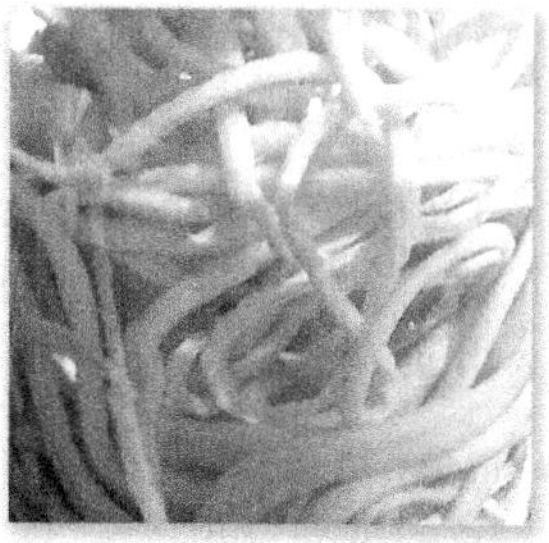

Roundworms

- **Hookworm** — these parasites evolve in a similar manner to roundworms and once in the intestines, attach to the intestine wall and live off the host's blood resulting in abdominal pain and poor appetite leading to protein and nutrient deficiencies.

- **Intestinal / Liver Fluke** — quite common and mainly inhabit the upper jejunum of the small intestine, but can also be found in the ileum, stomach and liver. Generally, the size (and look) of a blanched almond or white watermelon seed, various species can grow up to 7.5cm long (3 in). They cause abdominal pain, diarrhoea, anaemia, toxaemia, allergies and bowel obstructions.

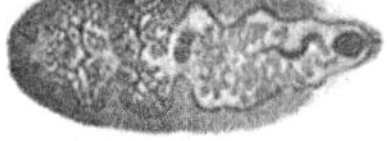

Intestinal fluke

  Because flukes are often found in the liver, it is a good idea to cleanse for parasites prior to a liver and gall bladder flush, otherwise you may end up flushing flukes instead of gallstones; a waste of a good flush.

- **Tapeworm** — infestation is mainly through cysts residing within under-cooked meat and once ingested, the cyst anchors to the colon wall (often near the cecum) and various species can grow to 2-8 metres long (6–26 feet) enabling it to reach into the transverse and descending colon, contracting at will (e.g. during colonoscopies). Tapeworms are white, flat, up to 1 cm (1/2 in) wide and once mature, break off in segments as small as 1cm or up to 10cm (4") or more, which can be seen in the faeces as they leave the host to reproduce. Tapeworms can successfully live in the colon in this manner for up to 20 years.

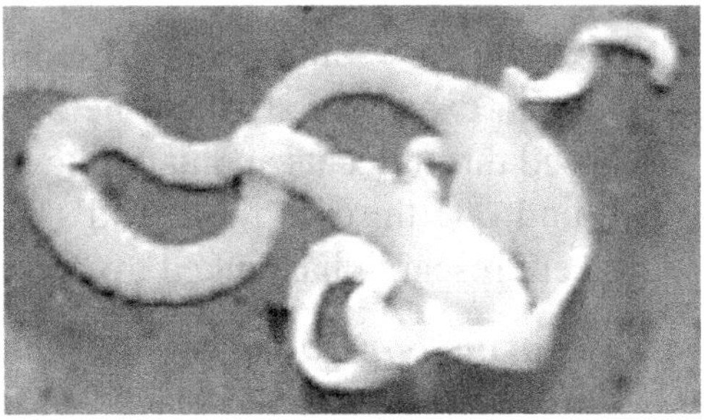

Tapeworm

  Cattle and pigs pass tapeworm segments through their faeces onto grass, where segments can live for several days and be ingested again by the next animal that eats grass in that area.

  Our family has a 'great affinity' with tapeworms — my wife released a two-metre tapeworm after taking AIM Herbal FiberBlend® early in our health journey *(see 'My Wife' previously)*.

- **Fungi** — fungal infections can occur mostly in people with weak immune systems, acid bodies, gut flora imbalance, diabetes and in women taking oral contraceptives. Candida albicans are commonly found in the mouth, ears, vagina and intestines and can proliferate when the fungi feeds on sugar and carbs and when eating excessive amounts of cheese/dairy.

Symptoms of Parasites

- Diarrhoea
- Loose, smelly stools with blood and mucus
- Nausea and vomiting
- Abdominal pain
- Flatulence and bloating
- Poor appetite and weight loss
- Fatigue and lethargy
- Foggy brain
- Visible parasites in stool

Many of the above symptoms are also typical of common bowel ailments, which mostly derive from constipation.

Managing Intestinal Parasites

Conventional medications generally contain a unique ingredient to treat specific parasites, therefore there are few 'all round' drugs that can treat several parasites at once, either resulting in some parasites remaining even though others have been killed or several different drugs being needed. Drugs all have side-effects such as depletion of gut flora, diarrhoea or both, and may require replacement of fluids.

One of the first things you can do to minimise your chances of hosting parasites is to remove their comfortable, intestinal home of stale, stagnant poop. Constipated, filth-clogged colons and intestines are ideal environments in which parasites can proliferate. There are several things you can do to remove their breeding bed. *(see 'How to Relieve Constipation' previously)*

You can also...

- Include traditionally recognised foods such as pumpkin seeds, garlic, beetroot, carrots, black walnut hulls, shavegrass, violet, barberry in your diet
- Include traditionally recognised herbs such as black walnut, wormwood, clove, garlic, sweet Annie
- Reduce sugar, processed food and dairy in your diet
- Alkalise your body and bring it back into balance
- Supplement with, or eat foods containing zinc and vitamins A and C to support your gut and immune system

- Take probiotics and enzymes daily to support correct balance of gut flora and improve absorption

Chronic Fatigue and Lethargy

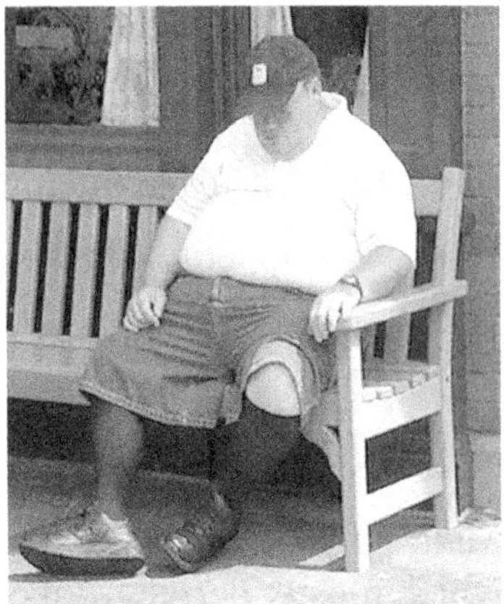
Chronically fatigued?

Chronic fatigue is noted when the body's fatigue situation is not improved by rest and may be worsened by physical or mental activity. With the processed, sugar-ladened food we ingest supplying the fuel to run our bodies, is it any wonder why many find themselves chronically fatigued? Other situations adding to fatigue are city tap water, parasites and their toxic excrement, chemicals, bad gut flora balance, low enzyme activity, clogged colons, alcohol, toxic livers, stress and anxiety (causing insomnia).

If you were to put diesel fuel in your car which should run on petrol, it would probably start, but would run roughly for a while and stop soon after. It's only when you clean out the fuel tank, filters and pipes and replace the diesel with the petrol meant for the car, that the car will run as designed — at peak performance. Your body operates in a similar way.

Causes of Chronic Fatigue
I believe a negative mind-set, poor diet and exercise regimes — leading to low stem cell circulation, constipation and an overwhelmed liver — are root causes of most chronic fatigue, lethargy (tiredness; laziness), nervous conditions and mental illness. *See Chapter 2*

Low probiotic and enzyme activity reduces absorption and fails to convert proteins into building-blocks for energy.

The longer toxic waste sits in the colon, the more toxic material is absorbed into the blood which is used as a foundation to build your body's cells; and the cells are acidic and depleted of oxygen, making you feel chronically fatigued, sick and mentally depressed.

CFS; a Nervous Condition
To support my claim, the World Health Organisation has classified chronic fatigue syndrome (CFS) as a disease of the nervous system, and the bowel supplies 95% of the body's serotonin (a neurotransmitter) for brain activity and communication between nerves.

Many symptoms of CFS like abdominal pain, bloating, diarrhoea, depression, anxiety, irritability and skin rashes are the same as many bowel disorders.

Clean up the colon, detox the liver, drink plenty of quality water, exercise regularly and eat a more plant and animal-based, wholefood diet and the fatigue and negative attitudes should diminish.

Allergies

The sickness industry has narrowed allergies down to two causes: a person's heritage (genes) and environmental factors – food, dust, chemicals, pollens.

Basically, allergies are a reflection (feedback) that the liver is somehow struggling due to its inheritance or degeneration from food and toxins being passed to it from the bowel, and it's calling for detoxing and cleansing. If the liver was in peak condition it should process allergens correctly without issue.

Whilst genes might provide the body with a predisposition for allergies, I feel it's more about the condition of the bowel and liver (often inherited from the mother, but can be degenerated through ongoing lifestyle choices), in combination with unsupportive food eaten (usually carbs) that triggers allergic reactions. This means you're not a victim — you have choices that can improve your situation.

Genetically modified organisms (GMOs) have changed the way our filtering and processing systems work (liver and kidneys) and if molecules from food can no longer be recognised by the liver, they will be treated as an invader, causing reactions (allergies). Injecting several vaccines in the first few months of birth have been shown to low the immune system which normally helps protect against allergens.

Supplementing over time with fibre, probiotics, enzymes and quality water significantly assist with allergy reactions. Studies have shown children with potentially fatal peanut allergies have resolved their issues with the addition of just one friendly bacteria to their gut.

At any time, you can choose to clean out your liver and improve your diet and lifestyle, which should improve your liver's function, decreasing your allergic reactions. Start now, because this process may take several years.

I also observe some people wear their allergies like a badge of honour — seeking special attention, announcing to everyone within ear-shot of all their food allergies, giving reasons why they can't... *(fill in this space),* causing chaos in the kitchens at restaurants and on airplanes. Their mothers should have given them much more attention when they were young.

DNA and Genes Can Change

DNA hair samples kept in a locket prior to World War Two and analysed afterwards showed different DNA (gene) make-up following a women's horrific internment in Auschwitz Concentration Camp under the Nazis. The high-stress situation over several years changed the woman's DNA, and subsequently, her daughter (born after the war) had the new, less supportive DNA structure, reflecting her mother's stress. The woman's granddaughter went on to inherit the new gene structure too.

Following birth, the body can only be built with what you eat, drink, breathe and think. How you react to situations filtered through your emotional responses matters and can be reflected through your offspring, giving children a predisposition to ailments and allergies. Perhaps this is why the incidence of allergies are increasing in children.

However, this is not the victim-situation it might seem! As the body can change its structure into a negative state according to the impact of stress (Sickness Cycle), the body can also improve its situation in a positive manner (Wellness Cycle) through cleansing, improved nutrition and supplementation and happier thoughts. Having a happier, grateful outlook on life is an incredibly powerful tool, as how you feel about any situation will be reflected in your choices of food and actions. You have control!

Australian Children at Greatest Risk

Recently in Australia there has been a great deal of media attention surrounding a four-fold increase in allergies in children over the past ten years. In fact, Australia has the highest rate of child food allergies in the world, which may lead to chronic illness as an adult.

Children who grow up on farms where they live closer to nature, and interact with bacteria daily, have seven times less chance of developing food allergies than city-based, metropolitan children.

Experts at the Murdoch Children's Research Institute have listed possible causes currently under research:

1. Excessive cleanliness (limited exposure to bacteria — not developing the immune system)
2. Concentration of toxins in the child
3. Medication given early in life that stresses or challenges the immune system (e.g. vaccination)
4. The epigenetic make-up (activated or deactivated genes) from the mother's, and grandmother's health situation (especially the liver)
5. Lack of sunlight and overuse of sunscreen
6. Artificial food colouring, preservatives and additives in food

7. Stimulants like caffeine and sugar (energy drinks, Coca Cola, chocolate)
8. Excessive consumption of sugar (food is fermented rather than digested)
9. Imbalance of gut flora
10. Low enzyme activity
11. Chemicals in drinking water (chlorine, fluoride, pesticides)
12. High use of antibiotics (medicines and food (dairy))
13. Sedentary lifestyle (computer and phone use, video games)

Stressed Liver

A stressed liver (resulting from a constipated, dysfunctional bowel) can't process toxins, proteins, pollens, chemicals, medicines, etc. the way nature intended and therefore the liver passes the unprocessed allergens through the bloodstream onto other organs to handle (or react), resulting in a reaction which mostly involves inflammation, production of mucus, rashes and swelling — resulting in a low immune system.

People who have allergies often describe ongoing regular symptoms like abdominal pain, bloating, diarrhoea, nausea, skin irritations, swelling, malnutrition, poor eyesight, headaches, circulatory problems and more. Again, many of these symptoms are similar to most bowel ailments which mostly derive originally from constipation.

A Natural Reaction

It's relatively natural to have some degree of **lactose** (a sugar) or **gluten** (a protein/starch combination) or casein (a protein in dairy) **intolerance**, as the body generally finds it difficult to process such molecules requiring large amounts of insulin from the pancreas to process. Basically, the digestive system is not designed to process large amounts of sugar, flour or dairy (especially GMO) — however these foods make up about 90% of the typical western diet. That's why so many people have chronic phlegm and blocked sinuses. To prove this to yourself, try eliminating such food from your diet for three days and notice the difference.

If you find it difficult to eliminate them completely from your diet, try supplementing with enzymes to support the absorption and processing of these allergens.

Glue-ten

When ingested, gluten turns into a type of glue (especially when mixed with sugar) which makes the system sluggish. *(see section on 'Cholesterol' previously)* Remember how glue was made as a child... you mixed white flour and water together. It seems lactose and gluten-intolerant people are simply more sensitive than most; it's more a matter of degrees of intolerance, so limit your intake whatever your situation. I'd go as far to say that most people are "Carb Intolerant"!

Recent research is showing that slowly introducing the allergen to the child along with good gut bacteria is achieving excellent results.

Haemorrhoids

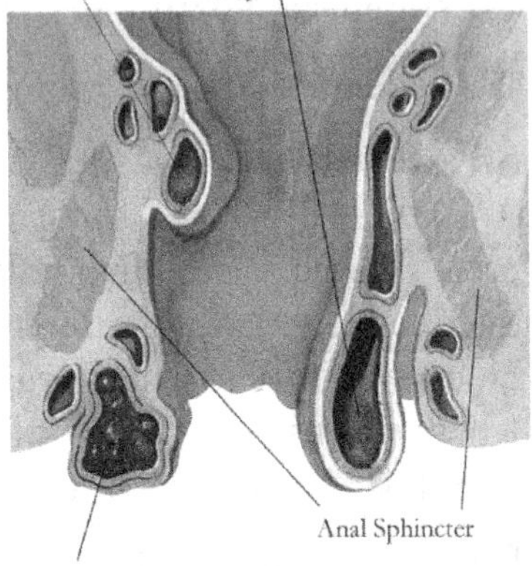

Haemorrhoids are dear to my heart... Having haemorrhoid surgery at just 17 years old, I have many painful memories of not being able to sit down comfortably (which was difficult as a draftsman), a continually irritated and itchy anus, embarrassing bleeding and pain whilst passing a motion.

Haemorrhoids (also known as piles) are blood veins around the rectum and anus that dilate and are forced to the surface due to internal pressure exerted mostly through constipation and excessive laxative dependency. Other contributing factors include pregnancy, aging and diarrhoea. The exposed blood veins can rupture at the most inopportune times and bleed profusely.

Problems such as fissures, fistulae, abscesses, irritation, itching have similar symptoms, however, can sometimes be incorrectly diagnosed as haemorrhoids.

Haemorrhoids can mostly be resolved through fixing constipation and diarrhoea issues through increasing fibre, friendly gut bacteria, enzymes bile flow and quality water in the diet as mentioned previously. Eating animal protein at the correct time, reducing carbs and drinking more quality water and more vegetables may help, along with supplementing the diet with psyllium husk or extra whole bran products like oats. *(see 'Fibre' previously)*

Simple nappy rash cream containing zinc and castor oil can help relieve irritations until the fibre makes a difference in irritation.

Varicose Veins

Surprisingly, constipation can contribute to varicose veins as the strain of the body pushing so hard to release faeces results in increased blood pressure causing surface veins around the legs (especially) to dilate, become swollen and rise to the surface.

Urine retention from an enlarged prostate, a chronic cough or any other conditions that cause strain for prolonged periods of time and cause an increase in the forces transmitted to the leg veins may also result in varicose veins.

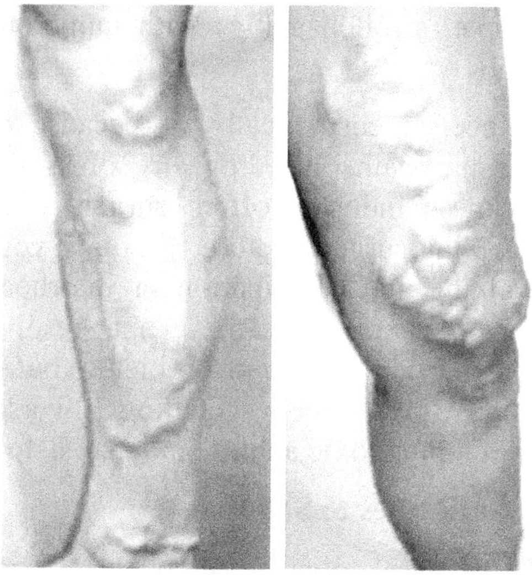

Varicose veins

Also, if you don't exercise regularly, the blood stagnates in the lower extremities and you risk varicose veins and other circulatory ailments. Veins carrying deoxygenated blood back to the heart rely on muscle contractions of the major muscle groups to push the blood along.

Blood veins in the legs have numerous 'non- return valves' known as leaflet valves that stop gravity allowing blood to drop to the lower part of the legs between muscle contractions as the blood is progressively pumped uphill (back) towards the heart.

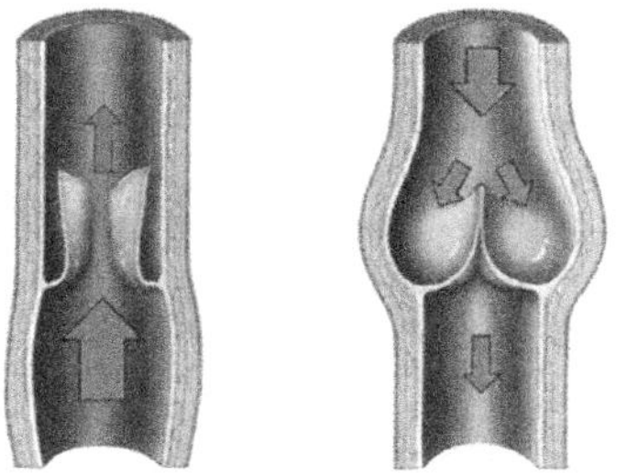

Valves open when muscles contract, allowing blood to return to the heart.

Valves close when muscles relax. Blood cannot flow backwards.

It's all pretty logical, the heart pumps from the largest arteries down to the smallest capillaries in the feet, therefore blood pressure is increased as it flows. However, the veins returning to the heart are pumping blood uphill from the smallest capillaries to the larger veins, dropping blood pressure on the way. That's why good hydration and regular walking is critical to keep the blood viscose and assist with the pumping action back to the heart.

Internal strain can push against these valves making them permanently dysfunctional, causing blood to flow downhill and gather permanently in the lower veins around the legs and ankles.

Besides cosmetic issues, varicose veins can also be painful (if standing for a long time) and can itch. Scratching them can cause bleeding and ulcers. Over the longer term, because some of the blood may remain stagnant and can't circulate from the lower legs, toxins can gather in the lower legs, which can develop into ulcers that won't heal — often a sign of diabetes. I observe many people at shopping centres with varicose veins, circulation problems and

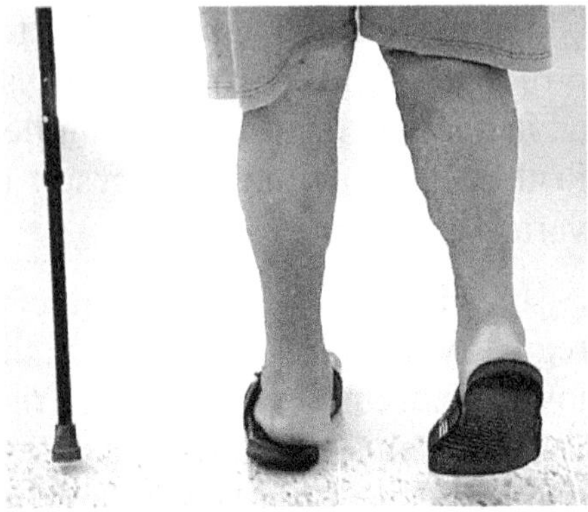

purple, swollen ankles with numerous scabs.

If needed cosmetically or because of chronic pain, bleeding or sores, the sickness industry offers surgery. Try avoiding surgery before resolving your walking and constipation or diarrhoea issues first. This may not resolve existing varicose vein problems, but it may stop them getting worse, developing toxic ankles, and may help with improved blood circulation.

Skin Rashes & Solutions

If the liver, colon or kidneys are dysfunctional, you have recently been exposed to toxins or the liver is detoxing, the body should do its best to eliminate waste through the colon, liver and kidneys. But when they become overwhelmed, the elimination of waste and toxins can be passed onto mucus, lungs, skin, or the eyes. Many people who suffer from skin irritations such as eczema, acne, psoriasis, boils and pimples can be actually trying to eliminate or detox.

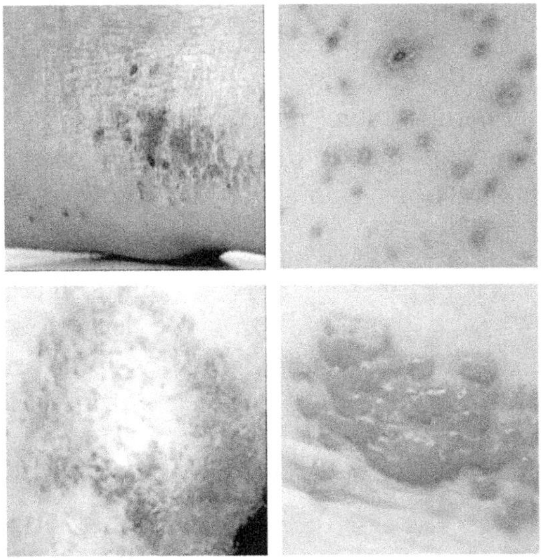

Skin rashes can appear in various forms and are often a result of a dysfunctional bowel and liver. Skin rashes can also be a symptom of detoxing.

Skin irritation can be a symptom of several bowel-related diseases like celiac, colitis, Crohn's disease, IBD, IBS, gut flora imbalance, leaky gut syndrome and autointoxication. Skin irritations can also appear with subsequent diseases like acidosis, diabetes, gallstones and liver cirrhosis.

Dermatologists recommend topical creams to ease symptoms which often only sooth and moisturise the irritation. I feel we need to deal with the cause, rather than only treating the symptoms. Clean out the colon and liver and your body should take the load away from the skin. Constipation can lead to situations that encourage skin irritations.

Skin Solutions

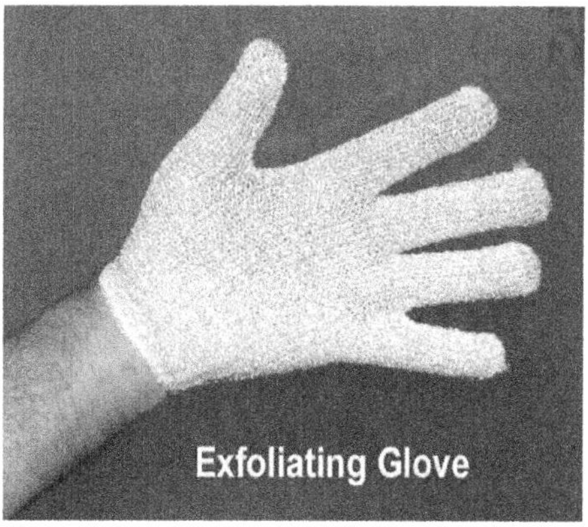

Because skin rashes can be a sign of toxic overload or detoxing, consider using **exfoliating gloves** in the shower once every week or two. Wet yourself, lather-up the gloves with quality soap, turn off the water and rub every part of your skin vigorously, then rinse. This removes the outer layer of toxin-ladened skin more quickly. I personally have found this extremely supportive in removing detoxing rashes, body odour and toxins.

Alternatively, daily dry skin brushing utilising a natural pig-bristle brush before showering is another option.

Having a clean colon, good nutrition and the correct amount of essential fatty acids (EFAs) daily can help ensure smoother, healthier skin as the body is supplied with the correct DNA molecules for cell renewal. Skin cells are replenished every 14 days, therefore by exfoliating regularly and supplying good nutrition, you can accelerate the detoxing process.

Some skin disorders may be a result of diseases like measles, chickenpox or shingles. This section doesn't relate to these issues.

Essential Fatty Acids (EFAs)

EFA's significantly assist with skin, eyes and circulation. There are three main EFAs; omega-3, 6 and 9. EFAs can't be stored in the body for long and need to be ingested daily. If the body is supplied with enough omega-3 and 6, then the body can make its own omega-9 and therefore omega-9 isn't really essential and doesn't <u>need</u> to be ingested, but it's okay to ingest.

Fatty acids are made up of carbon and hydrogen with a couple of oxygen atoms and exist in long-chains starting at the beginning (alpha) and finishing at the end (omega). Omega-3, 6 and 9 are so called due to their position along the chain; from the omega end. If a fat has no double bonds, it's a saturated fat. If it has just one double bond, it is monounsaturated (O-9). If it has two or more double bonds, it is referred to as polyunsaturated fat (O-3 and O-6).

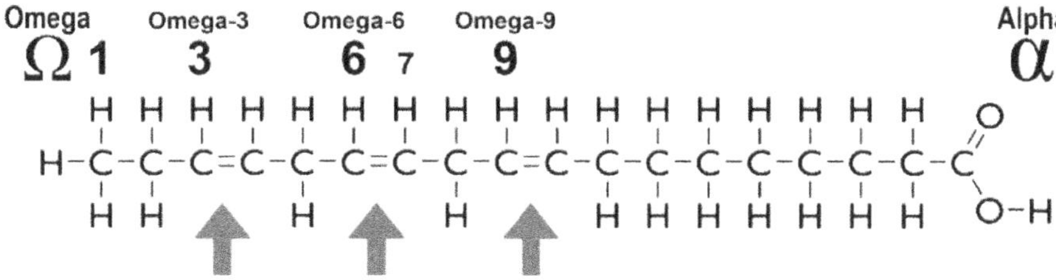

Omega-6 is **extremely** prevalent in today's modern processed food and vegetable/seed oils (as is omega-9). Products like biscuits, bread, margarine, snacks, chips, vegetable oils (which are seed oils) and oven-fried food all use oils containing omega-6 as a basic, cheap ingredient. Thus, supplementation of omega-6 is rarely necessary, however the quality of the oil may be low as omega-3 and 6 both degenerate when heated to cooking and processing temperatures.

In fact, the body is often extremely over supplied in omega-6 to its detriment. An overabundance of omega-6 is linked to heart disease, stroke, arthritis, asthma, diabetes, headaches, macular degeneration, menstrual cramps and tumours. Overabundance of omega-6 is especially a problem when there is **lack of omega-3** – the body's preferred EFA.

If there is an undersupply of omega-3, the body will utilise the more detrimental omega-6 in lieu. In this situation, omega-6, though essential, can become a destructive free radical causing sluggishness, solidification and inflammation, i.e. disease.

Omega-3 is like the mortar that holds the bricks together in the DNA. In that omega-3 is a foundation material for the regeneration of cells throughout the body. Omega-3 is very fast moving, morphs into any shape when combining with stem cells to renew a dead cell and if you have plenty of omega-3, your heart should beat properly, your blood should flow freely, your eyes should see clearly *(read below)* and you should make decisions faster - making for a more energetic, happier life.

When consuming food, try to eat an abundance of omega-3 based food and minimise food high in omega-6, carbs and sugar as per the chart shown in *the 'Losing It' section previously and available to download freely at www.cleanup-your-act.com.*

Remember all margarines are just a combination of chemicals and are very high in omega-6. Margarine is pale grey before manufacturers add yellow dye, so it looks like butter.

Most plant-based omegas contain all three EFAs omega-3, 6 and 9 in varying ratios. Leafy green vegetables contain higher ratios of omega-3. Seafood contains only omega-3.

The preferred ratio of ingested plant-based EFAs omega-3, 6 and 9 is 2:1:1 respectively. You can gain understanding of the need for the correct ratio if we equate omega-3, 6 and 9 to threading a necklace with two blue, one orange and one green bead respectively (2:1:1 ratio). If at any time during the threading process we are unable to provide a blue bead, but it is **essential** to continue to create the necklace with orange and green beads, the pattern will be broken and the necklace will be inferior to the requirements of the customer (your body) and you are more likely to lower the immune system and age more quickly. Once more blue beads are supplied, the correct pattern can be restored, and the customer is happier and supported — regaining health.

Flaxseed and hempseed oils are two of the better plant-based options for supplementation and is economical and easily available, but must be kept at low temperatures, out of light and stored in glass or is likely to degenerate quickly. Plant-based EFAs only contain the ALA form of Omega-3 and you would have to take 57 x 1,000mg Flaxseed Oil capsules a day to get the same value from 2 x 500mg Fish Oil capsules or 14 x 1,000mg Krill capsules.

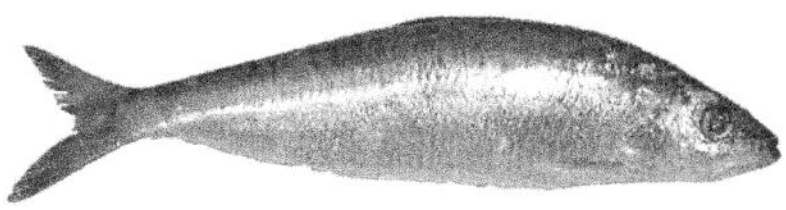

Fish oil is the best daily supplement that contains only omega-3 in EPA, DHA and GLA forms. If you're not concerned about vegan issues, it's worth considering taking omega-3, as your body gains enough omega-6 from other sources and therefore satisfies the above daily ingestion ratio requirements.

However, fish oil should be of high quality and ensure it doesn't contain heavy metal toxins and pesticides from the accumulative effect of top feeding fish such as shark, tuna, etc.

Every day, dozens of ships leave the harbours of (mainly) Asian ports and head out to sea for weeks on end. When the ships drop-nets and process their haul, their cheap labour quickly fillet the catch and freeze the fillets. The remaining guts, heads and skeletons are boiled in large vats and the fish oil floats to the top, skimmed off and capsulated in factories later. This is the cheapest method of harvesting fish oil which I have seen sold in supermarkets from as **cheap as $14.50 for 1,000 capsules** but is likely to contain **large amounts of toxins** and won't be very bio-available for your body to use.

Through my research and use, I have found only one fish oil that stands out from the rest. **Nordic Naturals** are the only company in the world that have complete control over every process from boat to bottle. Nordic have their own sustainable fisheries and only use their catch.

They then molecularly distil the oil to remove any toxins and pesticides that may be present. During this process the fish oils are concentrated beyond what is normally found in fish.

If the oil is left at this stage of the process (as is the case with most other brands who distil fish oil) it would only be about 60% absorbable for humans.

So, Nordic Naturals then have a final process called Re-Estification whereby they bring the oil back to a molecular structure that is at least 93% absorbable.

Just one capsule, twice a day, 12 hours apart will supply your body with enough quality omega-3.

Coconut oil, although not an omega-3 or omega-6 fat, is also an extremely beneficial dietary fat with an "embarrassment of riches" for your heart, metabolism, immune system, skin and thyroid. Coconut oil's health benefits derive from its special MCFAs (medium-chain fatty acids).

Coconut oil is available at most supermarkets and is one of the healthiest oils to use for cooking and a great alternative to vegetable (seed) oils. I encourage you to conduct your own research and find out more.

Eczema Relief...

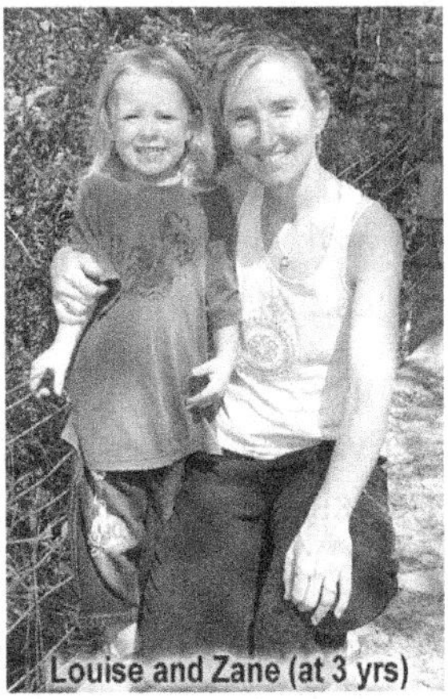

Louise and Zane (at 3 yrs)

"As I watched my youngest child climb and play on the jungle gym at school, I looked at his body covered in eczema, where he had enthusiastically scratched himself raw for so long trying to relieve the continuous itching and discomfort. I wondered could I ever help him find relief, or even a cure?

Zane had tolerated eczema for all his two short years on earth and continual itching and discomfort was all he knew. This led to a lack of sleep, which made him very irritable and did not help with feeding him. He also had continual reflux which meant he found it difficult to keep food down. His stools were runny, and he was under weight for his age and I was very concerned about his long-term health.

I had tried several doctors and what seemed like all the lotions ever made, but nothing helped — I was at my wits end. Then I was approached by Shakti, another mother at school, who said she had noticed Zane's rashes and raw skin (which was bleeding). Shakti seemed genuinely interested and wanted to help as she asked a few questions; "Does he eliminate regularly? Does he have reflux? How long does he sleep? What is his behaviour like?"

"What's this go to do with Zane's skin?" I thought. Shakti explained how parasites can infest the bowel, slowing digestion drastically and creating a toxic mix that is then excreted into the body and is often eliminated through the skin, because there is no other way to get toxins out of the body (as the bowel is too sluggish).

Zane would cringe at having a bath because it was too uncomfortable for him, which also eliminated him from swimming and the surf. Living on the Gold Coast, it was so regrettable that we could not enjoy the city's beautiful beaches.

The next day Shakti gave me some information and I soon purchased AIM Herbal FiberBlend® through her. Herbal FiberBlend is a mixture of natural fibres and herbs that assist the bowel to eliminate and make life very uncomfortable for parasites. Zane was not keen at first as I started him on just a quarter of a teaspoon twice a day, but I persevered and told him it would help stop the itching and help him sleep. As a result, his bowel motions became firmer, more regular and he started to have more sleep.

I had heard that often when treating something like eczema internally, it can become a lot worse before it gets better as the herbs deal with the cause rather than the symptoms, so I was expecting the worst. However, in Zane's case Herbal FiberBlend worked within four weeks and I watched in amazement as the eczema, rashes and dry, blotchy skin started to disappear. By now he was sleeping all night and his behaviour improved immensely, along with his appetite and he started gaining weight.

When I finished the first container of Herbal FiberBlend and Zane's skin had improved immensely, I thought he should have a rest from the product, but then the eczema reappeared. Apparently, it takes quite a while for the herbs to do their work at eliminating parasites and their eggs entirely out of the body. So, I bought another couple of containers and started giving half teaspoon servings of Herbal FiberBlend again and within weeks Zane's skin started to clear again.

Late 2006, Shakti introduced me to AIM BarleyLife® too, which is the powdered juice of young, green barley plants. With excellent nutrition, the tissue damage caused by parasites was repaired rapidly. I am comforted knowing he is receiving all the nutrients his body needs — every day.

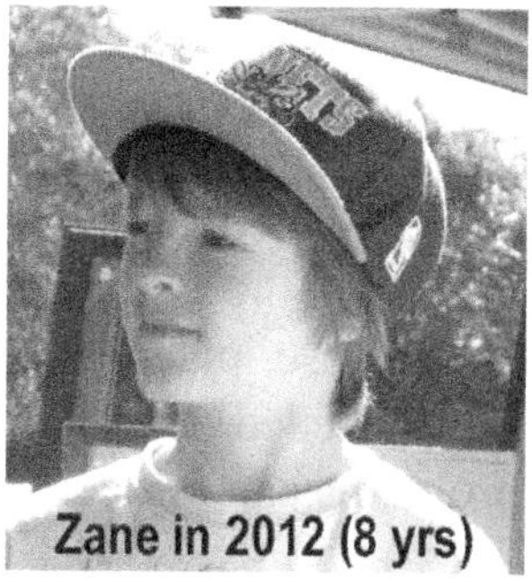
Zane in 2012 (8 yrs)

Zane is now three years old and finally I have a happy little boy who sleeps well, enjoys life and is fun to be with (and I love him so much)."

Louise L — Gold Coast Qld, Australia

Testimonials should not be construed as representing results everybody can achieve. Results may not be typical and may vary from person to person.

Macular Degeneration

Constipation can lead to toxic build up in the body. Toxins, excessive amounts of omega-6, sugar and fat produced by sugar and carbs float in the blood stream and can readily become trapped in the body's capillaries.

The finest capillaries are found in the retina of the eyes and when blocked from fat and toxins, eyesight declines. This is commonly known as macular degeneration, again a symptom of diabetes, which can ultimately lead to blindness.

EFA's and Macular Degeneration

Essential fatty acids (EFAs) consist of omega-3, 6 and 9, as mentioned above.

Omega-3 fats make up the light sensitive cells of the retina and are the most frequently replaced cells in our body. Each time the retina senses different light, the cells are replaced. Stem cells initiate the replacement process.

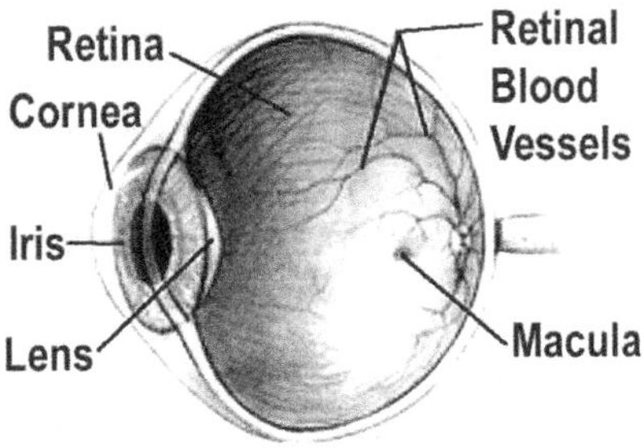

A lack of omega-3 in the body forces the eyes to utilise omega-6 in lieu. The waste produced by the retina after using omega-6 is more hazardous than if the eyes had used the preferred omega-3. Waste from omega-3 eye function is readily dispatched for expulsion in the bowel. The waste from omega-6 is not recognised by the eyes waste disposal function and accumulates over decades as waste deposits which lead to macular degeneration.

Therefore, supplement daily with omega-3s and eat a low-carb diet with plenty of high content omega-3 food from the chart mentioned above. This really matters if you want to see your grandchildren later on in life!

Fertility Problems

A constipated, ballooned, faecal-ladened colon can weigh as much as 5kg (11 lb) and in the female body especially, gravity can cause the transverse colon to prolapse, placing pressure on the uterus and ovaries, disrupting the blood flow needed for the natural menstrual cycle. Numerous gynaecological problems can arise from this situation.

By relieving constipation and having regular bowel movements, the weight of the colon is reduced, and the load taken off the reproductive organs, allowing regular blood flow which is conducive to supporting fertility.

My Journey Towards Health and Birth

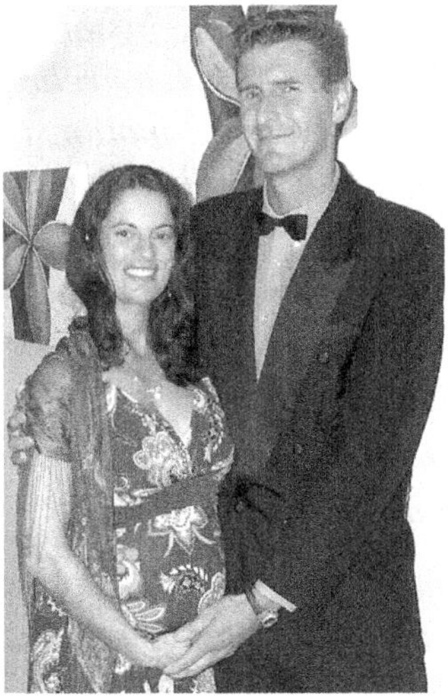

"At the age of 15 I had my first liver surgery to remove a hydatid cyst and a second surgery ten years later. I've had a slow colon from a young age, which became more intense after my surgeries. For many years, I was only passing one to two bowel motions every two to three weeks. Other symptoms included difficulty concentrating and remembering with a lack of motivation. My hands would shake, and I often felt itchy all over as if the itch was in my blood. I didn't sleep well at night (often waking at 3am to a stabbing pain in my kidneys) and I had lack of libido. Overall my mood was affected, and I felt irritable and internally angry.

To the outside world I looked happy and in control, however behind closed doors I was often emotional, tired and unhappy.

I had tried every conceivable option through orthodox and natural treatments to relieve my constipation. I tried every recommendation I was given, desperate for relief. As per my doctor's advice, I followed a healthy eating plan and exercised regularly and included more fibre in my diet after a colonoscopy. Eventually I was told I was a hypochondriac.

I was introduced to AIM Herbal FiberBlend® (HFB) by a friend after a healing session. I said I would consider taking it but wondered how HFB would be any different to everything else I had tried, so I put the details in a safe place! Three years on and our friend was staying with us for a short while. He then convinced me to try the HFB.

I quickly realised I suffered for those three years unnecessarily. After just a few days of taking HFB, AIM Composure® and the AIM Garden Trio (BarleyLife®, Just Carrots® and RediBeets®), I was a new person! It was hard to believe the results!

I was amazed when I started having bowel movements after the second day on the products. I was eliminating waste naturally two to three times each day by the end of the first week on the AIM products. My nerves had settled, I was sleeping through the night, I was able to focus and concentrate, I was calm, and my mind chatter had settled. And the most amazing outcome was that for the first time in my life I was having continual natural urges to eliminate. No effort, no pain and NO waiting required. Every day, I regained hours of my life back. I felt clean and alive. The results are still today remarkable!

HFB worked like a broom sweeping away old debris, and I believe by taking the Composure® just before bed, my whole body was helped to relax, including the muscles around my colon assisting the peristalsis motion to loosen and move years of stored waste. I slept soundly for the first time in many years and my husband was grateful for the changes he saw. Garden Trio boosted my energy and I drank two to three litres of filtered water each day. This was all a big part in my initial clean out. I stayed on the products for three months continually and took them as recommended.

After a few weeks, I started removing a darker, smelly, rope-like material, which I now know was putrefied mucus lining (plaque) off my colon wall.

I took Herbal Release® about 4 weeks after I started on HFB; I believe this product helped shift toxins from my lymph system as I was able to feel the changes.

Because of my previous health issues, I had resigned myself to never becoming pregnant, therefore was not on contraceptives. We weren't trying to fall pregnant; however, after eight weeks on AIM products, we were surprised with the news that we were going to have a baby.

I had an easy pregnancy with no morning sickness. My body craved Barley Life so I took it whenever I felt like it. During the last hours of giving birth, my midwife wanted me to eat. I clearly stated I only wanted Barley Life – so my husband called a friend to go home to get the canister. You don't argue with a birthing mother!

I took HFB on and off during pregnancy to help with the usual pregnancy constipation, then after giving birth, I went back onto HFB when I felt I needed it while nursing my son.

I now understand cleaning out my bowel took the weight of my uterus which allowed normal blood flow to happen, enabling me to become pregnant.

We are grateful every day for our healthy lifestyle and continued learning on natural health."

Jen B. – Mackay Qld

Testimonials should not be construed as representing results everybody can achieve. Results may not be typical and may vary from person to person.

In Men

Similarly in men, constipation can cause prostate problems as weight from the colon bears down on the prostate and urethra tube, affecting semen production and flow.

I know of a few women who became pregnant after resolving their constipation issues by taking AIM Composure®, AIM Herbal FiberBlend® AIM BarleyLife®, though this may not be typical for all women.

Prostate

The prostate is a male gland, about the size of a walnut, that sits below the bladder (surrounding the urethra) and its main function is to provide semen for sperm to travel within.

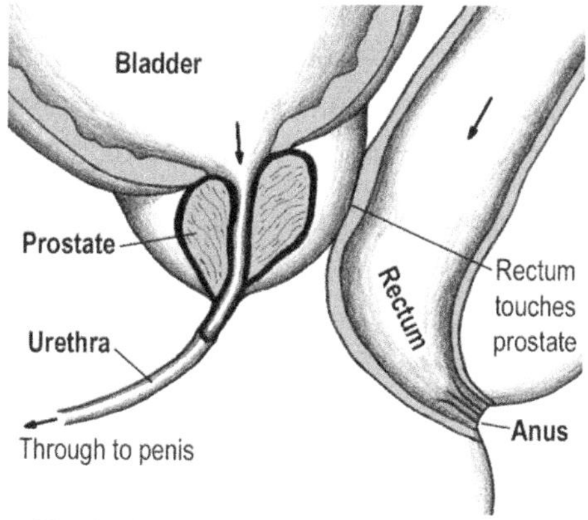

Showing the proximity of the prostate to the rectum

In cross-section (front to back through the body) the sigmoid of the colon is located directly next to (and touches) the prostate. Continual pressure on the bladder, prostate or both (from a prolapsed transverse colon on top and ballooned descending colon or sigmoid) can cause the prostate to distort or shift slightly, partially blocking the urethra, affecting urination.

Toxic leaching through the colon wall into the prostate from stale, toxic, stagnant faeces encourages inflammation and hardening of the prostate, which in turn can strangle and block the urethra, making it difficult to urinate and may lay the foundations for prostate cancer.

Prostate Cancer

The above situations may be a reason for the high rate of prostate cancer in Australia where 20,000 men are diagnosed each year. Prostate cancer is the third highest cancer killer in Australia, behind lung and bowel cancer and can sit for many years undetected, often taking over five years to kill the patient. Around 50% of men over 70 years have latent prostate cancer which is not yet causing discomfort.

The NNT (Number Needed to Treat – *see 'Statins' previously*) for surgical removal of the prostate gland in men as a cancer treatment is 49. Side-effects occur in 50% of patients and include impotence, erectile dysfunction, urinary and faecal incontinence, and rectal tearing. This means you are 25 times more likely to be harmed by prostate surgery than helped.

Drugs

Recently there has been an increase in men having recurrences (having previously been treated with medical drugs around ten years ago). Could this be because the drugs don't really deal with the cause, but rather exacerbate, the problem through various side-effects like constipation?

Dairy's Impact
A lifetime excess consumption of dairy products can provide a **four times greater chance** of contracting prostate cancer, compared to men who don't regularly consume dairy. A protein called 'casein' seems to be the culprit and makes up 87% of milk. Casein consumption has an impact on other cancer rates too, such as breast cancer in women. Supplementing with enzymes may alleviate some of the issues of consuming casein.

Ginger and Turmeric

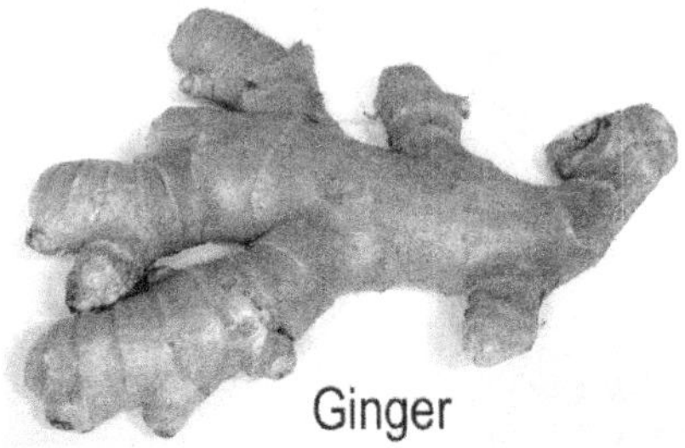

A combination of ginger and turmeric tea is one of the best natural anti-inflammatories. Thinly slice a thumb-sized piece of ginger and turmeric root and boil for ten minutes in two litres of filtered water (refrigerate after the first day). Drink two cups a day and you're likely to see prostate issues dissipate over coming months. I used to wake up three to four times a night to urinate, rarely sleeping soundly. After drinking ginger and turmeric tea regularly, I now mostly sleep through the night undisturbed.

Recent research confirms ginger's credentials too, finding that ginger regressed prostate cancer cells by 60%, without toxicity. As usual, Big Pharma are trying to isolate the specific active ingredients, synthesise them and sell them to you in a tablet, however the science is proving (again) that the synergistic sum of the whole ginger is greater than the individual active ingredients.

Diet and Sunlight
Coupled with the above solutions, optimise your vitamin 1,25D and K2 levels (which means sunlight and a clean, functioning colon, as discussed previously) and exercising regularly can help. Ensure **cauliflower, broccoli and green tea** are included in your diet. Avoid the usual suspects like sugar, grains, transfats and excessive dairy.

Diagnosis
If you notice pain or changes in your rate or need to urinate, you should contact your healthcare practitioner. Prostate cancer can be diagnosed from a simple blood test that checks for a prostate specific antigen (PSA) which often creates more concerns for patients than warranted, as the PSA test can show a high reading, even in patients without prostate cancer. However, patients diagnosed with prostate cancer, mostly have a higher PSA count.

Erectile Dysfunction
While we are down there, if there is a problem with obtaining a natural

erection, it's usually concerned around a few issues: nervous conditions (anxiety, stress, emotions, etc.), drugs, alcohol, toxins or circulation issues.

If you have impotence and it's identified as a circulation problem (that drugs like Viagra may resolve), take this as a timely 'tap on your shoulder'; an early warning that it may be supportive to change your lifestyle now before diabetes and heart disease take hold or you suffer a stroke.

If you don't make changes for the better, it's highly possible you could be diagnosed in the next few years with diabetes, heart disease and a fatty/toxic liver with diminishing eyesight as the small capillaries in the feet, eyes and penis are blocked with toxic fat caused by sugar and carbs.

Inflammation (Tissue, Muscle and Joint Pain)

Inflammation is general swelling of body tissue due to irritation or reactions to food, toxins, chemicals, infections, injury, pressure, constant rubbing, and the like. Many people in western society live most of their lives with general body inflammation becoming a normal part of life, due to unsupportive hypnotic habits and a resulting dysfunctional liver.

When inflammation occurs, chemicals from the body's white blood cells are released into the blood or affected tissues, attempting to protect an injury or rid the body of foreign substances. This release of these blood cell chemicals signals the need for stem cells to initiate repair and increases the blood flow to the area and may result in redness, swelling and warmth. The inflammatory process may stimulate nerves and cause pain.

With today's unsupportive lifestyle choices, most peoples' bodies have a continual low-grade general inflammation. General body inflammation is apparent in nearly all heart disease, high blood pressure, diabetes and dementia patients.

Following 7 years of research and clinical trials, an extract of spirulina called 'phycocyanin' has been identified to significantly reduce general body inflammation. Phycocyanin has been encapsulated in a product called 'Cyactiv' that can be found in the *resources section.*

Formulated for people specifically with joint inflammation 'Cyactiv Joint' *(see resources)* phycocyanin has been combined with eggshell membrane (cartilage strength), Boswellia Serrata extract (reduces swelling whilst increasing blood supply) and Tart Cherry extract (muscle support and recovery).

Snoring

General inflammation and the resulting build-up of mucus causes many people to snore, which (in itself) seems relatively harmless, but inconvenient to sleep partners around the world. However snoring presents a concerning situation, as the body is regularly deprived of oxygen (sleep apnoea) which can cause brain damage and prevents the snorer (and partner) from reaching the deep levels of sleep necessary to regenerate the immune system daily.

The lack of quality sleep for snorer and partner causes daytime drowsiness and irritability, resulting in increased stress for themselves and everyone around them. Studies have shown a correlation between loud snoring and risk of heart attack (about 34% chance) and stroke (about 67% chance). Snoring is often indicative of underlying obesity and other health issues.

Again, the sickness industry has invented numerous mouth guards, splints, surgery, nasal sprays, and pillows to alleviate snoring rather than working on the obvious — stop smoking, improve the diet, reduce alcohol, exercise and weight loss. Foods such as vegetable oils, grain, sugar, dairy and alcohol can inflame the mucus membrane around the throat and restrict airflow, causing snoring.

I have a friend, about 50, who was diagnosed with sleep apnoea and prescribed a machine with tubes that kept his mouth open with a constant feed of oxygen all night. He claimed instant success – a cure! He is a builder who drinks 4 large bottles of **Coke (5 litres) every day**. His body is permanently inflamed from over 100 teaspoons of sugar, plus caffeine every day.

I was surprised during a recent conversation between several friends to find that all the people involved in the conversation commented on their partner's snoring and how it disturbed their quality of sleep.

Sleep

If you don't get at least 7-9 hours' sleep, your metabolic rate will drop by 20% the next day. Therefore, you won't burn as much energy and will store more fat. Your appetite hormones will be deregulated – which makes you hungrier.

You're better to have at least 7 hours' sleep, than wake one hour early to exercise (and only get 6 hours' sleep).

How to Have a Better Night's Sleep...

- Prioritise sleep – make sleep important to you! Calculate when you need to be asleep to get your 7-9 hours. If you need to get up at 6 am to eat, exercise, shower and go to work, then be asleep by 11 pm, i.e. go to bed at 10 pm.
- Develop a routine every night. Eat early 5pm–7pm. Avoid eating, snacking, alcohol, computers or exercise within 3 hours before sleeping.

- Avoid Alcohol – alcohol will send you to sleep quickly but will wake you (4-5 hours) later and deprive you of valuable, replenishing REM sleep. Alcohol also distracts the liver from metabolising fat, toxins and body-waste overnight.
- Change into bed attire and brush teeth earlier to avoid snacking and drinking.
- Avoid Sleeping Pills – they have toxic side effects and deprive you of quality REM sleep and you may become reliant.
- Take herbal relaxants like camomile tea or AIM Composure®, or StemEnhance Ultra before bed. Rub lavender essential oil on your feet and temple areas on your head.
- Stop thinking, worrying and/or working at least 1 ½ hours before bed ~ still the mind. Write notes for action tomorrow and let it go.
- No Computers or Mobile Phones 1 ½ hours before (their blue light wave stimulates brain). Most phones have blue light filters within their settings.
- Avoid having electronic equipment near your head at night. This includes digital clocks, radios and charging phones. Lamps are okay. Electronic equipment gives off Electro-Magnetic Frequencies (EMFs) which disturb brain rhythms. Don't use electric blankets.
- Have dim lights in the evening and a darken your bedroom – Melatonin (sleep hormone) needs dim lights to activate.
- Play relaxation music - No Lyrics, No Rhythm.
- Repeat in your mind, *"My mind is still, my mind is blank, I am at peace"* Let go of any tension in the gut upon the word "peace".
- Check the position of your bed-head. What's on the other side of the wall? Is there an electrical meter box or TV, sound equipment, phone charging station, etc.? Sometimes, depending on EMFs from underground streams, rocks, minerals etc, moving your bed from N-S to E-W can change the energy and help you sleep. Visit orgoneffectsaustralia.com.au and check out your place.

5G and EMFs

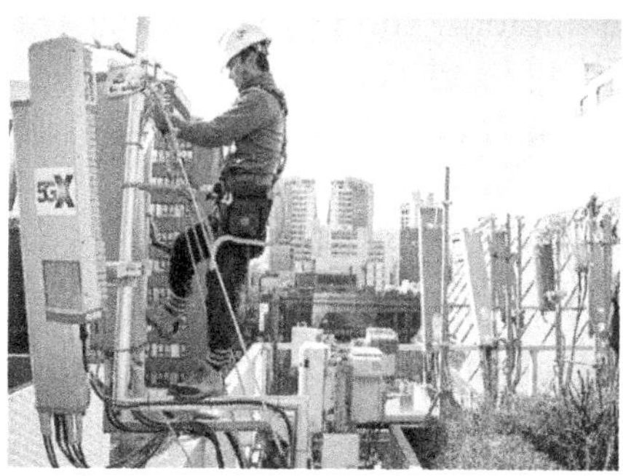

We live in an electromagnetic universe created by torus fields on a magnetic planet that humans, animals, insects and plants have evolved to handle over millennia. Our cells are made of atoms that are made of neutrons and electrons, therefore at a quantum level, we are 99% space and energy, therefore we emit a frequency. Brain activity is easily measured by an EEG machine, or an ECG for the heart. Therefore, what happens around us with electromagnetic frequencies (EMFs) impacts our brain, heart and body, as well as our food chain.

There have been greater concerns about the impact of EMFs on humans since the advent of mobile phones (cell phones) in the 1990s. Each generation of mobile phone signal from 1G, 2G, 3G and 4G have had increasing levels of EMFs impact.

The next generation of mobile data signal is 5G NR (New Radio, commonly termed simply 5G), which uses entirely different technology and meters able to read 1G-4G are not able to read 5G because of this difference.

5G sprung from military technology called the 'Active Denial System' which sends a focused beam of millimetre frequency EMF at the enemy and heats the surface of their skin and disperses combatants from activity. The pulse can simply be annoying or turned all the way up to burn. Operated through a joystick, the pulse can target one person in a group, or the entire group.

The pulse can change emotional state of a person, therefore the quality of their choices. This technology has been used in crowd control to disperse protestors, activists, etc.

5G EMFs for mobile phones have been turned down significantly, however delivers 1000+ MBPS download speeds, and there have been **no** long-term biological safety tests on humans, therefore <u>we are the experiment</u>.

The larger bandwidth, high frequency (millimetre wavelength) and high level of pulsation means signals from transmitters don't travel very far, only a few hundred metres, and are easily blocked by trees, buildings, fences or screens. This means many, many more towers or nodes (every 100m on buildings in the CBD or every 1km in most places). This generates more low-level background radio frequency radiation, especially if you live or work in or near one of the buildings upon which a node or tower is installed.

Symptoms known to be associated with EMF exposure are nose bleeds, cheek pain, headaches, eye pain, nausea, vomiting, dizziness, fatigue, flu-like symptoms, irritability, anxiety, tinnitus, insomnia and nervous system signalling issues. Diseases associated with long-term EMF exposure are diabetes, infertility, cancer, psychiatric disorders and depression.

5G is slowly being rolled out "for our convenience" to make us more interconnected utilising the artificial intelligence (AI) of Google, Facebook, YouTube, Netflix, etc. Besides the EMF issues mentioned, there are social implications, like the easy implementation of Social Credit Scoring (SCS) which is already happening in China and is being experimented with in Darwin, Australia. With SCS, if you cross the street on a red light, you will be scored down… and a higher score allows better access for your children's education, better banking interest rates, travel rights, queue positions, etc. The technology can also quell rebellion by blocking phone signals, platforms, etc, especially if the government is corrupt and your protest is legitimate.

Besides the EMF issues, there are numerous privacy and security issues as well. Ultimately, the purpose if 5G is to do away with having to carry a device (phone) and simply rely on the system "Big Brother" (AI) to provide your requirements and handle payments. The technology is already sophisticated enough in China to simply speak the words, e.g. "Hey Google - Uber", and your driverless ride will appear, you will be taken to your destination and Uber will be paid without needing a phone. Your Uber ride will go onto your SCS and record. Imagine the impact on your privacy if you are talking to friends alfresco and AI doesn't like some of the keywords it is sensing, therefore your SCS is scored down and/or you are arrested for subversion. Extremely dangerous depending on the morals and ethics of those in control.

On the EMF level, don't place your body between a phone tower signal or your Wi-Fi modem and your phone. When downloading or receiving a signal, the signal travels in a straight line in an invisible tube-like channel directly from the source to your phone. Don't use Bluetooth earpieces, instead utilise earphones when communicating and avoid having your phone in your pocket when doing so. Turn off your Wi-Fi setting when you leave home, so your phone doesn't continually scan for Wi-Fi signals. Also, don't leave phones on charge in your bedroom overnight and consider what is on the other side of your bedroom wall, relative to your body position when lying in bed.

If you don't want to be part of the grand 5G experiment and want to protect yourself against the existing 4G and future 5G radiation – for over a decade, we have utilised the expertise and protection of orgoneffectsaustralia.com.au. *see the resources section later*

Information for this topic has be gathered from Dr Anthony Miller MD, Prof (Emeritus) Uni of Toronto, Dr Magda Havas PhD, Dr Riina Bray MD and Chemical Engineer, Frank Clegg, former president of Microsoft Canada, Dr Martin Pall, Prof (Emeritus) Washington State Uni, Gerard Bini, founder of Orgone Effects Australia orgoneffectsaustralia.com.au

Arthritis and Gout

In some autoimmune diseases, the body's defence-immune system inappropriately triggers an inflammatory response when there are no foreign invaders to fight off and the body's normally protective immune system causes damage to its own tissue.

According to *The China Study*, foreign invaders that enter the body are protein molecules called antigens, which can be bacterium, viruses or molecules of food. One of these food antigens commonly consumed is cow's milk, which contains a protein called casein (87% of milk) which mimics the body's own healthy proteins. Some antigens can leak through the bowel wall without going through the proper digestion and liver filtering processes to produce amino acids. The immune system makes 'moulds' to identify and remember unsupportive antigens, but under some conditions (like overconsumption of dairy with sugar and carbs) the mould can be seen to fit the body's own similar proteins and white blood cells start attacking the body in error.

Overconsumption of **dairy with carbs and sugar** creates an acidic body and an excess production of uric acid from the kidneys. The excess uric acid gathers in joints causing inflammation — swelling and painful movement.

Overconsumption of **omega-6** (vegetable or seed oils found in packaged food) and insufficient omega-3 ingestion can cause joint inflammation too.

Doctors may prescribe anti-inflammatory drugs for arthritis, which come with their cocktail of negative side-effects. I remember how many pharmaceutical drugs Mum took to try to relieve her rheumatoid arthritis. I also recall having to lift Mum out of bed some mornings and rubbing her joints to get her going for the day, despite the drugs prescribed.

A few years ago, when I started observing and feeling signs of arthritis and gout, **I cleaned up my act** and worked hard on changing my diet. I supplemented, exercised and alkalised my system…

Methyl Sulphonyl Methane (MSM – a biologically-active form of the mineral sulphur) is another supportive supplement. Sulphur is the fourth most plentiful mineral in the body and is found in every cell. Sulphur plays a particularly important role in tissue structure. As a form of sulphur, MSM contributes to healthy joints.

Research has shown that individuals with arthritis are deficient in sulphur and supplementing with MSM may reduce inflammation and repair joints.

If your **fibre** intake is low, this may result in increasing your blood sugar levels, cholesterol or triglycerides which can result in an inflammatory response. See Fibre Boosts Immune System. Soluble fibre changes the characteristics of immune cells — they go from being pro-inflammatory, angry cells to anti-inflammatory, healing cells.

Gout Relief

Gout can be a prelude to arthritis and is caused through lifestyle choices. The usual suspects; excessive omega-6, sugar, grain products and alcohol.

Reversing Inflammation

Reduce the consumption of the above foods. Improving your diet, whilst alkalising the body and cleaning out the colon and liver, will reduce inflammation.

Ginger and turmeric tea is one of the best natural anti-inflammatories. Thinly slice a thumb-sized piece of ginger and/or turmeric and add boiling water in a cup. If the taste is too strong, add a squeeze of lemon juice.

In addition, take **omega-3** supplements daily. Omega-3 significantly decreases inflammation as the body prefers omega-3 to the over-ingested omega-6 and carbs as discussed previously.

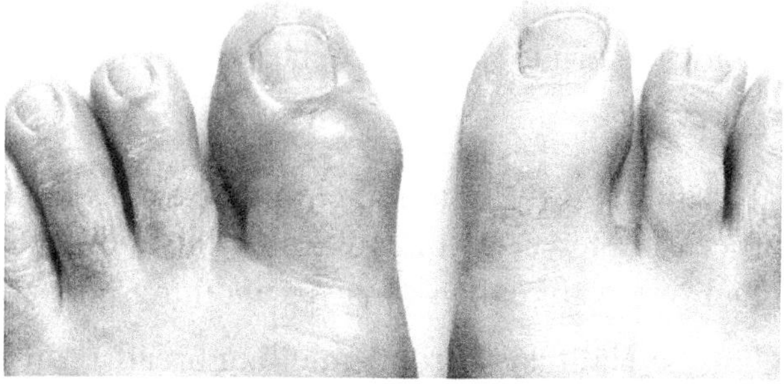

GOUT in left big toe - May 2012

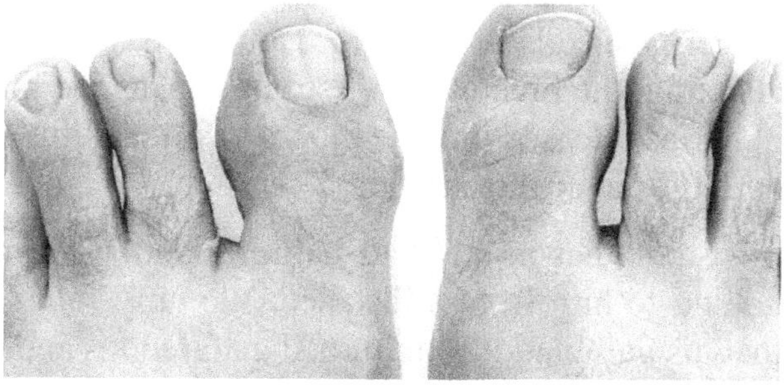

Toes after taking double doses of AIM BarleyLife® - August 2012
BarleyLife assists in alkalising the body, which may reduce the acidic pain and swelling of Gout

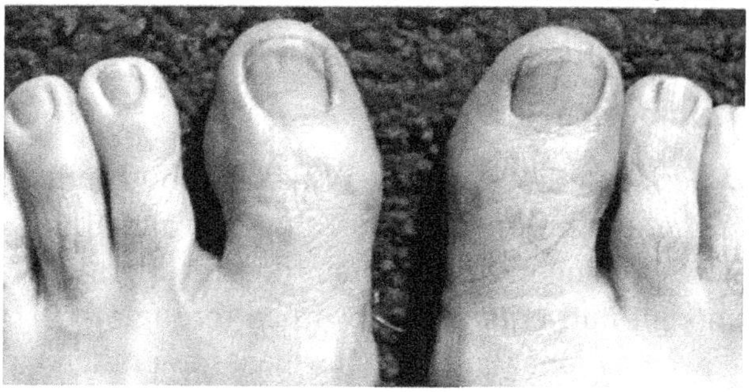

Toes after taking StemEnhance Ultra, PlasmaFlo & Cyactiv for 1 yr - Nov 2019
Toes & feet back to normal after increasing stem cells, blood flow & inflammation

Barley Grass Juice Powder

I found that increasing my servings of AIM BarleyLife® to my daily supplementation helped balance my body's pH and combat inflammation *(see photos),* with the added advantage of supplying countless combinations of vitamins, minerals, antioxidants, phytonutrients, chlorophyll and enzymes.

Alkalise the body with practitioner-grade bicarbonate soda (as mentioned previously), may reduce inflammation by neutralising uric acid in joints.

Natural Stem Cells, Anti-inflammatories and Circulation Boosters

Lastly, increasing the number of adult stem cells in circulation using stem cell nutrition is one of my recent discoveries. *See photos above and resources at back.* Cerule also have two natural products, one that aids the body to reduce overall body inflammation and the other that specifically supports joints. The combination of these products and Cerule's circulation booster, really helped my toes return to normal. A cheap investment to be able to walk freely again.

Halitosis

The failure of the colon to eliminate toxins due to constipation, and the liver processing fewer toxins, can cause the body to try to eliminate toxins through other organs like the skin, eyes and lungs.

Causes: Halitosis (strong-smelling breath) can be an indication that your gut organs are diseased or dysfunctional and holding onto toxins. Poor dental hygiene can also be a cause but is easily identified and repaired. When detoxing, the breath can be strong too, as the body tries to expel an overload of toxins released into the bloodstream. Halitosis with a 'sweetish' aroma can derive from cirrhosis of the liver.

My stepfather-in-law had halitosis and we handled it by being polite and talking to him from a distance. We only found out, just before his passing, that his gall bladder had turned gangrenous and infected other organs and his strong breath was actually the smell of gut organs rotting within. If we knew then what we know now, we could have guided him towards a better quality and longer life – but he wasn't one to listen to advice.

Malnourished Obese

When your diet is mostly processed food and sugar, the colon becomes sluggish and the liver dysfunctional, which doesn't permit enough nutrients to be absorbed through the bowel, as sugar and carbs ferment rather than digest. Therefore, the body 'screams out' for genuine nutrition (energy) to continue functioning as it should. Unfortunately, our habits mistake this signal as "I need to feel full," encouraging cravings (triggered by unfriendly gut bacteria and emotions) for any easy junk or comfort food to fill the stomach and satisfy the urges.

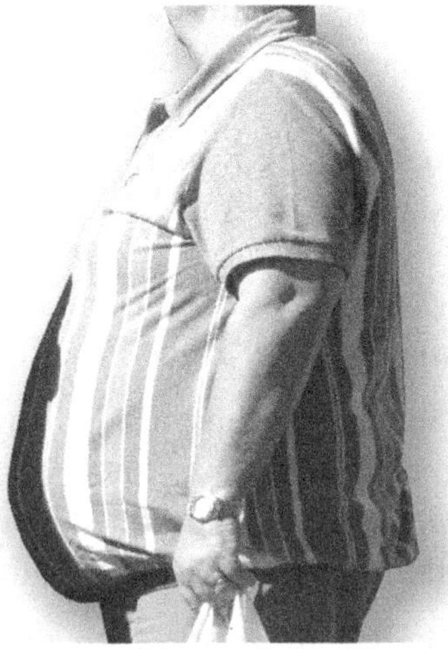

Highly processed junk food might contain only 20% of the nutrients the body needs at that time, therefore the body signals to keep eating to gain another 20% to get closer to satisfying its needs. However, the excess food has plenty of Calories too, and when we eat in this manner daily, the body adapts and stores the excess food as fat and toxins to be dealt with later. But there is no 'later' as fat is continually stacked on.

The body adapts to crave the basic flavours of salt, fat, sour and sweet and our cravings for flavour prevails over our need for nutrition. MSG is added to most spicy packet and fast food which enhances flavour but encourages cravings *(see 'MSG — the Hidden Additive' previously).* You really don't need what the body craves — you have already had enough.

Sometimes when we are **tired, upset, angry, exhausted or emotionally-triggered**, we tend to revert to old ways in an endeavour to feel better — to escape. Be aware of this, take time-out, rest, sleep, eat some protein, etc, rather than binging on sugar and carbs.

While the body is feeling continually full from overeating several times a day and is overburdening the liver and colon to process and eliminate the unused waste material, the body is nutritionally deprived.

If you can override your craving habits and listen to what your body needs, rather than what you want (or crave), and satisfy your body nutritionally through a clean bowel, functional liver, supportive food and supplementation, then cravings should subside. Mostly overriding cravings is about releasing the emotional triggers that incite the cravings, through The Emotion Code or Body Code work – *see resources later.*

The Root Cause of Craving

Besides the unfriendly gut bacteria and biochemical impacts of addictions that produce cravings (that should dissipate within about three days if not ingested) the root cause of most cravings are the **need for your soul to identify who you really are** (not the personality you've evolved to handle your world, but the real you) and the need to identify **"why aren't I happy?"**

When you make changes and live more in the moment, go with the flow and take notice of how you feel in the heart and gut about issues arising, you begin to let go of negative thoughts and focus on what makes you happy. The happier your thoughts, the happier you are.

You become more in touch with who you really are and feel much better about yourself, which reduces cravings. The **need** to be happy diminishes, because you are happy from the inside. Become happy and all your problems will go away.

How I Handle Cravings

I've worked for many years on finding out who I really am and I'm quite content with that situation now. I'm continuously working on improving my fulfillment and happiness level daily and this has made a considerable difference in my life, following the previous struggles our family had.

When I have biological cravings, for something sweet for example, I go somewhere quiet, close my eyes for two minutes and remember the image I have in my head of myself in perfect health, fit and slim. Then I focus on the energy of that craving in my belly. I don't judge it or tell it to go away, I simply observe until the craving energy naturally dissipates. Immediately after, find some other activity (other than eating) to distract yourself.

Quantum physics demonstrates scientifically that the simple act of observation changes the physical particles (atoms) surrounding that energy.

You can also eat protein (beef jerky, hard-boiled eggs, cheese, chicken, etc). Protein won't trigger a large insulin response and takes away the craving by feeling satisfied, nutritionally.

Remember, eat to live — don't live to eat.

Everything I think I need to do
is all in order to propel me
to some place that when I get there,
I think I will be happier.

So, everything I am doing;
all of my rights and wrongs...
are all about getting to a manifestation that
I believe I will then be happier...

So why don't I take a short cut
and just go get happy?

Abraham Hicks

Chapter 8

Solutions

How We Can Heal Chronic Toxicity and Disease

Imagine the dark napkins represent 20–50 years of constant toxic build-up in the colon and liver from eating excessive amounts of sugar, white flour, dairy, junk-food, coffee, alcohol and soft drink on top of chemical toxins from work, garden sprays, cleaning products, cosmetics, pharmaceutical drugs and negative thoughts.

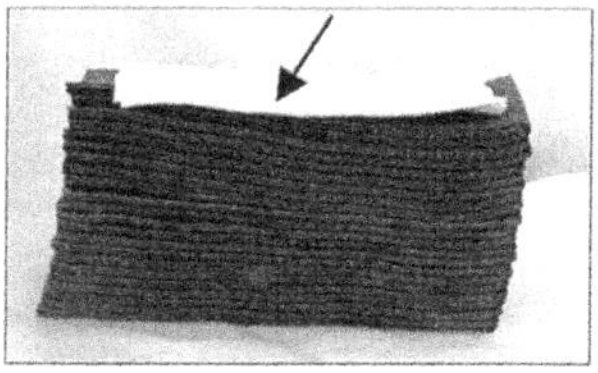

1. The build-up of toxins is potentially your future chronic disease that could reduce your quality of life and shorten your time on earth by around 15 years unless they are removed through cleansing the bowel and liver, correction of diet and supplementation or both. Some of the toxins are carcinogenic and are starting to spread throughout your body. The white layer represents the toxins from the junk food you ate today.

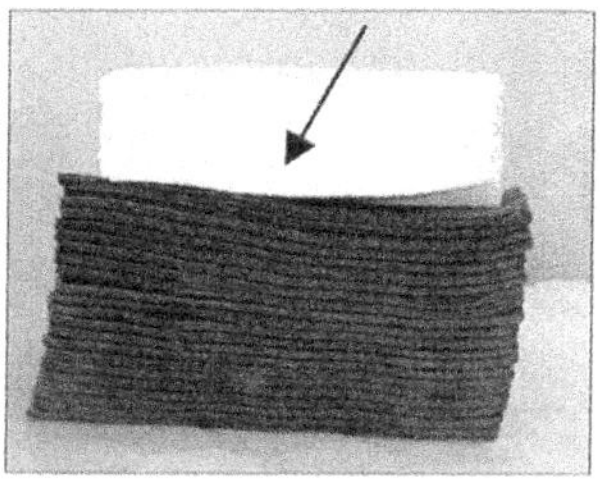

2. Let's imagine you continue eating in this manner, laying down more layers of toxins from unsupportive habits (represented by white napkins). Now your body has to deal with your recently introduced toxins, before it can get to the dark toxins, therefore your chronic illness continues and you feel more lethargic and chronically fatigued as you tolerate joint pain and headaches.

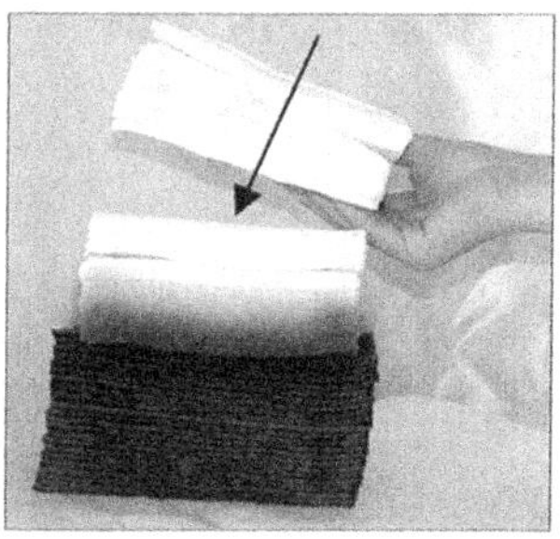

3. As you lay down more and more layers of new toxins (white napkins), the white napkins laid down previously begin to decay and turn dark, becoming more toxic, adding to your chronic illness. You feel fatigued all the time and your memory fades with bouts of depression and anger, and you find it difficult to sleep, so you take sleeping pills, adding to your toxic mix.

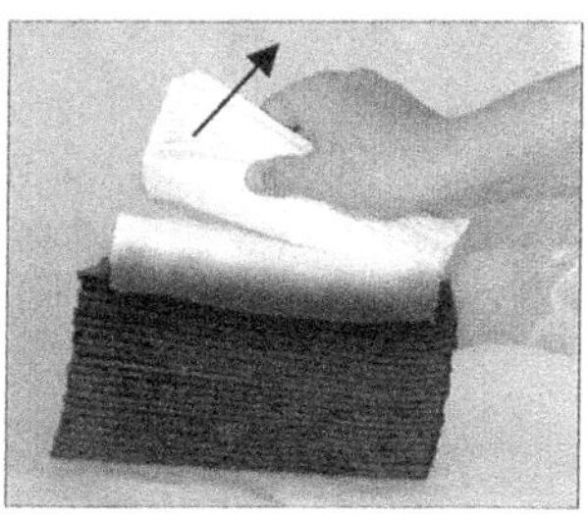

4. If you start eating better and exercising daily. You stop laying down new toxins and your body begins to burn up the newly-laid layers through exercise and improved metabolism. You are now getting closer to dealing with and alleviating your chronic illness and pain — looking forward to a healthier future.

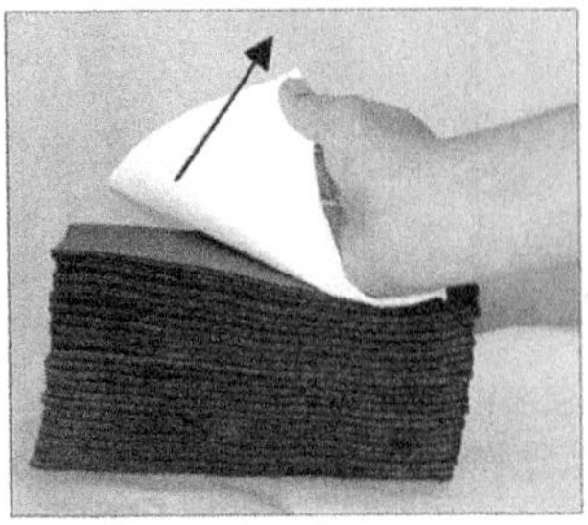

5. Finally you release all your newly-laid toxins and start releasing the darker, more insidious toxins by continuing your cleansing, exercise, supportive eating and supplementation. Detox symptoms appear occasionally, but you are able to deal with them as you know what you are doing is for your highest good over the long-term.

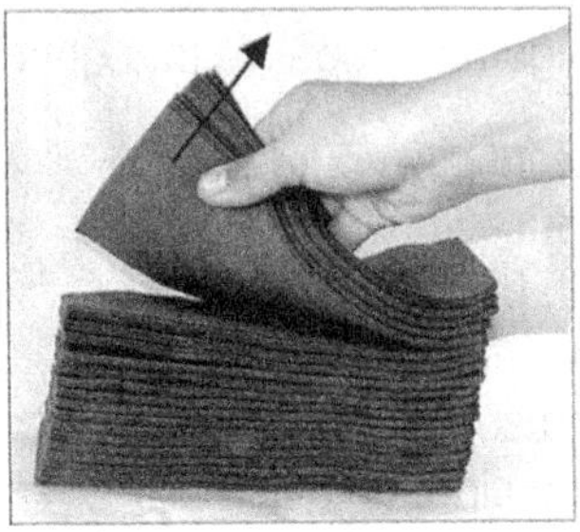

6. You continue diligently on your quest to release your build-up of toxins. Your liver begins to regenerate and repair itself. Your colon releases plaque and blockages and you finally start digesting food properly, gaining more energy. Chronic inflammation throughout the body is reduced and your blood pressure and blood sugar levels begin to return to normal.

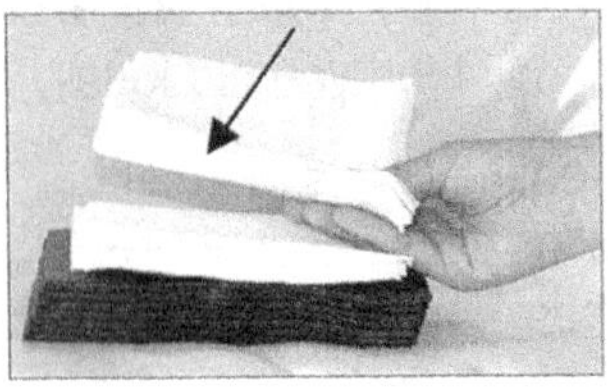

7. If you slip back, and start eating poorly again, you begin to lay down new layers of toxins again, and your body has to deal with these first before dealing with the ongoing cleansing previously started. Your energy levels drop again, headaches return, you feel depressed, fatigued and tired all the time.

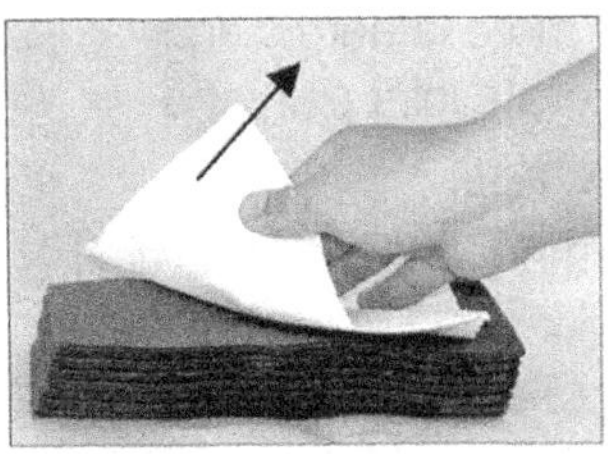

8. You get back on track and start eating better and exercising again. You can begin releasing those chronic, toxic dark layers again. Your energy levels being to pick up and you feel on top of the world with your new positive attitude.

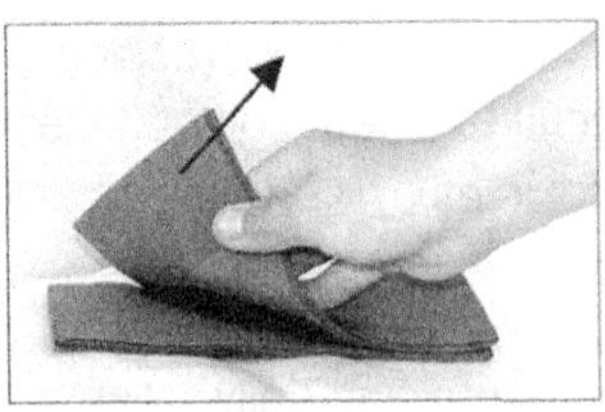

9. Well done, you have removed most of the insidious, carcinogenic dark layers. Your liver and colon are functioning properly and you naturally begin to eat less. Your energy and quality of life has greatly improved and you have possibly added an extra 10–20 years to your life.

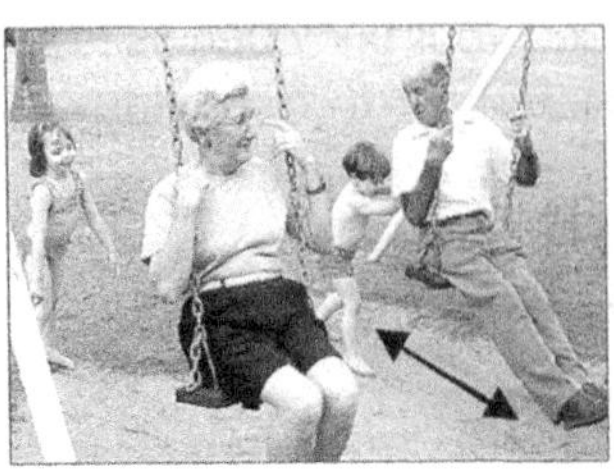

10. You feel more positive about your future and begin to look for opportunities. Though it has taken a number of years and you've had to tolerate some detox symptoms, you realise it has been worthwhile as you now have the energy to play with your grandchildren.

Stem Cell Nutrition ~ the Secret is Out!

The body needs 60 minerals, 16 vitamins, 12 amino acids & 3 essential fatty acids (91 nutrients total) to function optimally. The fact is, without full utilisation of all 91 nutrients, some part of your body will be in decline. However, even if you're ingesting enough nutrients daily, they can still sit around (dormant) like labourers having an extended 'smoko' on a building site, until the boss comes along and tells them where to go and what to do. Nutrients are simply building materials (timber, bricks, mortar and glass) used in construction and they need instructions and guidance to be fully utilised.

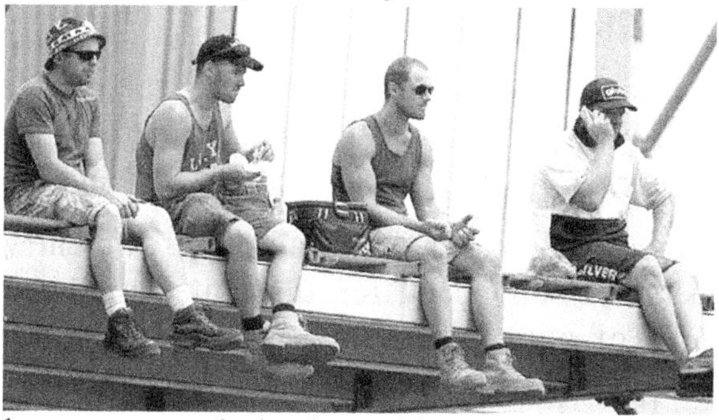

The body's supreme and most versatile leader (the boss) is the stem cell. The stem cell duplicates incredibly fast and its role is to listen for, and identify injuries and requirements, then initiate the correct nutrients and distribution for repair and replacement of old, dead and damaged cells. With enough stem cells circulating, the body can mitigate disease, repair damage and slow down the aging process.

Every day, 40 billion cells die and are passed out the bladder and bowel as one third of your faeces (if you eat enough fibre and water). Every 5 days the intestinal lining is replaced, 4 months the blood, 1 year the brain and every 3 years the liver and pancreas. If there is an injury or inflammation, your body may send around 40% more stem cells to that area until the issue is resolved. Adult stem cells also morph into any new cell required – cells such as brain, heart, lungs, blood, gut microbiome, cartilage, nerves, eyes, skin, hair, etc. Through this process, stem cells naturally repair and renew your body daily, but only if you have enough in circulation.

From around 25 years when the body ceases its growing phase, stem cells are reduced in circulation by around 5% per year. By the age of 65, the body only has about 10% of the adult stem cells circulating. A sticky molecule called 'L-selectin' is the culprit and locks adult stem cells inside the bone marrow. When more cells die than are renewed during this natural attrition process, we call this disease, illness, degenerative, aging, etc and is one of the main reasons the body degenerates as we age.

Having more stem cells circulating around your body **must benefit** your body, health and overall wellbeing.

How do we get More Stem Cells?

Over 30 year's research started with embryonic stem cells, however there were ethical issues with taking embryos to supply the medical industry with embryonic stem cells. This is where stem cells initially gained a bad name in the 1980/90s.

Research progressed onto umbilical cord and placental stem cells from afterbirth. Next, liposuction and treatment of fat cells which were processed, sterilised, frozen, transported, thawed and injected into areas of injury.

Liposuction progressed into day-treatment where fat was extracted from a person's body, centrifuged, isolated and injected back into the same person's area of injury. The above treatments externally introduced around 10-25 million new stem cells into an injury but may have side-effects like rejection and mutated growth and were very expensive – between $5000 - $10,000 per treatment. Such treatments are still conducted today and are often require repeated treatments every 3-6-12 months depending on the situation.

Breakthrough in Stem Cell Nutrition

To quote Dr Steven Cohen, MD, Plastic Surgeon (San Diego, USA) *"Maybe we need to create a pill that helps the body push out their stem cells more effectively."* That "pill" StemEnhance Ultra (SEU) arrived several years ago in the form of a capsule combining a patented blend of two specific algae and an extract of spirulina – *see 'My Recovery' previously and resources later.*

SEU has been scientifically proven to block the action of L-selectin, utilising 'L-selectin ligand,' which inhibits the locking away stem cells and releases more stem cells freely into the bloodstream. This increases the circulation of adult stem cells around the body by up to 60% (4-10 million) within two hours of ingesting just 2 capsules.

Take two capsules twice a day and you can increase the number of stem cells circulating in the body by 8-20 million per day – comparable to the above therapies for less than the price of a cup of coffee, with no side-effects.

A considerable bonus of SEU is that it naturally contains Phenylethylamine (PEA). PEA is the chemical produced in the brain when a person is in love and is said to put a woman in the mood for love. PEA is commonly found in its highest concentration in chocolate, and that's why chocolate is often linked to romance and love. Chocolate can become very addictive due to the search for self-love, recognition and inclusiveness that may be missing in one's life.

SEU supplies PEA to the brain and 'relaxes' the nervous system and brain, relieving stress, providing more harmony, peace, acceptance and tolerance; therefore, greater happiness.

Personally, I have found taking SEU on a regular basis for over a year has improved my mood, mind-clarity, sleep and energy. Injuries heal quickly, and my circulation improved with more flexibility. As mentioned previously, my face rash I endured for two years cleared up within weeks of stem cell nutrition.

Hundreds more testimonies from all parts of the world also testify to SEU's effectiveness as a master nutrient. I am walking proof that the body will take what you provide and utilise it to optimise the body and work on repairing what isn't functioning properly.

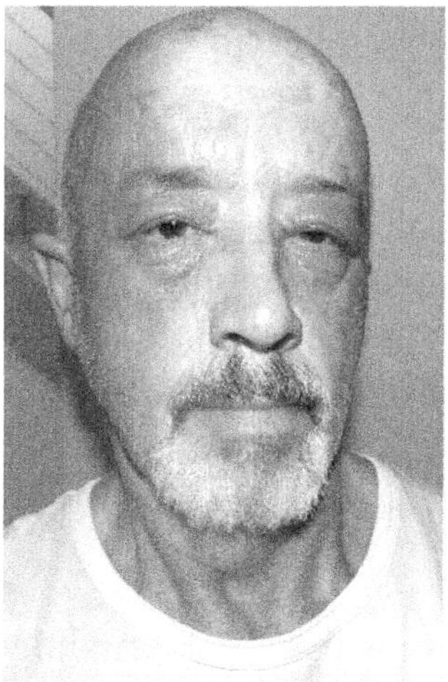

June 2016

9 months after root canal removal

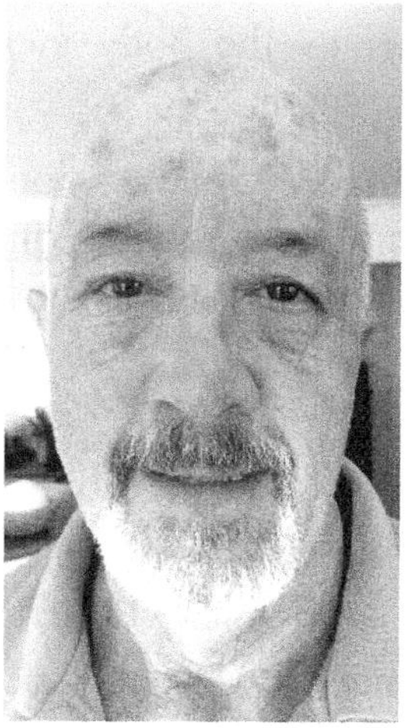

July 2017

1 year later

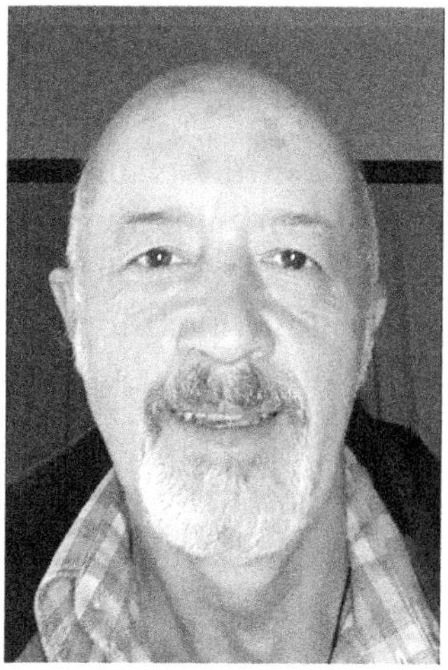

Aug 2018

After 3 weeks of Stem Cell Nutrition

Your Natural Digestive Rhythm

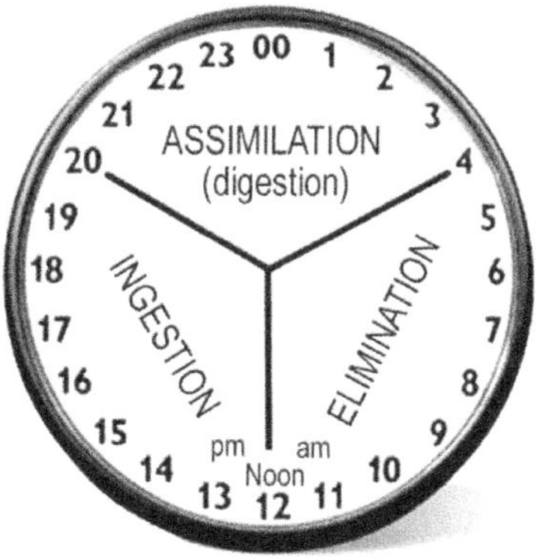

The body has a natural digestive rhythm and if you can work with it, you can better overcome cravings, reduce weight, gently detox, feel more vibrant and save a lot of money by not eating so much.

From 12 noon through to 8 pm is the best time to **eat**. This should be mostly based around one main meal with 60-70% fat, 20% protein, 15-20% steamed or raw veggies from the garden which includes carbohydrates. Included in the above carb intake – grains, fruit or sugar should be no more than 5%.

From 8 pm through to 4 am is the **assimilation** process, when the intestines digest and the liver processes food. Bile is sent through the body to collect waste and dead cells. Generally, you should not eat during this time and ingest mostly water, herbal teas and supplements.

From 4 am through to 12 noon is **elimination** time, when the food and waste the body has gathered overnight is eliminated. As per the previously mentioned *'Losing It' section*, avoid eating breakfast or snacking.

If you eat traditional grain, sugar and dairy (high carb) breakfasts early in the morning while the body is in the elimination cycle, the body may be inclined to stop eliminating and **store the waste as fat** — creating toxic fat. The body is less likely to **eliminate**, as the body switches over to digesting and processing the food recently eaten.

Because of the changes in habit, you may notice you could have a stronger body odour with unpleasant breath and may initially experience some detox symptoms (headache, lethargy) in the mornings until you more fully detox. Attuning yourself to your natural digestive rhythms can take a few weeks to feel comfortable, but stick with it — it is worth the effort.

You may not be able to follow your digestive rhythms all the time, but even if you partially work towards it or do it most of the time, your weight and health should improve.

It's okay to go out for dinner with friends occasionally and overindulge — that is about the occasion — don't feel guilty — it's good for you. It's also okay initially to splurge a little on the weekend, but for at least 5-6 days a week, try to follow your natural rhythms.

Detoxing

Detoxification is the term used to describe the process your body goes through to get rid of toxins. It's recommended that you generally detox every day through lifestyle recommendations in this book, rather than go through one great 'detox flush' and resume your unsupportive habits again next week.

There are **three phases** to detoxing:

Phase 1
Starts the breakdown of toxins by changing them into an even more toxic mix that can be up to 60 times more toxic than the original substance.

For phase 1 to work successfully, your body needs A, C, D, E and B vitamins, glutathione, amino acids, antioxidants, copper, zinc and magnesium.

If you are especially reactive to caffeine, alcohol, cleaning products or strong smells like perfumes or incense; it's possible that phase 1 is not working properly during digestion. You should seriously consider probiotic and enzyme supplementation.

Phase 2

Must immediately follow Phase 1, where the liver requires six different enzymes to convert proteins into a water-soluble form so toxins can be excreted through six linked pathways in the body; liver, bowel, bladder, lungs, lymphatic system and skin.

To complete this task, the body needs B vitamins, amino acids, glutathione, molybdenum, flavonoids, iron, iodine, magnesium and selenium. If the body is low in any of these elements or nutrients, toxins will be less-neutralised and have an ongoing negative impact, causing faster aging and disease.

Without **animal protein**, phases 1 and 2 slow down, or can't be performed, and autointoxication is more likely to occur. The body especially needs **glutathione and amino acids,** and animal protein contributes to building such amino acids which combine carbon, oxygen, hydrogen and nitrogen to form over 50 different proteins that perform phases 1 and 2.

Plant protein and fibre alone can't perform this function satisfactorily.

If you have asthma, strong smelling urine or had toxaemia or jaundice during pregnancy, it's possible that phase 2 isn't working correctly and again, supplementing with probiotics and enzymes are recommended.

Phase 3

The now neutralised substances are passed out of the body via the above-mentioned systems. Phase 3 requires fibre, moderate exercise and lots of quality water to function.

Detox Symptoms

Detoxification symptoms — both physical and mental — may appear when you improve your lifestyle by starting something new such as changing your diet or exercising, or by discontinuing a current habit, such as eating chocolate or drinking coffee or alcohol.

As you begin to make changes, you may experience detox symptoms as your body rids itself of old toxic matter that may have been accumulating for decades. You may experience symptoms for three days or more, however this may not happen to everyone. But, it's helpful to know what could happen...

Your body will always favour higher quality nutrients over toxins and waste, therefore as natural cell attrition occurs, the discarded 40 billion cells per day (containing toxins and waste) move into the bloodstream and may make you feel unwell in the short-term. You are potentially releasing toxins that may contribute to a long-term terminal illness, so it's worth doing. Often, the worse you feel during this period is an indication of just how many toxins you may be shifting and how sick you could have been in the future.

The quickest, most efficient way to release such toxins from your body is through the bladder and the bowel which requires plenty of fibre and plenty of quality water, along with consistent moderate exercise.

Detox symptoms may include **tummy cramps, diarrhoea, rashes, pimples, boils, skin peeling, swollen glands, nausea, headaches, eye irritation and blurred vision, irritability, anxiety, intolerance, muscle and joint pain, lethargy, fatigue, tiredness, dizziness, flu-like symptoms, night fevers and pain in areas of old injuries.** Often people will blame supplements for how they feel, but this is not accurate. Mostly all you need is to halve the serving for a week or less, rest as much as possible and/or to increase your daily fibre and water intake.

Because symptoms are similar to symptoms that show up in certain illnesses, changing your diet or lifestyle can result in misunderstanding, *"If I am doing something that is supposed to be good for me, why do I have these symptoms? Why do I feel worse, and not better?"*

Understanding this apparent paradox is perhaps the **first and most important hurdle** you must get over when making a dietary or lifestyle change.

It may have taken decades for your bowel to become clogged, chronically inflamed and dysfunctional. Every time you have chosen to do or taken something unsupportive to your body, you incurred a debt to your future health. Detoxing is the quickest and easy way to relinquish that debt without going through the pain of chronic illness for decades to come.

Give any recommendation for change at least 3-4 months to assist your body in its healing. It takes 4 months for your body to fully renew its blood, and blood carries all nutrients, toxins and waste.

Allergies are a sign of a dysfunctional liver, so clean out your bowel and liver. Persist; it's definitely worthwhile for your future health, happiness and quality of life. Life is miserable without health, no matter how wealthy you are.

When symptoms are severe, water and coffee enemas are the most powerful tool for toxin clearance and relief. Please trust me on this, I've been there, done that — I speak from experience.

What can you do during this period?

The hardest thing for many people to do is accept that they are not sick and realise that the body is cleansing itself.

1. **Rest** as much as possible but include some moderate exercise to assist

with circulation.

2. Eat light foods that are easy to digest; consume **meat, fat and vegetables** and drink plenty of water. Supplement with **probiotics**.
3. Take **extra fibre and water**. Fibre and water are the vehicles your toxins will utilise to exit your body.
4. Avoid pain relieving medications like paracetamol as they are injurious to the liver and will slow the toxin-filtering process.
5. The **most effective way** of relieving symptoms of detoxing are water and **coffee enemas**. There have been times when suffering detox symptoms that I have conducted a coffee enema and found immediate relief within 20 minutes. Coffee taken as an enema dilates the blood vessels in the liver and allows for more a rapid release of the toxins *(see 'Enemas' later)*.
6. **Skin brushing** before showering or exfoliating in the shower once a week can help speed up the detox process, as it helps to remove the outer layer of toxin-ladened skin.
7. Have deep-tissue massage and lymphatic drainage to move toxins through more quickly.
8. Take supplements to support your body. If taking supplements was the original trigger of your detox symptoms, then halve your servings for a few days, then resume your original servings once you are feeling better.
9. Turning upside-down on an **inversion bed** daily may help the liver and gut organs drain, then flush and release toxins. The inversion bed also allows your spine, neck and hips to come into correct alignment daily, which I have found beneficial.

For me, Personally...

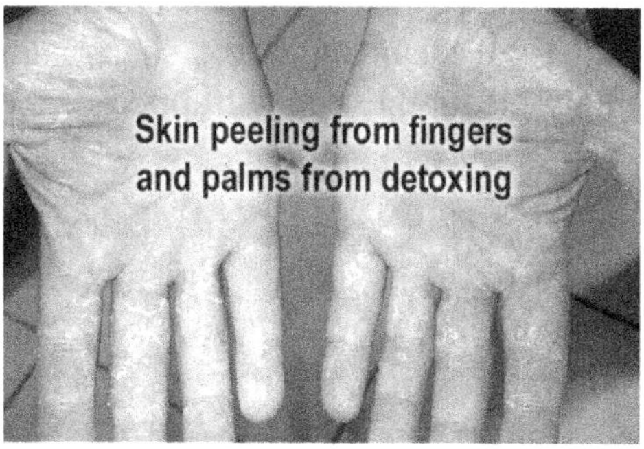

Please note that this section relates to symptoms I experienced over a total period of **seven to eight years**, so they are **not as intense** as it might first appear.

When I detox, I tend to have strong-smelling urine, faeces, breath and body odour. I often have temporary pain or twitching in my liver, headaches and flu-like symptoms. At times, specific muscles twitch for two to four days and I have even lost 80% of my hearing one time for a couple of days. My eyesight has been temporarily degraded with occasional blind spots but improves within hours. I occasionally have skin abrasions appear on my face that feel as if they are from burns, but these eventually turn into patches of skin discolouration (commonly known as liver spots).

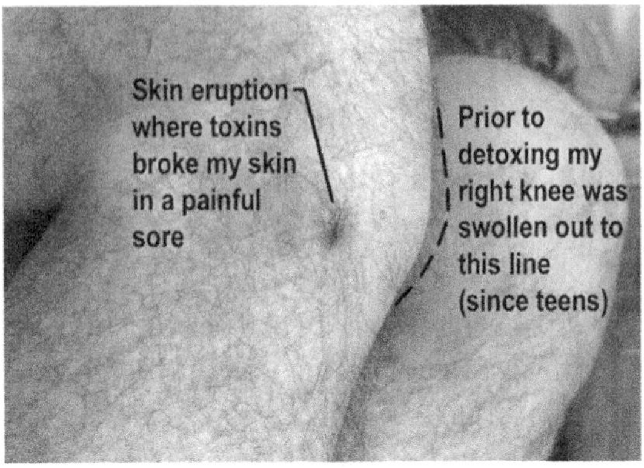

At one time in early 2011, I felt lethargic for months with ongoing headaches and joint pain. During this period, I increased my coffee enemas, reduced my exercise to what I could handle, rested more, ate better and increased my supplementation until I came out the other end feeling better and more switched on. If you're as highly toxic as I was, it takes a lot of understanding and resilience to push through and have faith in the process.

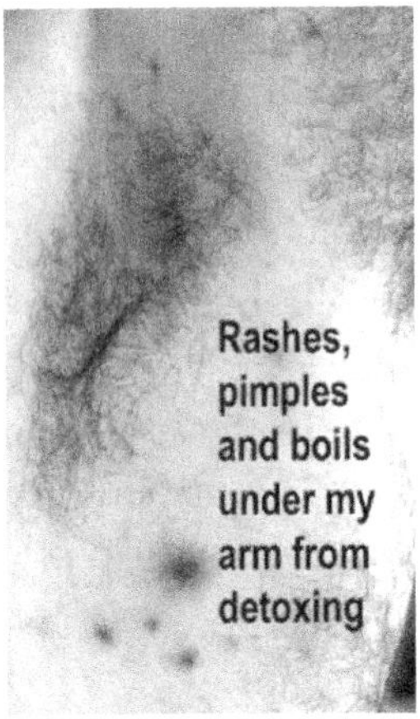

My thinking became clouded and foggy, making silly mistakes, often finding it hard to remember a friend's name, or recall information. But again, this clears up and I begin to think more clearly than before. The sickness industry might say that these are early signs of dementia, but I see it as reassurance of my theory that toxins in the bloodstream contribute significantly to mental disease. If my symptoms were early signs of dementia, I would not have regained my mental and cognitive faculties.

I have also had pangs of pain in places where I've had previous injury. Over the years I've had a couple of serious injuries including breaking my left fibula. During detox, sharp pain can be felt in areas of old injury as my body clears the toxins trapped in the fracture points.

The most telling detox features in my body are skin rashes, boils under my arms (near lymph glands) and skin peeling from my hands and feet *(see pictures)*. Also, I sometimes get swelling and pain in elbow and toe joints for a few months as the toxins dissipate.

Keep in mind that these symptoms may not be typical for everyone and may vary from person to person depending on your heritage, work and previous lifestyle choices.

It's worth it!

I know it may sound painful and a lot of work, temporarily reducing your quality of life through detoxing, but I believe **I've removed toxins that were the foundations of my future terminal illnesses**: rheumatoid arthritis (as per my mother); and heart disease, and bowel and liver cancer (as per my father). I believe a little short-term pain for a better quality and extension of life is well worth the effort.

Remember it's probably taken 4-5 decades of ignorance and neglect to clog your colon and build up toxins in your liver and body until most of your organs become inefficient and blocked. Please allow a couple of years of consistent effort to release these toxins, repair your body and replace damaged cells with better ones. If you are taking supplements to support your changes, please give them **at least** **3-4 months** to assist your body in its healing.

The alternative is to possibly continue along the old journey towards lower quality of life, drugs, surgery, dependence and possibly premature passing.

A Possible Future Scenario?

If ever there was a sudden shortage of fuel (for example), and we couldn't drive and goods couldn't be delivered to local supermarkets, and as a result we weren't to be able to gain access to 95% of our normal supermarket food or fast food stores, what would happen?

We'd be forced to eat from our own garden or local markets by necessity, and the result would be a mass-community detox as people trundle off to their doctors for prescriptions to resolve their (flu-like) symptoms. It's unlikely they will understand that they're actually detoxing.

Exercise

"People who don't find time for exercise, sooner or later will have to find time for illness," 15th Earl of Derby.

As mentioned previously, if you don't work physically hard, exercise is necessary to support the body in numerous ways, especially through the mature stages of life. Not only does it strengthen muscles, bones, tendons, ligaments and cartilage, but also keeps joints and the skeleton in line.

Exercise helps preserve memory and reduces the risk of developing dementia. US research found walking for 40 minutes a few times a week boosts the hippocampus, an area of the brain that creates memories. This small amount of exercise also extends life by an additional two years — for free☺.

A Canadian study conducted by Eric Larose of the 'Institut Universitaire de Cardiologie et de Pneumologie de Quebec and Universite Laval' concluded that regular exercise decreases your cardiovascular risk by a factor of two or three. At the other end of the scale, overdoing exercise, for example running marathons, can increase risk factors by seven (during the run). Moderation, regularity and balance are required to support your body best.

Exercise also supplies extra oxygen to cells throughout the body, assisting in alkalising the body — something a sedentary person is deprived of. When sitting, we only use the top two thirds of the lungs. However, the lower third of the lungs supplies two thirds of the body's oxygen and is fully utilised during exercise. Oxygen stimulates white blood cell production; white blood cells are the foundation of the immune system.

Veins carrying deoxygenated blood back to the heart rely on muscle contractions of the major muscle groups to push the blood along. If you don't exercise regularly, the blood stagnates in the lower extremities of the limbs and you risk varicose veins and other circulatory ailments.

Added bonuses of exercise are the 'feel-good' and supportive hormones produced that assist your mental health too:

- **Growth hormone** — Released from the pituitary gland in the brain, growth hormones burn fat and help keep blood glucose at normal levels. It strengthens bones, tendons, and ligaments through stimulating natural protein production.
- **Endorphins** — Again released from the pituitary gland, numerous endorphins block pain, decrease appetite, reduces anxiety and make you feel happier.
- **Oestrogen** — Oestradiol increases fat breakdown, metabolism and libido, and elevates mood.
- **Testosterone** — Maintains muscle tone, strength and volume in both sexes. Increases metabolism and elevates confidence.
- **Adrenaline** — Breaks down fat and glycogen (stored carbohydrates) in muscles and liver.
- **Thyroxine (T4)** — Produced in the thyroid, increases metabolic rate and calorie burn.
- **Insulin** — Decreases blood sugar levels and reduces appetite.
- **Glucagon** — Initiates the release of blood sugar and fat from the liver.

My Exercise Regime

I endeavour to exercise for 45–60 mins every morning, six days a week, followed by the inversion bed. Occasionally when I have appointments, it's raining or am not feeling up to it, I'll do less or skip a day.

Monday — walk 4km (2 ½ miles) 45 mins.

Tuesday — gym workout to maintain strength in the upper body and quads

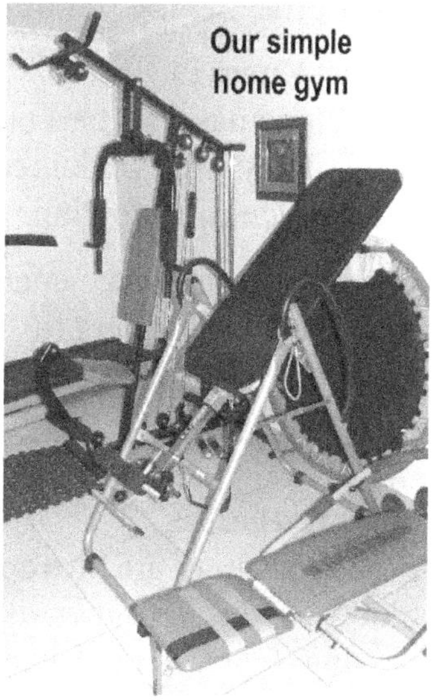

Wednesday & Thursday — walk 4km

Friday — gym workout

Saturday — walk 4km

Sun — rest

Do whatever you can do, to your capacity and level of fitness. Once you get into the routine, you'll look forward to exercising and you'll find it easier to climb stairs, bend over and more.

When I exercise, I listen to audio books and podcasts through my phone so I am gaining education as I walk and time passes quickly.

Chapter 9

Colon Cleansing Treatments

Enemas and Colonics
Colon cleansing through enemas and colonics has been recorded in history since 600 BC as noted in Babylonian inscriptions. Enemas were a normal part of medical treatment up to the 1950s. So, it's not new; you simply haven't kept up!

Colon Hydrotherapy
Colonic hydrotherapy is different to enemas as you will soon read.

Also known as colonic irrigation. Under controlled conditions, a therapist inserts a catheter into the anus and moves water into the colon at varying temperature and pressure via a tube. The colon is 'flushed' several times and the results can be seen through a clear viewing tube exhibiting the removed mucus, parasites, undigested food, deep-seated faecal matter and dead tissue. The procedure takes around 45 minutes.

By removing unwanted material from the colon wall, the peristaltic action can function uninhibited and if the colon has been distorted by segmentation or strictures, it allows the colon to come back into shape of its own accord. Colonics also stimulates reflex points in the colon that relate to all organs in the body.

I've had several colonics and found them relaxing, worthwhile and I felt good afterwards, having removed a great deal of mucus and old faecal matter.

Water Enemas

Water enemas can be conducted by one's self in a bathroom, near a toilet bowl. They are conducted in a similar manner to the details in the coffee enema section following.

Filtered, warm water enemas are most common; however other ingredients can be added for benefit. Enemas can be helpful on occasions when you are experiencing severe constipation.

Coffee Enemas (Taking your Coffee the Right Way)

Why Bother?

Coffee enemas are extremely supportive for detoxing the liver by dilating blood vessels and increasing bile flow, releasing toxins into the bowel for passing. Coffee enemas also increase glutathione production in the liver and therefore reducing free radicals. I believe so much in the power of coffee enemas that I have devoted this chapter to fully inform you, so you can be confident in trying it.

Easy Detoxing

One of the most rewarding techniques I've used to remove toxins and assist with feeling better from detox symptoms is having coffee enemas. Whenever I have pain in the liver, headache, aching joints, feeling foggy brained, continually fatigued, tired or lethargic (detox symptoms), I conduct a coffee enema in my bathroom — usually in the morning. These days I have a coffee enema daily after exercise.

I know the thought of having enemas might sound gross to some readers and you won't even go there, but believe me, after your first experience (which you may find somewhat awkward until you establish your own technique and rhythm) you will look forward to each experience as a meditative and cleansing experience.

If your mind won't even contemplate an enema, try to open your thinking and allow new experiences into your life. You need to change something for change to happen in our health. Or you could do nothing and continue complaining and whinging☹.

The History of Coffee Enemas

Coffee enemas evolved from World War I, when medical supplies were low and a nurse wanted to relieve the pain of soldiers in hospital. The nurse, having some experience in simple water enemas, which were regularly used by medical staff in those days, used coffee left over from her doctor's use (to keep the doctors awake). Her thinking was, "if it's good for the doctors, it is probably good for the patient". She found that the coffee enema relieved the soldiers' pain, headaches and lifted their overall feeling of wellbeing. Water enemas were generally ordered for each soldier following surgery anyway.

How Coffee Enemas Work

When coffee is taken through the rectum, caffeine from the coffee is taken up via the haemorrhoidal blood vessels, then through the portal vein, directly to the liver and proceeds to dilate (open-up, expand) blood vessels and capillaries rather than shrinking them, like when coffee is ingested through the mouth. In doing so, the liver releases toxins into the blood and bile that may have been trapped in the liver's filtering process. It also stimulates the flow of bile (which is the body's alkaliser and cleaner). The bile carries the toxins via the bile duct into the duodenum, then into the small intestine for passing. The increase of bile in the small intestines dramatically increases the production of a major hormone called **glutathione S-transferase (GST) by up to 700%.** GST gobbles up free radicals, assisting to alkalise the body. *(see 'Glutathione' previously).*

Remembering that the entire body's blood is filtered through the liver every three minutes; the end result is that many toxins are shifted from storage in the liver for release through the bowel. This can leave you feeling instantly refreshed, energised and less grumpy (yes, occasionally men get grumpy). I have even experienced instant relief from headache and pain, and an increase in focus and energy on many occasions.

Key Points

1. Always endeavour to have a natural bowel motion **before** your coffee enema. Because of the regularity of my own coffee enemas, I find my body triggers (stimulates) my motion forward as I'm setting up for my enema. Your body is part of your mind — it knows what to do. "Do it and --it will come," maybe not at first, but with regularity, your body will adjust.

2. If you can't have a natural bowel motion prior, conduct a simple water enema prior to the coffee enema. If you don't release the stored faeces from the colon, there will be little space for the diluted coffee liquid to be held.

3. Use **organic ground coffee beans**, <u>not instant coffee</u>. Sounds obvious, however, we know of a few of people who didn't read the details and used instant coffee.

4. Generally, you can have a coffee enema one to three times per week. If you are detoxing or suffering from pain, headaches, or similar, you can

take a coffee enema daily. If you have a major disease like cancer, you can have coffee enemas up to three times a day according to Dr Max Gerson, the originator of the internationally recognised Gerson Therapy that has saved many terminally ill patients in natural ways.

5. If you are having several enemas in one day, it is difficult to have natural motions between, but take plenty of fibre and probiotics and try have at least one natural motion before your first enema, so the muscles performing the peristalsis action in the colon are naturally exercised.
6. Keep everything clean and as sterile as possible.
7. Occasionally (maybe once a month or weekly at the most) you can add a few **Magnesium Chloride** flakes and ¼ teaspoon of practitioner-grade **Bicarbonate Soda** to the mix. This will alkalise the coffee mix. As mentioned earlier, the bowel and friendly gut bacteria operate best in an acid environment, so feeding an alkaline coffee mix into the liver (via the bowel) stirs things up and can release a lot more toxins and built-up waste. Ensure you have a good probiotic afterwards to replace the gut bacteria that may have been displaced by the alkalinity.
8. Enema kits are for one person only and should not be shared, however you can purchase an extra catheter for personal use and share the use of the remainder of the kit. Choose a kit with a plastic jug/bowl at the top, not a closed bag. They can be difficult to clean over time, that's why I suggest a cheaper plastic model. We've found the best value on eBay and use my image as a guide and ensure it holds at least 1 litre.

The Coffee Enema Process

I will describe how I set up my space for a coffee enema. This works for me, but remember, everyone's bathroom layout, facilities and bodies are different. You might want to adapt to suit your situation.

Bathroom Space

- Privacy! You can't relax adequately if you know you might be disturbed by your partner, children, pets, phones, emails, couriers, etc. Ensure you create a space and time to relax. Post a note on your front door if needed.
- Timing? Allow 30-45 minutes to fully prepare and clean up afterwards.
- You will need somewhere to hang your enema kit at about doorknob/towel rack height or top of the shower partition. The higher you hang the enema kit, the greater the flow. The hanging place is best to be in front of you when you lie on your right-hand side, on the floor with your knees bent. This allows you to easily manage the opening and closing of the tube valve.
- You need access to a toilet bowl either in the same bathroom or next room

— ensure no one else will be using it and you can move from room to room without embarrassment. Over several years, I have enjoyed coffee enemas in numerous houses with different bathroom layouts and they've all worked fine.

- One of the most difficult places I enjoyed coffee enemas was on a boat cruise where I used 2 double-shot espresso as a base, then added bottled water. The bathroom was so small, I had to hang my feet out the door, but the regular enemas helped me cope with the rich food and good times that boat cruises offer.

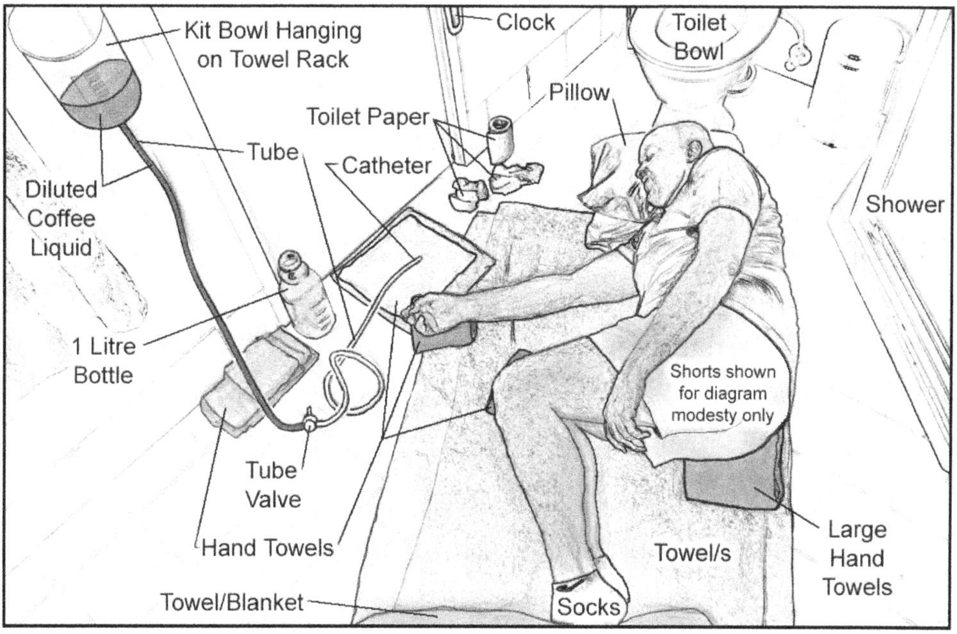

Coffee Enema — 'Must Have' Equipment:

- Enema kit. Note; over time, the valve (being plastic) may break or stop working. If this happens, use a large bulldog (or fold-back) clip, bend the main tube (not the catheter) then clamp it.
- Hook
- Clock or timer
- Bathroom towel
- Pillow
- Small hand towels
- 1-metre-long (3 ft) piece of toilet paper or tissues — scrunched
- 1-litre bottle or jug marked at 250ml, 500ml, 750ml and1 litre increments

- 250 ml (1 cup) of prepared coffee liquid (see next)
- 250 ml (1 cup) hot water
- 200–500 ml (1–2 cups) filtered cold water
- Olive oil (or similar lubricating oil or nappy-rash cream)
- Hydrogen peroxide (for occasional sterilising)
- Note — if you need to have a simple water enema prior, you will need a second bottle or jug and another 250 ml (1 cup) of hot water, plus another 500–750 ml (2–3 cups) of filtered cold water.

Coffee Enema — 'Nice to Have' Equipment:

- Socks for your feet in cooler weather
- Heater or fan (for a comfortable temperature)
- Relaxation music. Avoid phone calls, texting and Facebook
- An extra bath towel or yoga mat to place under you, which will help insulate you from cold bathroom tiles
- If it's cold, a large towel to act as a blanket

Coffee Liquid Preparation

- Large pot with a lid to make 2 litres
- 250g (12oz) of organic ground coffee. Don't use instant coffee!
- 2 litres (8 cups) of filtered, boiling water
- 2-litre storage bottle or jug
- Strainer or sieve

1. Place the ground coffee and boiling water into the pot and bring to boil. Once boiling, **simmer for 30 minutes**. Ideally, leave this mixture to cool and settle for a day. If you need to use the coffee liquid sooner, you can do so, but know that the water will be hot and there will be some sediment suspended in the liquid regardless of how much you filter.
2. Once cooled and settled, use the strainer over the storage bottle to filter the coffee liquid and discard the sediment in the garden. If you find that some of the water has evaporated during the boiling process, simply top up with filtered water to make two litres.
3. This process will make enough liquid for eight enema procedures and should be kept in the refrigerator.

Coffee Enema Preparation

Diluted Coffee Liquid for Enema

1. Pour 250-350 ml (1 cup) of coffee liquid into a 1 litre (2 pints) jug.
2. Then add 150–250 ml (5–8 oz) of filtered hot water. Adjust the amount of hot water to about the temperature that matches your body or less. If you accidentally make your mixture too hot, simply add a few ice cubes to cool it down quickly without adding excessive water. It is okay to use the liquid at room temperature if you like.
3. Top up with filtered water to make a total of 500+ ml (2 cups) of diluted coffee liquid, but if this is too much for the size of your colon, reduce to around 250 ml (1 cup). Everybody's colon holds a different amount; adjust to what suits you. Personally, I use 700 ml (just over 2 cups).
4. As you become more familiar with the process and if it's comfortable, you can use up to 1 litre (2 pints) of liquid, but start small. The main advantage of taking the maximum liquid for your colon is that the liquid should travel further towards the transverse colon where more caffeine is likely to be absorbed — there is less absorption in the descending colon. In having more liquid, the extra liquid is simply extra water; the amount of coffee stays the same.
5. It's better to take less and keep it held longer than taking more and must release too quickly.

Bathroom Preparation

- Whilst preparing, in your mind, start thinking about passing a motion.
- Lay the towel/s on the floor with the long side facing the hanging point for the enema kit.
- Place a folded large hand towel in the position where your hip will lie on the towel to catch any spillage.
- Place your pillow at the headspace.
- Place your hand towels on the floor in front of you for easy access.
- If you are using the large towel as a blanket, have that ready at your feet.
- Scrunch your 1-metre-long (3 ft) toilet tissue and have it on the floor within easy access to your hands.
- Place your clock, timer or phone on the floor in front of you so you can easily see the time.
- For easy access, the toilet bowl seat should be down, with the lid up. If your toilet is separate from your bathroom, ensure the door is open and

there is a roll of toilet paper handy.

- Have your bottle of diluted coffee liquid ready for use.
- Have your lubricating oil handy.
- Hang your enema kit on your towel rack, doorknob or similar. Ensure the **tube valve is closed**.
- At about this time, I usually allow my body to pass a natural bowel motion. Prior, I often hold from urinating from around 30 minutes before, which tends to intensify the release of a motion at my desired timing. I usually have my enema after my morning walk, which stimulates the bowel too. You have more control over your body than most realise.
- **If a natural bowel motion is not forthcoming**, or you have not had a bowel release within the previous two to three hours, then it's helpful to conduct a simple water enema which follows similar lines to the coffee enema, but without the coffee liquid *(see 'Water Enema' previously)*. You should allow as much water liquid into the colon as you need to release any stools waiting. Hold the water inside for as long as you can (often around 5–10 mins) and enjoy a relaxing release. Then proceed to enjoy your coffee enema.
- **If you have a natural bowel motion**, then proceed onward...
- Pour the diluted coffee liquid into the enema container (kit bowl)
- Hold the end of the catheter up higher than the kit bowl
- Place a few drops of oil on one finger and wipe it over the end of the catheter and wipe the residue around your anus. This lubricates for insertion. Then wash your hands.
- Ensure your bladder is empty before you proceed. You want to avoid getting up to urinate during the process.

Taking your Coffee Enema

Now you are ready to enjoy your 'long black' ☺

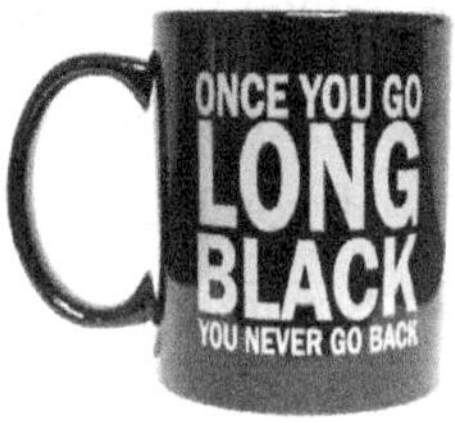

- Lie on the floor on your right side on the towel/s. Your liver is on the right side of your body and gravity helps feed the coffee liquid along the transverse colon.
- Ensure you are lying comfortably with your hips on the folded hand towel
- Place a couple of hand towels (or a cushion) between your knees
- If you have a large towel acting as a blanket, have this pulled over your ankles so it is easy to simply pull up if needed

- Lay your head on the pillow
- Reach over and grab the end of the lubricated catheter and insert it into your anus between 10-30 cm (4-12").
- Open the valve and drain the diluted coffee liquid from the tube into your anus, then turn the valve off and remove the tube from your anus.
- Place the end of the catheter on a hand towel or toilet paper where leaking residue will be absorbed.
- Wipe your anal area with some scrunched toilet paper or tissue
- Take note of the time
- **How long should you hold the liquid?** As mentioned earlier, your liver filters all your body's blood every three minutes. So, try to hold the liquid in multiples of three minutes and for at least 12–15 minutes. Try to make 21 minutes if you can, or 30 minutes if possible. If you can't make 12 minutes, have a release, then set up again and add on the extra minutes you missed. The time you can hold varies from time to time, especially if you are new to this process. Tests have shown that the maximum amount of caffeine is taken up within 12–15 minutes. If it is comfortable to hold the diluted coffee liquid, I enjoy the extra 10–15 minutes.
- Pull up your large towel/blanket and relax — meditate. Listen to relaxation music or learn by watching videos on BitChute, TED, YouTube, etc.
- If bowel pressure builds to a point where you just have to release, there are a couple of things you can do. Hold the scrunched toilet paper at your anus with finger pressure towards your anus. Sometimes gas can be trapped within pockets of the colon, so moving your abdominal muscles around to stimulate the release of the trapped gas and helps tremendously. Next time reduce the amount of liquid you use.
- At the end of the process, usually one bowel release will occur, but a couple is also normal.
- On the same day I have a coffee enema, and often for days afterwards, I can feel my liver continually moving toxins through for release. Sometimes the flatulence I release afterwards can be extremely sulphurous and putrid, indicating some old toxins have been released.
- After your bowel release, study your motion, which is a good habit. Studying your poo gives you great feedback on how your digestive and elimination system is operating. Look for parasites, blood, mucus, undigested matter like corn, carrots or peas. Some gallstones may have even been released.

- I usually have a shower afterwards, but the process is clean enough to not need a shower.
- If necessary, apply just a dab of nappy-rash cream (containing zinc and castor oil) to your anus to help ease any irritation.

Immediately After

Now that you have removed most of the matter from your colon, you need to have a glass of **water, good bacteria (probiotics) and fibre** to assist building your next motion that should move through in the next 8–12 hours.

Clean Up

- Use any leftover scrunched toilet paper to clean the underside of the toilet seat and around the top of the toilet bowl, then flush.
- Wash any soiled towels
- Wash the enema kit with warm water and hang to dry. Ensure it is dry before storing. It's important to maintain good hygiene practices – allowing bacteria to grow in your enema kit could transfer the unsupportive bacteria to the bowel causing illness.
- You can use 3–6% hydrogen peroxide in water to clean your enema kit
- Occasionally, every few weeks, I run a metre-long, thin pipe cleaner through the tubes (pipe cleaners can be difficult to source; I adapt ours from items purchased off eBay). Then, I fill the whole tube with hydrogen peroxide and leave it to sit for a day. A large paper clip is useful to clamp the tube at the right height so that all the tube is filled. I have found hydrogen peroxide to be one of the best killers of unsupportive bacteria since the year dot. We use it on open cuts, infections, and the like — often avoiding the use of antibiotics. Peroxide is available at most pharmacies and supermarkets in the healthcare section.

Disclaimer: You should always consult your natural health practitioner prior to treatment. The supplier of this information is not responsible for any unexpected outcomes or consequences from this treatment. Treatment is your choice; I have simply explained what I do.

Your life is an expression of your mind.
The quality of your life is brought about
by the quality of your thinking -
Think about that…
Thoughts Produce Actions
Look at what you are Thinking

From the 'Theme from Time'

Chapter 10

Taking Responsibility for Your Health!

Big Pharma and the Sickness Industrial Complex

The medical industrial complex uses "care" as a marketing tool, not motivation!

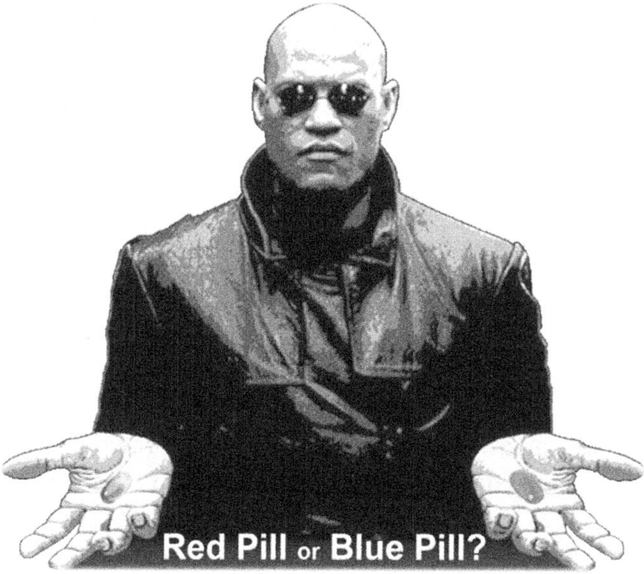

Remember the 1999 movie trilogy, "The Matrix"

Morpheus offers Neo the blue pill and he will continue in a world that has been pulled over his eyes to blind him from the truth – that he is a slave to the physical matrix. Or take the red pill and go down the rabbit hole and see what's really happening behind the illusion called life.

This is your red pill moment…

Who Do You Listen To?

My intent in writing on this topic is not to conduct a massive exposé on the sickness industrial complex. There are already plenty of books and documentaries on this topic. It's my intention to provide enough references to inspire you to check the facts for yourself. You'll find the following information hard to believe at first, as I did initially, so you're more likely to believe the facts when you check for yourself.

You might be surprised to know that the only thing that can **legally treat a disease are pharmaceutical drugs** – that's how successful Big Pharma lobbyists have been at influencing governments.

I want to make the point that the sickness industry also does a great deal of good work for trauma patients, correctional procedures, and more. I feel most practitioners and nurses are doing their best for their patients, but are unknowingly too close (and too busy) to observe the system and realise they're unwittingly part of a corrupt system — their work paradigm is normal to them and they won't be aligned with my information because their livelihood is linked to the system and therefore will mostly be critical.

Your Choice

Self-responsibility health crusaders like Del Bigtree (The Highwire – YouTube) and Elaine Hollingsworth (www.doctorsaredangerous.com) have been exposing such information for decades without one legal challenge, because their information is factual and accurate and Big Pharma don't want to create headlines that are unsupportive to their subversive cause.

Something that spurs me on in my quest to communicate knowledge and logic to the public to empower them to take control of their own health is Mahatma Gandhi's quote, "When I despair, I remember that all through history the way of truth and love has always won. There have been tyrants and murderers and for a time they can seem invincible, but in the end the always fall... always!"

We were all raised as children to know that, 'doctors and scientists are wise people who know everything — whatever they say is true'. If a doctor makes a statement, we believe it to be true — it's in our social consciousness. Even governments will not challenge medical statements from doctors.

However, recent history regarding the over prescription of antibiotics, opioids and statins has shown that doctors are neither always right nor trustworthy. Society has also found similar issues with clergy, bankers, CEOs and lawyers.

The 'qualified,' educated elite will often be quoted to prove a point and give information credibility. Indeed, I have used this tactic in my books too. However, I have also researched several outlets, provided links and encouraged you to do your own research.

If you are ever challenged with medical, life changing decisions, I urge you to **always obtain a second (or third) opinion, take your time,** seek the opinion of someone **trusted in the natural healing field** too and research the internet, but **avoid** the medically-biased **Google** search engine.

Open your mind to the possibility that your doctor may believe what s/he is saying, but the information may not be up-to-date or accurate as they can only repeat what they have remembered through Big Pharma's teaching system. I have made numerous mentions of how our family have been treated for ailments that were incorrectly diagnosed.

Often doctors qualify as doctors because they have good memories. They are intelligent and have invested hundreds of thousands of dollars and the best part of a decade to **learn through institution-tuition rather than intuition.** Doctors will often hold their ground and be un-swaying to alternative evidence presented to justify their position; a sort of cognitive dissonance. Therefore, doctors will mostly never be interested if you tell them about natural remedies, food or supplements you've been using to treat your condition with success. They won't want to rock the boat of the establishment.

You may not have heard of the NNT (Number Needed to Treat) which is a medical term for the number of people who need to be treated (drugs, surgery, etc.) before one single person gains benefit; the lower the number – the better.

Big Pharma giant GlaxoSmithKline (GSK) themselves calculate that 90% of all drugs only work in 50% of the people. You should ask your doctor what is the NNT for the treatment they are prescribing for your situation.

I have a 22-year-old friend from Ireland who was diagnosed with a brain tumour. He conducted his own research and supplemented with iodine. A year later, scans showed the tumour had shrunk dramatically. He expected his doctor to celebrate and tell the medical community of this new 'cure' for this type of cancer. Instead, his doctor said that he must follow 'the script' and only recommend treatment that he was taught at medical college, otherwise his doctor was open to being disbarred by the sickness system and being sued by his patients.

Doctors are taught basic anatomy for the first few years, then told what drugs to prescribe to treat specific ailments, after which they do an internship at a hospital to 'practice.' If they don't follow what they have been taught, they can be open to a negligence lawsuit, so are keen to flow with the system. There are a few rogue doctors who have stepped out of the system to expose some of Big Pharma's tricks (like Dr Mercola).

Doctors are **not** trained extensively in nutrition, digestion or elimination and therefore may make conservative, safe decisions when answering your questions about food, herbs or constipation. Instead of saying, "I don't know", doctors may tell you what they have been told to say through their medical training like, "It's probably a virus". Doctors don't understand that a disease is not really a disease; it's symptoms of the body's adaption to a toxic, deficient environment.

Symptoms are simply the result of an imbalance that has existed for years. Symptoms are like the oil warning light in your car, you can simply fix the symptom by covering it up with tape, but the underlying condition remains, and your engine will eventually blow up. Taking medication (painkillers) to cover up the symptom (pain) without fixing the cause, will allow your body to (most likely) eventually present a terminal illness.

Government Administration

Big Pharma is the colloquial name given to large, multi-national pharmaceutical companies either singularly or collectively, or the self-supporting system surrounding the sickness industry. The government medical bureaucrats — the TGA (Therapeutic Goods Administration) in Australia and the FDA (Food and Drug Administration) in the US — give the appearance of being somewhat tainted and compromised by the fact that they receive most of their funding through approvals of drugs and procedures from Big Pharma. Therefore any person working within the administration (or within Big Pharma) knows the game they must play to keep their job and sustain a multi-trillion dollar industry that involves factories, hospitals, universities, doctors, nurses, clinics, pharmacists, receptionists, clerks, accountants, couriers, sales reps, bureaucrats, ambulance drivers, equipment manufacturers and suppliers, warehouse distribution, pathology labs, nursing homes, rehabilitation centres, the construction industry, advertising, printing, newspapers, radio, TV, even charities, hotels and restaurants.

In the US, the FDA receives around 75% of its funding from Big Pharma. The lamestream media receives over $25-billion per year in advertising from Big Pharma, that's why the media give natural therapies a hard time. The World Health Organisation (WHO) receives 50% of its funding from Big Pharma, mostly for vaccination programs.

Big Pharma appears to lobby governments to create laws that limit the promotion and distribution of natural remedies (*can't* be patented — low profit) and promote the sale their synthetic chemical-based drugs (*can* be patented — high profit). Using arguments that initially seem logical, they advise the government to legislate for scientific proof for the effectiveness of natural therapies, herbs and products (despite hundreds or thousands of year's history). At the same time, government bureaucrats believe Big Pharma has "done the research" in their own labs and proved their drug works better than the previous situation, or that the "benefits outweigh the risks" (side-effects). The bureaucrats don't actually check or confirm the clinical study results presented by Big Pharma — it would be too costly. If a company is paying for scientific research, they want a viable result they can profit from and the 'in-house' research is at times biased towards the company's needs, corrupted and shouldn't be trusted. That's why audited, triple blind placebo studies are so important.

The administration has expert panels to approve drug applications and panels consist of mostly professionals with financial links to Big Pharma. It's like asking the fox to make decisions regarding the structure of a hen house.

Big Pharma may then continue to lobby the government for the inclusion of their expensive drug on the Pharmaceutical Benefits Scheme (PBS) medicine list – the 'Holy Grail'. The PBS is a list of 'perceived', necessary chemical drugs or procedures that are subsidised by the government – you, the taxpayer. The list runs at about 140 applications per year from fifty or so Big Pharma companies in Australia, allowing the Australian government to pay over $8.3 billion per year of our tax money to Big Pharma *(see 'Medicines Australia' inset later)* in the form of public subsidies.

There are over 560,000 patented drugs (made from chemicals which may be toxic to the body) and every drug has an average of 70 side-effects.

Most active (chemical) ingredients used in drugs can have up to 75 different brand names and may be prescribed for over 300 different diseases.

As evidence that Big Pharma don't always conduct extensive and accurate, clinical testing of drugs, try searching (but not on Google) these products: Voltaren, Vioxx, Avandia, Ketek, Prexige and Zelnorm (for IBS) which have all been withdrawn from sale because of significant side-effects or death. A quick search on the internet should reveal some further sixty-plus approved drugs that have been withdrawn. Bureaucrats are moving away from time-consuming, expensive clinical, triple blind, placebo studies in lieu of gene history and computer modelling, adjusting product approvals as the public reacts with negative side-effects (or as deaths occur) to new drugs — dangerous territory, I feel.

Big Pharma funds medical students' activities, parties, doctors' training, education events, hospitals, universities, lobbyists, and research in an effective, self-serving system.

There seems to be a cosy, co-dependent web of convenience between Big Pharma, institutions (charities and associations), administrations and government (bureaucracy) with staff often swapping jobs between organisations and government departments.

The main purpose of a public company is to raise capital, minimise liability and maximise profits for shareholders. Laws place little emphasis on social, health outcomes or environmental consequences from their actions. Laws do however limit or negate litigation towards pharmaceutical companies regarding some products like vaccines.

In 1982 Dr Richard Crout, FDA's director of the Bureau of Drugs said, "I never have and never will approve a new drug to an individual, but only to a large pharmaceutical firm with unlimited finances." What chance do small companies or individuals have for discovery, innovation or testing herbs?

And the laws passed by the government are enforced with bias and passion – some at gunpoint. Remember 2003 in Australia when Pan Pharmaceuticals was raided and closed by an overzealous TGA? At lightning speed, within six months of the raid, a liquidator (who consults to Big Pharma) was engaged and Pan (worth $500 million) was sold for just $20 million and closed.

The TGA found themselves in court and was fined $50 million plus a further $67.5 million in a following class action by Pan's wholesalers. Keep in mind that this is government money paying the fines — your taxes. It was a cheap way of ridding the market of independent competition that didn't play Big Pharma's game.

There were no deaths caused from Pan's single batch of faulty pharmaceutical drug that was voluntarily withdrawn prior to the raid, unlike the 55,000 American deaths Vioxx caused before its withdrawal. And the TGA has never done an investigation regarding Vioxx in Australia.

The problem for Big Pharma was that Pan was one of the last privately-owned pharmaceutical companies in the world and was large enough to direct sales strategies within Australia (including complimentary medicines); Pan was affecting Big Pharma's profits and ideology. Pan no longer exists and the owner (Jim Selim) died of cancer in 2008, but Big Pharma rolls on. Such is the ruthlessness of pharmaceutical companies when you threaten their profit.

To witness an even more bizarre US version, search for "Burzynski Movie" — Dr Burzynski discovered, tested and patented antineoplaston with a 50-60% success rate of curing cancer (far better than chemo or radiation) from his privately-owned Texas facility. Dr Burzynski is one of the rare survivors who fought Big Pharma and won, but it took him 15 years, millions of dollars while US government agencies spent over $100 million of taxpayer's money to fight him.

To quote a couple of Nobel Prize Laureates... *"The [US] National Cancer Program is a bunch of shit",* Dr James Watson, discoverer of DNA, 1975 (pardon the language, but that's what he said). And *"Everyone should know that cancer research is largely fraud",* Dr Linus Pauling, 1986.

"Truth is incontrovertible;
malice may attack it and ignorance may deride it,
but, in the end, there it is"

Sir Winston Churchill

MEDICINES Australia

HOME | ABOUT US | MEDIA | EVENTS | ISSUES | INFORMATION | CODE OF CONDUCT | LINKS

Key industry facts medicinesaustralia.com.au/code-of-conduct/education-events-reports

- In 2008/09 there were 14,042 people employed in human pharmaceutical and medicinal product manufacturing, which had sales and service income of $8.2 billion and paid $1.1 billion in wages and salaries. [1]
- Australian pharmaceutical businesses invested $1023 million on research and development in 2008/09. [2]
- In the 12 months to 30 June 2010, medicinal and pharmaceuticals worth over $ 4.1 billion were exported from Australia, making Pharmaceuticals the largest hi-technology Australian export. [3]
- The Pharmaceutical Benefits Scheme paid $8.3 billion in benefits for listed medicines in 2009/10. [4]
- The Pharmaceutical Benefits Advisory Committee recommended 124 items for listing on the PBS in 2009/10 and 146 items for listing on the PBS in 2008/09. [5]
- 77,800 medical practitioners, 229,100 nurses [6], 77,800 medical practitioners, 229,100 nurses 6, and 19,200 pharmacists were employed in Australia in 2008. [7]

Company Reports Summary

Company Reports Summary 1 October 2010 – 30 March 2011	
Number of reports	38
Number of events	13,873
Number of attendees	* 370,048
Education hours	27,775
Hospitality cost	$13,354,696.13
Average cost of hospitality per head	$36.09
Total cost of events	* $27,424,115.10
Average cost of event per head	$74.11

Vaccination is NOT Science-Based

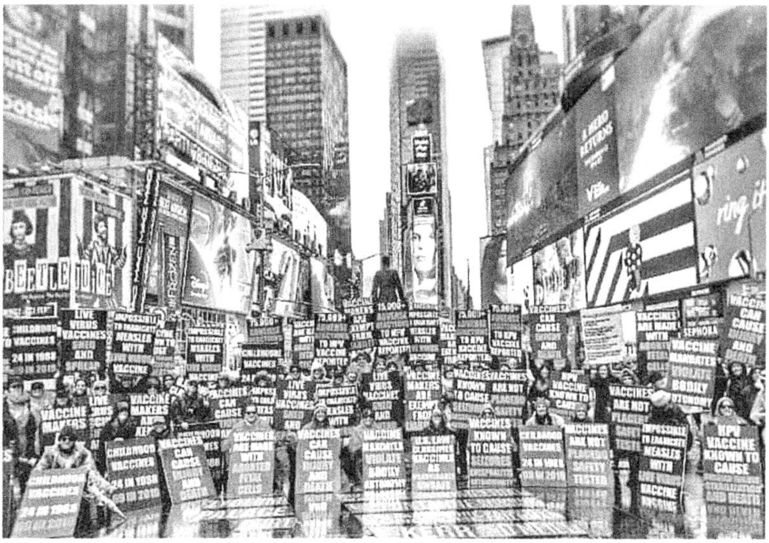

<u>YOU ARE NOT ALONE!</u>

< Vaccination protest in Time Square, New York.

You can fool some of the people some of the time, but not all the people, all the time.

To alleviate unbearable guilt and regret; and before parents decide to vaccinate, the ultimate questions every parent must ask regarding vaccination is... if my child is unlucky enough to be one of the tens of thousands of children permanently damaged every year from vaccination...

1. **Is there anything I could have done to prevent their injury?**
2. **Am I prepared to support my child for the rest of his/her/my life?**

YES, you could have opened your mind and investigated your truth more thoroughly right now (rather than blindly follow to mainstream spiel). This is your opportunity. The evidence is compelling. Please read on...

For the past two print runs of this book, I've declined to mention my view regarding vaccination as it is so divisive in the community. However, Big Pharma have recently tripled-down and persuaded governments to legislate for mandatory vaccination in some countries and I want to encourage you to investigate and find your truth and not just blindly follow – because this really matters. Our ill-informed mainstream sickness industry has manipulated innocent 'sheeple' into bullying, condemnation and isolation of parents that choose to make an informed, science-based choice for their children.

Big Pharma's first tool is to ALWAYS attack the messenger, never discuss the science and make a blanket statement that "vaccines are safe" (trust us – what do they know)? Informed parents simply want to rely on science and facts, and to have the right to choose what goes into their own body, and the bodies of their children. Big Pharma manipulate through basic censoring and propaganda #101 via lamestream news, entertainment, governments, doctors, biased Google, Facebook, Twitter, Wikipedia and YouTube searches.

Don't believe me? Try searching Google for "Dr John Bergman" and see if you can find his website www.drjohnbergman.com on the first two pages. It should appear first on page one, but doesn't appear until half way down on page three (at the time of publishing).

In 1997 we chose not to vaccinate our two children and went through all the isolation and discrimination involved at the time. Both our children have grown to be healthy, mentally strong individuals with strong immune systems. We were ground breakers at the time and (thankfully) we were quietly guided by our

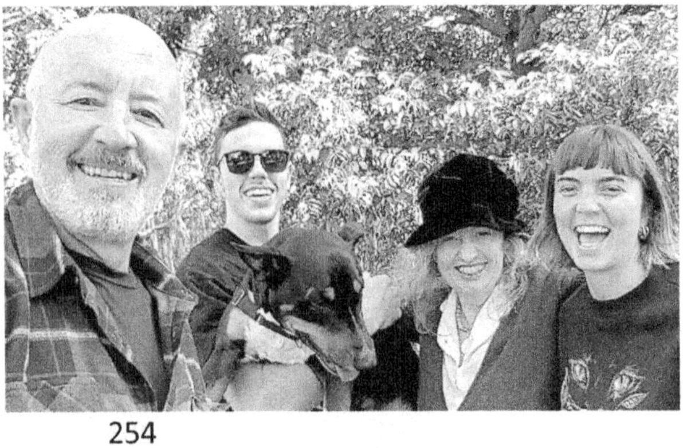

midwife who had seen too many unreported negative events from vaccination.

The science simply has not been done to support the mainstream view and when challenged to produce scientific evidence of the safety and effectiveness of vaccines, at every post the sickness industry comes up short. Government health departments, namely the CDC (Centres for Disease Control and Prevention) in the US have been shown to officially distort, falsify, omit and lie about vaccination facts *(see the movie 'Vaxxed' and 'Vaxxed II').*

According to www.globalresearch.ca the vaccine industry has a US$24 billion annual market, making up around 20% of Big Pharma's profits (mostly funded by taxpayers), therefore vaccination is too big for Big Pharma to let go, regardless of negative health implications on families.

According to Robert F Kennedy Jr (yes, the son of RFK),

- The US Institute of Medicine and the FDA admit that over 150 different injuries are caused by vaccines and those injuries are listed on the inserts of every vaccine vile to protect the company, not the patient (as you don't get to read the inserts and you are not told about the likelihood of injury).
- Since 2009, the four major manufacturers of vaccines in the world have collectively paid over US$35 billion in fines for defrauding government regulators, falsifying science, bribing doctors and lying. Can they be trusted to be telling the truth about vaccines?
- Vaccines are not officially 'medicine', they are called 'biologics' and therefore don't need proof of effectiveness or safety. Vaccine manufacturers are (by law) exempt from liability from injury, death and safety testing of their vaccines.
- No vaccine has been scientifically tested against an audited, triple-blind placebo study and published in peer-reviewed journals, as required for other medical interventions, yet vaccines are essentially forced onto our community as 'safe'.

I am not an "anti-vaxxer" as the lamestream media would like to label me, I am simply "**pro-science**". I want robust science and a choice based on truth and scientific evidence. Choice without coercion and not linked to welfare payments. I want independent regulators to carry out research and swear the truth on oath or risk perjury.

If the truth is what we're currently been told today, then why do lamestream media outlets like NBC in the US falsely alter stock images to spread lies and build fear campaigns about regular "measles epidemics" that don't exist.

December 2019 in **Samoa**, headlines went around the world about their "measles epidemic". But what if you knew the facts and science:

2018

- **July**, a qualified nurse made a big mistake and incorrectly vaccinated two babies with a mix-up of the MMR vaccine and the children tragically died.
- Immediately vaccination stopped until the case was investigated, and new procedures put in place.

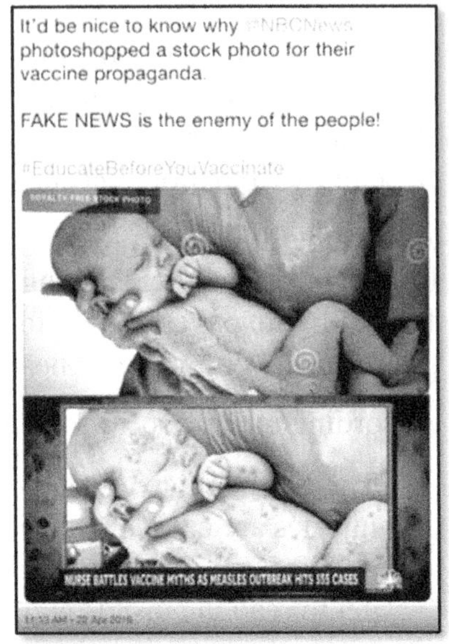

2019

- **April**, vaccination resumes in Samoa.
- **October 1**, UNICEF delivered 115,000 doses of measles vaccine to Samoa – at the time; unfunded, and there was no outbreak.
- **October 12**, the World Bank grants US$34 million for a measles outbreak that was non-existent – it hadn't happened yet, but this was to pay for administering the 115,000 doses of vaccines.
- **November 15**, Samoa declares a 'State of Emergency' over a measles outbreak that gave their government extraordinary powers to force vaccination onto every child.
- **December 9** the World Bank issues a press release announcing they will immediately send an emergency grant of US$34 million. You know, the grant they issued two months ago.
- **Around 30%** of the measles cases were of the particular strain that could have only derive from a vaccine. In other words, the vaccine children were given caused some of the measles cases.

Gardasil

There is too much information to conduct a deep-dive into the Gardasil vaccine here. Gardasil is promoted as a prevention for cervical cancer. Suffices to say the vaccine is given to both girls and boys (boys don't have a cervix) and there is no evidence that it works, and it can possibly cause harm.

Before taking a chance with your teenagers, search Dr Sherri Tenpenny or watch The HighWire episode to become more informed.

Parental Pressure

There is so much pressure on today's young parents with vaccination linked with welfare payments, playgroup, day-care, school, etc. My advice to young parents… Why be normal, why be average? Work smart and become wealthy so you don't need welfare and can pay the price for childcare and schooling of your choice – schooling that doesn't discriminate, even if it's home schooling. Make this goal your primary driver in life and **you will achieve it**.

We've learned over the last few decades that if you don't pay the price now to give your children enough attention and teach them to be free thinkers and develop their natural immune system the way nature intended, you'll pay the price later in medical, disability support, housing and legal fees.

To quote Del Bigtree (producer of the movie "Vaxxed" 1 and 2), *"Since 1988, HHS has been required to submit to Congress details of safety improvements made to vaccines. By filing a FOIA (freedom of information) request, we have learned HHS has failed to file these reports for 30 years!*

To make matters worse, Congress passed protections for Big Pharma, so even if those reports showed the dangers of vaccines, the industry would not be held responsible! Instead, USA taxpayers have been put on the hook for more than $4 billion of vaccine injuries since 1986."

If Big Pharma's corrupt agenda doesn't change soon, we will end up in a few decades with a small group of informed, intelligent, unvaccinated families leading the way in society with purpose and a future, whilst the ill-informed system followers languish behind overcoming autism and illness by taking medically prescribed drugs and treatments. A nice closed-loop system to keep the minions employed but producing nothing as our economy languishes.

From a Family of Medical Professionals…

"I am an MD... My wife was an R.N (Registered Nurse) ... My 2 brothers were MDs... My mother and sister were both RNs... We were all taught the cartoonish CDC version about vaccines 'that all vaccines are safe and effective and do not cause side-effects and vaccines saved the world'... The next thing doctors and nurses are taught/ordered to do is to give all vaccines on the CDC list, just as the CDC's arbitrary schedule dictates, and to tell all of our patients to take all of our vaccines... Our paediatrician talked us into vaccinating our baby son with 3-4 vaccines on the same day... Our healthy, happy, precocious, active, creative, talkative, loving, 2-year-old son was injured by his 4 vaccines and regressed starting that night... The paediatrician said it was NOT from the vaccines, BUT, I was an eye-witness to that immediate problem as his parent... My baby brother (the MD) died from paralysis (Guillain-Barre) after his flu shot... It was a long, agonizing

8-weeks of suffering in the ICU, hooked up to breathing machines, tubes, monitors, and in diapers until he died... The doctors, all specialists and consults, could not tell us what "just happened" but said it was NOT from the vaccine... The US Vaccine Court disagreed and paid the family because they ruled that the vaccine killed him... and Folks, my mother was a RN who was the Head Nurse and ran the largest ER in our medical centre... They "discovered" that she was not current with the CDC's newest list of vaccines and had her take 8-9 vaccines to "catch-up" with the "updated" CDC schedule to keep her job... She could not refuse, or she would lose her job... She then got severe "brain fog" within days, then lost her ability to dial her phone or push the elevator buttons or start her car... She went into diapers and then had to be hospitalized and then died a terrible, tragic, prolonged death drooling and unable to walk, talk, eat or recognised any of her family... None of the specialists and consults could tell her or us what "just happened" but they told us it was "NOT" from those vaccines... It was called the "worst case of aggressive dementia" of "unknown cause" the doctors "had ever seen"... Folks, what killed our mother just weeks after her vaccines was all from her fatal doses of neurotoxic aluminium and mercury ingredients from those vaccines... She left behind her husband, 5 children, 4 grandchildren, and now 7 great-grandchildren..."

From a Head Nurse Whistle-Blower…

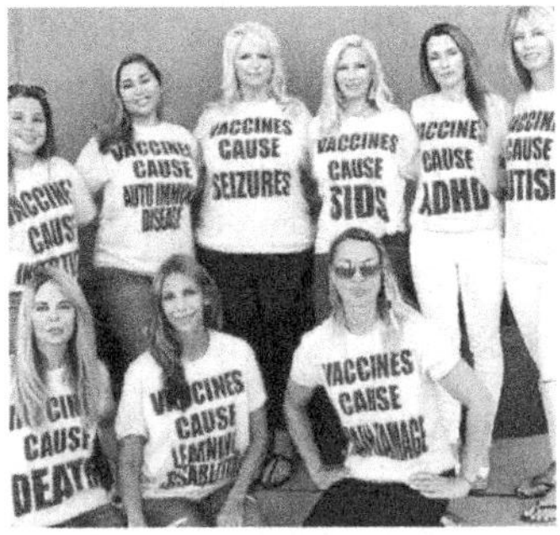
VACCINES CAUSE SEIZURES
VACCINES CAUSE SIDS
CAUSE ADHD
VACCINES CAUSE

"I've been a hospital nurse for 25 years. I got out of floor nursing because of vaccines. I was the charge nurse of 66 telemetry patients, 12 nurses, 3 halls and I have over 400 stories and I'm not exaggerating about vaccines reactions.

I've watched seizures, death, anaphylactic shock, abortions, patients collapsing to the floor because their legs won't work and flaccid arms.

Brilliant nurses in the profession for 20+ years are changing their views on vaccines. To be blunt, they're powerless toxic chemical cocktails.

You want to debate me? I've got 20 years of research behind me. I've been to court and I've lived on the battlefield."

Resources for Research

From the website of Stephanie Messenger

"So how does a mother feel when her baby is dead from vaccines and all she hears from doctors, the government and media is that vaccines are safe and effective?

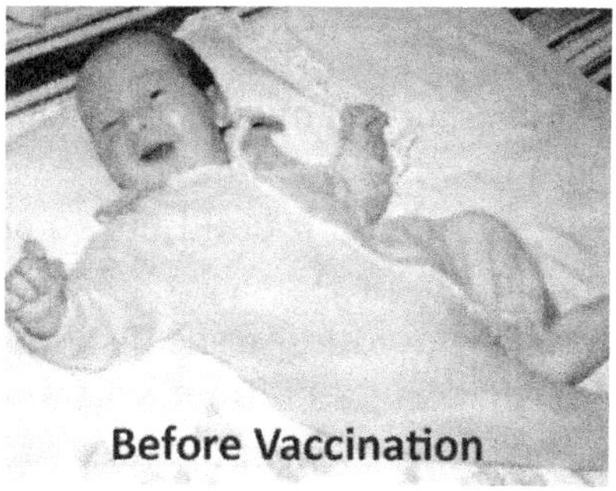
Before Vaccination

I can't say I believed in vaccination. I knew nothing about it, but had it done anyway. It's what you do, right? You do what doctors and baby health clinics tell you and what your parents and the media advise you to do. Well I did it, without so much as a question or thought into it. Within moments of my son receiving his immunisations he was screaming. This continued for most of the day and when he wasn't screaming, he was crying. This was unusual as he was a very happy, placid baby, who was already rolling over at 8 weeks and gooing and gahing at the first sight of his mother. The doctor told me his reactions were 'normal' and he'd be OK in a couple of days.

After the first day he had almost recovered with only some irritability and restlessness noticeable. As the weeks passed, he continued to reach milestones, and all appeared Ok.

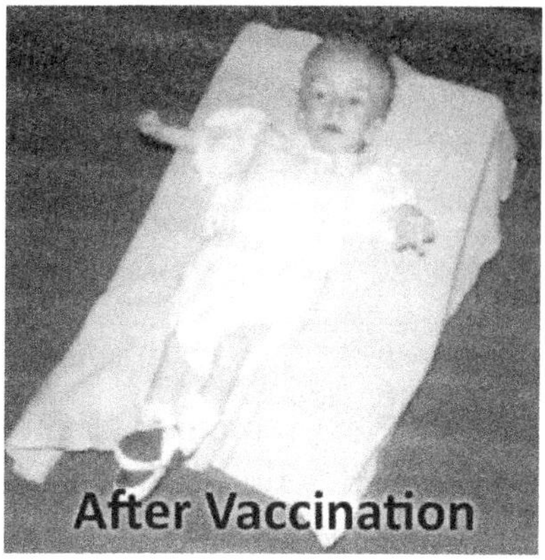
After Vaccination

At 4 months of age I dutifully took him for his next round of vaccinations. This time he screamed louder, and I could not console him at all. I would breastfeed him, only to have him projectile vomit it back up and still the screaming continued. He had never before vomited at all, ever. After he had vomited 2 feeds, I called the doctor and told her what was happening, and she said to stop breastfeeding and give him juice only. He kept some of it down but still vomited often.

The next day I called the doctor and told her I think the vaccines have done this and she told me, "no, it's just a coincidence," but to bring him back in, which I did. She referred me to a specialist. While waiting for the specialist appointment in a few days, my baby boy started doing strange things. He started arching his back and crying out in pain. He was as stiff as a board. His eyes would roll into the back of his head. He didn't have a temperature. He had also started shuddering, but he wasn't cold. (I later learnt from the doctor these were convulsions and seizures). The vomiting continued and I was convinced to give up breastfeeding by the clinic sister. He vomited up the formula also. I was getting very scared."

Go to http://naturematters.info/ *and read the rest of Stephanie's tragic story.*

Luck of the Draw

I don't know anyone who has won lotto, but unfortunately, I know several parents whose children have been permanently injured by vaccination. After vaccinating their children, some cannot speak, some have been diagnosed on the autism or Asperger's spectrum, some are 'couch potatoes' for life, some have behavioural issues, some are permanently depressed, some are dead. I feel the chances of injury from vaccination is higher than the official narrative – **do your research!**

Vaccination Research Websites:

- https://avn.org.au/
- http://naturematters.info/
- https://drjohnbergman.com/
- http://www.thinktwice.com
- http://www.whale.to
- http://www.nvic.org
- http://vactruth.com/2012/01/19/baby-dies-after-first-shots/?utm_source=The
- http://www.ageofautism.com/2010/04/i-am-josh-a-boy-after-his-mmr.html
- https://www.youtube.com/channel/UCq6oOuhSx7ESreh6m9LGy6Q
  (search YouTube for 'The Highwire' with Del Bigtree)

What's Next from our 'Experts'…

At the WHO Global Vaccine Safety Summit in Geneva, Switzerland, in Dec 2019, Prof. Heidi Larson PhD tried to sell the idea that it **wasn't the chemical contents** of the vaccines that were causing tens of thousands of vaccine injuries around the world – in fact, **it was the experience** of having the vaccine. I.e. psychosomatic reactions, or the stress of going to the doctor and being injected causes autism, etc ☹ Really!!! – show us the science!

Prof Larsen is paid by the WHO as Prof of Anthropology, Risk and Decision Scientist Director with the Vaccination Confidence Project and may have tarnished the medical profession forever with this tripe.

The reaction was branded Immunisation Stress Related Responses (ISRR). I'm sure you will hear more about ISRR in the news soon – that's the system.

Opioid Addiction

Opioids (pain relief medication) derive from one of the original medicines, opium. Opioid addiction is now literally a bigger problem than illegal drugs.

Here's one doctor's observation of Big Pharma's opioid addiction system: problem/pain > pain medication (opioid) > anti-inflammatories > opioid > anti-inflammatories > surgery > opioid/chemo/radiation > anti-inflammatories > opioid > sorry it's not working any more > doctors don't know what else to do > you must have the bad gene > patient is still in pain and addicted to opioids > start covertly obtaining opioids > nursing home > palliative care. All the time employing millions of people and charging for every service, paid by health insurance.

Big Pharma's System

Big Pharma has perfected a system and are very patient; sometimes embarking on a ten-year plan to introduce a particular category of drugs.

The sickness industry utilises a classic formula to control the narrative:

1. **Attack the messenger** – never address the science or facts
2. **Exclusivity** – only scientists, doctors and professors know
3. **TRUST US** – as we are the authority, what would they know?
4. **Opacity** – the true facts and truth are kept secret from the public
5. **Reductionism** – only small amounts of information are released piece-meal, to explain complex issues
6. **Centralisation** – information is created and distributed from one source
7. **Censorship** – information from other sources is censored or hidden
8. **Depersonalisation** – the individual doesn't matter, only the group matters

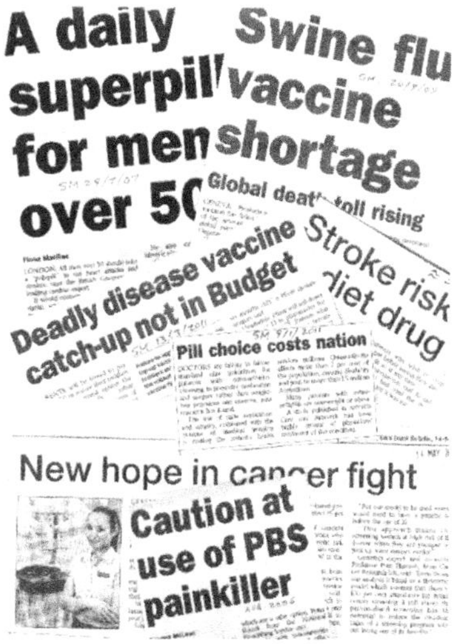
A daily
superpill
for men
Swine flu
vaccine
shortage
Global death toll rising
Stroke risk
Deadly disease vaccine
catch-up not in Budget
Pill choice costs nation
Caution at
use of PBS
painkiller

1. They start with "HOPE", a co-ordinated and consistent TV/radio/web ad or news items, weekday current affairs programs, newspaper articles or social media ads and clickbait. You've seen, read or heard them before; the "latest research shows...", "lab tests may lead to...", "possible cure for cancer with new research…", "gene research may lead to a cure for...", "wonder drug is not on the PBS list and look at all the suffering this causes...", "quit smoking, see your doctor...", "could your doctor help you lose weight?" etc. Or it might be a list of symptoms (disease) that a specific demographic display, explaining that 45% of the population

suffer from this ailment and don't know it (like diabetes, obesity, fatigue, ADHD, IBS). This is to arouse public interest and encourage discussion, neurosis and fear. It's particularly designed to get people to visit their doctor and ask questions, expecting an instant solution for their symptoms via prescribed drugs.

2. Today's negative, fear-based newsfeed (or script) is delivered electronically around the world to newsrooms at 4 am every morning mostly by news agencies, Associated Press (AP) and Reuters, or by a medical association's PR department, Big Pharma directly or 'charity' foundations. Newsrooms love this because it's easy work for them; it comes from a credentialed source; it evokes emotion and human interest and they don't have to check the facts. That's why nearly every news outlet broadcasts similar stories on the same day – they are reading from a script or use common keywords to anchor their story. Often the press release will be complete with pictures or a film package with expert or victim interviews that can go straight to air. Or they might sight a recent biased survey or suggest several experts (media doctors) who are open to be interviewed, to give variety to the story that's been sent to all news outlets. Usually each disease/topic will have a 'key opinion leader' heading most stories. Such experts usually have a long-running financial association with media and Big Pharma. How often have you seen the same medical story on different TV channels on the same day, after you've read it in a morning paper and heard it on the radio? Day after day, Big Pharma's medicine dependent health paradigm is reinforced — unless you are aware.

3. Coupled with the above stories are the 'fear campaigns' and pandemics like SARS, bird flu, swine flu, this year's virus or flu, measles or asthma outbreaks, allergy research, and on and on. Remember swine flu in 2009 when the Australian Government stockpiled over AU$1 billion worth of Tamiflu (which was not proven to work against swine flu) from Roche Pharmaceuticals after the public was shocked by visions of the mass slaughter of pigs in Europe and Asia. Despite offering Tamiflu vaccine freely to the public, very few Australians took up the government's offer and most of the vaccine had to be destroyed after its use-by-date expired. And look — no pandemic; in fact, the truth

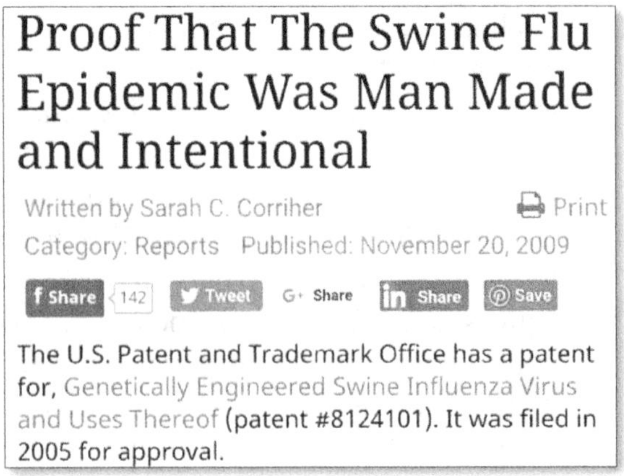
Proof That The Swine Flu Epidemic Was Man Made and Intentional

Written by Sarah C. Corriher Print

Category: Reports Published: November 20, 2009

f Share 142 Tweet G+ Share in Share Save

The U.S. Patent and Trademark Office has a patent for, Genetically Engineered Swine Influenza Virus and Uses Thereof (patent #8124101). It was filed in 2005 for approval.

was later revealed. US patent #8124101 was taken out for Swine Flu in 2005, four years before it hit in 2009, indicating Swine Flu was man made. Search "swine flu hoax" for more info.

Also go to patents.justia.com and search for recent epidemics and/or 'Pirbright Institute' and you will find numerous patents for mutant variants of animal viruses which may cross the animal/human divide. Pirbright's patented products may also be used for vaccines for **Coronavirus** (2015), Foot and Mouth Disease, Swine Fever, etc. Caveat; these patents may not be for the same strain of disease as recent "epidemics", as I haven't had time to go down that rabbit hole yet. Take home message; this is basic marketing; create the problem – provide the solution – make the money.

4. At the same time, Big Pharma may court doctors directly, inviting them to free dinners at the best restaurants, conferences at resorts (holidays), seminars including flights, meals and accommodation. This happens over 13,800 times every year in Australia under the guise of 'educational events', to over 370,000 participants at a cost of over $27 million (see 'Medicines Australia' inset previously).
5. Big Pharma sponsor and influence medical physicians' conferences and offer 'suggestions' for topics and speakers.
6. In 2019, Facebook, Google, YouTube, Instagram, Pinterest, Netflix, Amazon, etc lost consumer trust when they adjusted algorithms bypassing natural health websites and videos that present facts and alternative views and remedies. Now the public only receive lamestream's version of truth. Instead of being platforms, they have become biased publishers with a socio-political propagandists' twist, compromising everyone's freedom to learn, experience and think. Over time, this reorients public perception as George Orwell's 1984 arrives. There are currently several legal cases, plus the US Department of Justice are pursuing tech-giants via Anti-Trust Legislation for breaching the 1st Amendment (freedom of speech), and we know truth (rather than money) will ultimately prevail as it always does.
7. Meanwhile, the various cancer, diabetes and heart foundations (often established by Big Pharma) assist by lobbying the government at the same time and issuing their own news stories in a similar manner. Of course, they will also be promoting their annual daffodil, red nose, pink/white/blue/yellow ribbon fundraising day or week. This money goes towards keeping their staff employed, not necessarily creating results from research. Such associations may also sell their 'tick of approval' for food products (for a fee) as a source of income.
8. Now when 'Joe Public' visits the doctor regarding the symptoms he's seen

on TV or the internet, the doctor knows just the product to prescribe. If enough products are dispensed from that doctor's surgery, the doctor might receive rewards or incentives like more educational events.

9. You won't hear about this in the lamestream media as they have too much to lose should Big Pharma, government departments and charities pull the plug on advertising. Instead they prop-up the system (and bank accounts) with biased headlines like "Natural Medicine a Time Bomb", as published by Brisbane's Sunday Mail, 25 Sept 2011.

10. There is currently a concerted campaign by Big Pharma to discredit complimentary medicine and natural or alternative therapies via TV, news and newspaper stories. The campaign is working towards withdrawing teaching of alternative therapies in universities. The public perceive – if it's taught in universities, it must have credibility, which it does.

11. The TGA and FDA usually require complaints to start an investigation into advertising, products and therapies. Often complaints are made anonymously by companies who have something to gain from an investigation into someone else's business and want to maximise their own profits at someone else's expense. This does not allow for transparency in the process.

One Intelligent View from One Professor

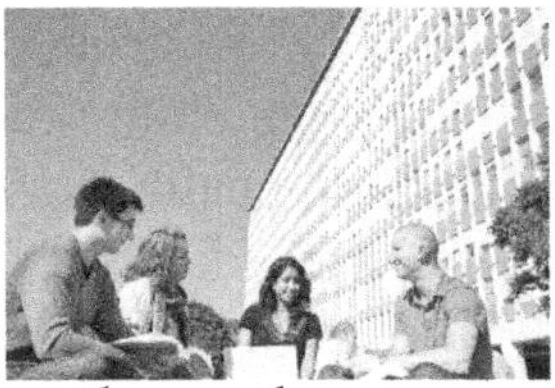

Medicine has long been the subject of vigorous debate about the control of social resources. The formation of modern medicine in the mid-19th century was itself the result of a century long fight for legitimacy among many contending groups. At that time, those who won out – the physicians, the surgeons and those who prepared and sold medicines – had no more evidence to support them than those they defeated. They succeeded on the basis of politics, not of evidence.

Since then, western medicine has grown into a key social institution supported by an elaborate scientific infrastructure. But the battle to defend its status, authority and access to wealth continues unabated.

On the one hand, doctors and their professional organisations are engaged in regular disputes with government about the control of fees and budgets, disciplinary practices and accreditation and the extent of their decision-making power. On the other hand, there is a persistent need to defend the boundaries against opposing forms of healthcare – so-called "complementary" medicine. The latter haven't died out, despite the undisputed success of medicine. Indeed, estimates show that in most developed countries, including Australia, about half the population regularly use health practices outside the mainstream.

By and large, most people would agree that this is unproblematic and regard it as just part of the rough and tumble of democratic life. What's more, the current arrangements are regarded as broadly satisfactory. The ability of individuals to choose their own forms of health care is maintained, subject to some limits on what practitioners can do: in the case of complementary therapists, for example, there are rules – admittedly, not always enforced – to protect vulnerable people from unscrupulous, unfounded and dangerous practices and restrictions on the kinds of claims that can be made in advertising and promotional materials.

Western vs Complementary Medicine

Debates about complementary medicine's place in society have traditionally been vigorous, but reasoned, with the proponents of medicine calling on the authority of science, and their opponents either appealing to their own evidence, which may be derived from traditional practices, or to philosophical theories, or drawing attention to perceived limitations of western medicine.

But there is a current tendency in Australia that may have crossed the line from reasoned discussion to the inappropriate use of power and authority. A group referring to itself as the "Friends of Science in Medicine", made up of senior doctors and scientists, has set itself up to "counter the growth" of what it regards as "pseudoscience in medicine", where "true science" is defined as a set of practices characterised by "an experimental, evidence- based approach".

The strategy of the group is to apply pressure on government and educational institutions through advertisements, the use of the media and sometimes personal criticisms of individuals to withdraw or prohibit funding for complementary health practices. The organisation models itself on groups in the United States and the United Kingdom that have succeeded in having funding removed from certain "alternative medicine" courses.

Philosophically and ethically, the approach of the group is questionable. As any practitioner knows, the role of empirical evidence in determining a particular clinical decision is, at best, partial and tentative. What we do is pose hypotheses on the basis of laboratory or clinical studies, which we then test through careful observation and assessment of outcomes. Each decision is conditioned by the unique circumstances of the individual involved, including his or her personal medical history, goals, values and preferences. It's about opening up possibilities, not closing them down.

The role of universities

The key places in our society where science is conducted are the universities.

These should therefore be protected as sites where unpopular ideas and theories can be examined. They must foster criticisms of orthodoxy, especially those embedded in the institutions of power and authority. Both western medical practitioners and scientists – like myself – and their interlocutors must be challenged and called to account for their claims and judgements.

What is objectionable about Friends of Science in Medicine is their lack of respect for the fragile balance on which genuine dialogues about knowledge and ethics depend, and their readiness to resort to the use of power and authority to win an intellectual debate. Of course, the medical research and teaching budgets are in the hundreds of millions of dollars, so the power is on their side. Although they may therefore win the battle, the trouble is that control of wealth and the institutions of authority does not generate truth.

Clear thinking

None of this means that there are not problems, either with complementary medicines or with aspects of western medicine. In both cases, vulnerable members of the community need to be protected from exaggerated or misleading claims. In both cases, the evidence – in all its forms – needs to be scrutinised and presented clearly and fairly to patients. And in both cases, the process of communication must be open, respectful and free of contamination with power or self-interest.

In the spirit and tradition of science, if there is a disagreement, let it be resolved in the crucible of public discourse. We do not need intellectual vigilantes patrolling the corridors of our institutions looking for theories or ideas with which they disagree to drive them out from our midst.

Paul Komesaroff, Professor of Medicine, Monash University.

Article as published in the Medical Journal of Australia.

Studies, Surveys and Statistics

Don't take too much notice of just one specific study! Check who funded the study, who participated, participant's other lifestyle choices, and if the researchers stand to gain financially from the results. The best studies are 'meta-analyses' which are reviews of several studies on a particular topic, taking into account biases, sample sizes, demographics, results, and so on.

There are also many online and public relations (PR) companies who pay participants to fill in regular surveys for payment. Their results are not reliable or representative of a true cross-section of society. However, PR firms often utilise their information with headlines like, "A recent survey has shown..." to justify news stories and interviews mentioned above.

Astroturf Groups

Not all associations are genuine, independent, victim-based, grassroots associations or councils. Some are what is known as "AstroTurf" groups (no grassroots) set up by Big Pharma as a window front to dispense their chemical-based information.

The 'Boomer Coalition' https://www.meetup.com/topics/boomer/ is a group started by Pfizer, but having no roots, only has 147 members worldwide.

Sick Enough?

Big Pharma don't really want you to die, however they would prefer you to be sick enough to go to your doctor, purchase repeat prescriptions, be referred to a specialist or check into hospital. The idea is to simply relieve your symptoms, but suggest you are still sick enough that you need to return to your doctor repeatedly.

Death is Death — Whatever the Cause

There are about 328,000 deaths each year in the US from FDA-approved and correctly prescribed medicines and around 200,000 in Europe. The total number of deaths caused by medical errors in the US is between 250,000 and 440,000 annually. This makes the medical system the third-leading cause of death in America, behind heart disease and cancer, according to www.ethics.harvard.edu and CNBC News.

Ron Law (former Director of the National Nutritional Foods Assoc NZ) said, "One in five [20%] deaths in Australia and New Zealand are caused by TGA-approved drugs and medical error", though statistics in Australia are difficult to find and I can't confirm this statement.

"Between 85,000 and 110,000 people over the age of 65 are admitted to hospital each year because of the adverse effects of their medication — and that is just the tip of the iceberg", *Sydney Morning Herald*, 18 Aug 2007.

And we remember the public deaths of celebrities like Michael Jackson, Heath Ledger, Amy Winehouse, Whitney Houston and Prince who died whilst under the care of doctors and taking prescription drugs.

To put this into perspective, **"officially"** 262 people died globally of bird flu and 79,009 from swine flu as of July 2010. This is a total figure for the whole world, not annually for one nation.

Food Industry

A similar situation happens in the food industry too, as the various dairy, beef, sugarcane and grain-grower groups lobby the government for industry-supportive laws and subsidies. Well-known media doctors can regularly be heard on radio and TV spruiking the interests of dairy, sugar, wheat and meat.

As a demonstration of the food lobby's impact on government policy, the Australian government (along with those of the US, Canada and EU) are **calling for the deletion** of the following paragraph — taken from a recently-released draft of the United Nations Health Initiative Sept 2011 — which calls on countries to implement "... *cost-effective interventions ... to reduce saturated and transfats in food ... reduce salt and refined sugars in foods, including through discouraging the production and marketing ... of unhealthy foods ...*" so that the food industry can continue to produce and market food containing these ingredients. Meanwhile, the Australian government has established the National Preventative Health Agency to **give the appearance** of making an effort to combat obesity and support healthy eating.

Big Pharma are currently trying to classify obesity as a disease, so it can legally prescribe drugs and have them registered on the PBS for up to 65% of the population.

Psychiatric Bible

The Diagnostic and Statistical Manual of Mental Disorders, or DSM (commonly known as the Psychiatric Bible) has been used by physicians since the 1950s to diagnose, name and therefore medically justify the prescription of drugs to treat named conditions.

The 2013 version five (V) known as DMS V included simple, everyday events like mood swings, grief and children's temper tantrums as pathological conditions so that psychiatrists can justify prescribing drugs, reaping big profits for Big Pharma.

Psychiatry remains such an inexact science that labelling behavioural symptoms without clear biological causes can lead to misdiagnosis and the misuse of drugs. For example, in Australia, prescription of anti-depressants has doubled, and antipsychotics has tripled over the past decade.

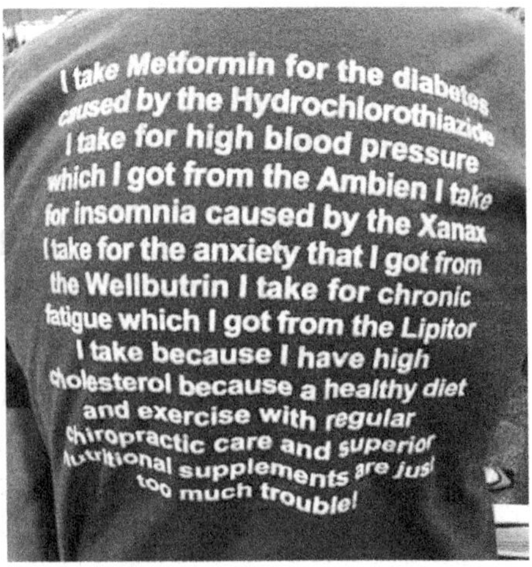

It almost seems as though the longer you stay in the system, the more diagnoses you get. Many symptoms are the result of side-effects caused by previously prescribed drugs.

As a demonstration of the DSM's past credibility, it used to list homosexuality as a mental illness in the 1970s.

The DSM was first launched in 1952 with 106 conditions identified. Over the past 60 years, the number of mental illnesses for which there is now a diagnosis has increased to near 350.

I'm Sorry

Sorry, but I've now handed you a dilemma: believe what I've written or continue trusting Big Pharma and the advice of your doctor without checking. Personally, I don't stand to gain a lot from your choice either way — I've already made my choices, which I believe saved my life.

The future of your health will be based on your choices from here on; you have your own free-will. I encourage you to become more educated and take responsibility for your own health and check all information provided from any source — including mine.

Remember <u>when researching</u>, **don't trust Google, YouTube, Facebook or Twitter** as they are biased and skew search results in favour of the sickness industry that supports them. Google's algorithm is so advanced that two people searching the exact same topic will receive different results based on their location, search history and the current political agenda of lamestream.

Your doctor is unlikely to encourage you to check their information, become more educated or take responsibility for your own health. In fact, they will probably discourage it.

Your Truth — Chart your Progress

Whether my truth about health is correct or not, over time, the truth must be revealed. Either western society is getting sicker from corporate-based, profit-minded diseases of affluence, or we are thriving from advances in medical technology and farming methods. At the moment, I feel the former is winning, indicating we as a society are heading in the wrong direction and need to make change.

Take a snapshot of where you are today, make some changes and note what changes you made, then compare how you feel in the sort-term ~ 3 months and in the long-term ~ 3-5 years.

I want you to **prove to yourself** that change is worthwhile and that you have power and control over your health and how you feel every day. I don't want to sell you anything, I want you to want to invest in your future.

Here is a couple of simple tables to help with this. Copy them or make up your own table/s on spreadsheets.

We are what we repeatedly do.
Excellence then is not an act, but a habit

Aristotle

1. **Fulfillment and Happiness**
   (Attitude and Responsibility)
2. **Quality of Life**
   (Health Span, Energy and Mind)
3. **Everything Else**
   (Positive Habitual Living)

Ramiah J Selwood

Short-Term

	Start	Wk 2	Mth 1	Mth 2	Mth 3	Mth 4	Mth 5	Mth 6
Date:								
Changes I've Made:								
Energy Levels								
Stress / **Mood** Levels								
Mental Focus								
Headaches								
Eye Sight / Vision								
Cravings / Addictions								
Workout **Recovery**								
Sleep Quality								
Muscle Comfort								
Joint Comfort								
Bowel Movements								
Bladder								
Skin / Hair / Nails								
TOTAL:								
Waist Measurement								
Weight								

1 = Very Bad   3 = Bad   5 = OK   7 = Good   10 = Excellent

Long-Term

5 Year Challenge

	Start	3 Months	6 Months	1 Year	2 Years	3 Years	4 Years	5 Years
Date:								
Energy Levels								
Stress Levels								
Mental Focus								
Workout **Recovery**								
Sleep Quality								
Muscle Comfort								
Joint Comfort								
Other								
TOTAL:								
Waist Measurment								
Weight								

0 = Very Bad   3 = Bad   5 = OK   7 = Good   10 = Very Good

www.cleanup-your-act.com

Finding your truth means taking responsibility

Bran Nue Dae... *(from the Aussie movie)*

Imagine waking tomorrow morning to a brand-new day; a brand-new life. Imagine you're no longer a son, daughter, sibling, parent, husband or wife. No longer are you aboriginal, indigenous, white, black, Asian, Australian or American. Imagine you're not your sexual orientation, not male nor female or LGBTQ. You're not classified by your disease, illness, addiction, personality, employment, wealth, education or politics. You're no longer Catholic, Christian, Muslim, Buddhist, Jew or atheist, so you're free to communicate to your own higher dimensional energy if believe, and if you choose – you no longer must connect via a priest.

From tomorrow morning you wake up simply as a person living on your piece of land – a free spirit with no possessions. A person who takes responsibility for their actions and whose sole purpose today is to be in the moment and fulfill every moment. You are happy and you are going to shine and will be the best person you can possibly be whilst considering others around you. You give unconditional help, love and support according to your heart, whilst achieving fair income for your effort, investment and skills.

Your past and history are simply that – history. You now take responsibility for your previous actions with love and create good karma. From tomorrow morning you no longer involve yourself in other peoples' drama – no judging, no categorising, you simply observe. You accept and only connect with family and friends who support your life. You are no longer obligated to your habits or to anyone else. You utilise your family's traditions of culture, dress, food, rituals and celebrations to add to your life, not rule it.

Imagine observing and questioning everything you've been indoctrinated with since childhood via the physical matrix; all the science, education, medicine, finance, debt, religion, culture, government, wars, laws, authority, technology, manners and especially the news, media and entertainment. Now you have more space to experience true learning, fulfillment and love.

From tomorrow morning and every morning after, you are no longer in the physical matrix and you are your own reality, but only if you choose.

Remember; you create your own reality, so take responsibility!

You are free to choose your thoughts and in so doing, you choose freedom.

John Lennon wrote a song about this 50 years ago… Image ☺

Good Vibes...

References

Books

Acidophilus and Colon Health by David Webster

Anatomy of an Illness by Norman Cousins

The China Study by Colon Campbell PhD (nutrition, genes, cancer, Big Pharma)

The Chemical Maze by Bill Statham (food additive codes)

Cleansing the Body and Colon for a Happier and Healthier You by Teresa Schumacher

Colon Health by Dr Norman Walker

Crohn's Disease and Ulcerative Colitis by Dr Fred Saibil

A Cure for All Diseases by Dr Hulda Clark

Excitotoxins: the Taste that Kills by Dr Russell Blaylock (MSG)

Green Leaves of Barley by Dr Mary Ruth Swope (barley grass and nutrition)

Happiness is a Regular Complete Bowel Motion by Peter Edwards

The Hidden Messages in Water by Dr Masaru Emoto

How Doctors Think by Jerome Groopman MD

Join Our Escape from Death Row – Cancer Jail by Barry Thomson

Oriental Secrets to a Thin and Healthy Body by Dr Stephen Chang

Sweet Poison by David Gillespie (sugar)

Lies My Doctor Told Me by Ken Berry MD

Sex, Lies and Pharmaceuticals by Ray Moynihan

Selling Sickness by Ray Moynihan

Tissue Cleansing Through Bowel Management by Bernard Jensen PhD

Take Control of Your Health by Elaine Hollingsworth

The Slow Poisoning of America by John Erb (MSG)

Understanding Your Gall Bladder by Dr Katie Ellard

Brain Food by Dr Karl Kruszelnicki

The Slight Edge by Jeff Olsen

Outwitting the Devil by Napoleon Hill

Videos and Documentaries

- *One Answer to Cancer*
- *Cancer is Curable Now*
- *Burzynski Movie*

- *Puncture*
- *Is Binge Drinking Really Bad?~ BBC Horizon*
- *Catalyst: Gut Reaction (Parts 1 & 2) ~ ABC TV Aust.*
- *Vaxxed and Vaxxed II Movies*
- *Root Cause (root canals) ~ Vimeo*

An excellent resource for health documentaries is:

www.documentarywire.com/category/health

Websites & Alternative Media

- abc.net.au
- ageofautism.com (vaccination)
- anoasisofhealing.com
- avn.org.au (vaccination - Australia)
- beyondblue.org.au
- budwigcenter.com
- burtongoldberg.com
- colonhealthinfo.com
- edwardtufte.com
- enemainfo.com
- ext.colostate.edu
- doctor-natasha.com
- doctoroz.com
- doctorsaredangerous.com
- drberg.com
- drconnealy.com
- drbradleynelson.com (emotion code)
- dr-gonzalez.com
- drjohnbergman.com
- healthranger.org
- howmuchsugar.com
- hugorodier.com
- iacvf-melb.com (International Assn of Cancer Victors and Friends)
- innerbody.com
- kenberrymd.com
- mercola.com
- naturematters.info (vaccination story)
- naturopath4you.com
- ncepod.org.uk
- nvic.org (vaccination)
- oasisofhope.com
- parasiteinfo.com
- puncture-the-movie.com
- reganhillyer.com (abundance code)
- rlrouse.com/colon

- thefatemperor.com (Ivor Cummins)
- The HighWire with Del Bigtree (YouTube – science-based vaccination choice)
- thinktwice.com (vaccination)
- topnews.in wellbeing.com.au
- vactruth.com (vaccination)
- whale.to (vaccination)
- whitehousedrugpolicy.gov/drugfact/prescriptn_drg

Resources

The AIM Companies

Information and Distributor Contact Details:

www.myaimstore.com/quantumknowledge

Ph: 0427 443 302 (Australia)

quantumk88@gmail.com

Sponsor ID # **9916901**

Note:

AIM products mentioned throughout this book marked * (e.g. AIM Fit 'n Fiber®*) may not be available for purchase from AIM Australia, however, may be purchased from AIM's NZ office for personal use once you are a member of AIM Australia. Contact the above distributor for more information and assistance.

AIM products are also available in the USA, UK, Europe, NZ, Africa and Canada.

- **BarleyLife** In 1982, the world's first all-natural, green barley juice powder concentrate helps provide the daily nutrition you need to develop a strong foundation for good health and is abundant in enzymes, essential amino acids, and rich in antioxidant ability, anti-inflammatory activity, and immune system support. Available in powder, vegetarian capsules, single-serving packets, and great-tasting **BarleyLife Xtra** with 18 different fruit and vegetable powders for 34% of your RDI of vitamin C per serving.

- **CoCoa LeafGreens** delivers the luscious taste and antioxidant activity of cocoa combined with four leaf juice powders – **spinach, field pea, faba bean, and barley – and broccoli sprout** powder to work synergistically for optimal health benefits. Great way to covertly provide your children with the nutrition they need in the form of chocolate smoothies.

- **Composure** a combination of relaxing herbs, helps to maintain your neuro health, especially regarding dealing efficiently with stress. Relaxes you without making you drowsy but allows the body to relax for sleep.

- **Fit 'n Fiber*** is an everyday fibre for safe, effective, consistent results. Featuring three complementary fibre ingredients— psyllium, konjac and oat—along with seven other synergistic fibre and herb ingredients, Fit 'n Fiber contains the effective nutrients to help keep you regular, stem your appetite and encourage a healthy weight.

- **Frame Essentials*** which combines a glucosamine complex with **MSM** and **boswellia** extract, helps maintain healthy joints.
- **Garden Trio** (**BarleyLife**, a juice powder of young barley plants; **Just Carrots**, a carrot juice powder; and **RediBeets**, a beet juice powder), provides us with an optimum nutritional base and is necessary to maintain whole body health. If you are missing important nutrients in your day (especially when travelling) this is for you – it's like having the nutrition of 3 garden salads in one blast.
- **Herbal FiberBlend** a combination of **soluble** and **insoluble psyllium fibre** and cleansing herbs, helps maintain bowel regularity, provides dietary fibre, and leads to detoxification. Available in unflavoured or natural raspberry powder.

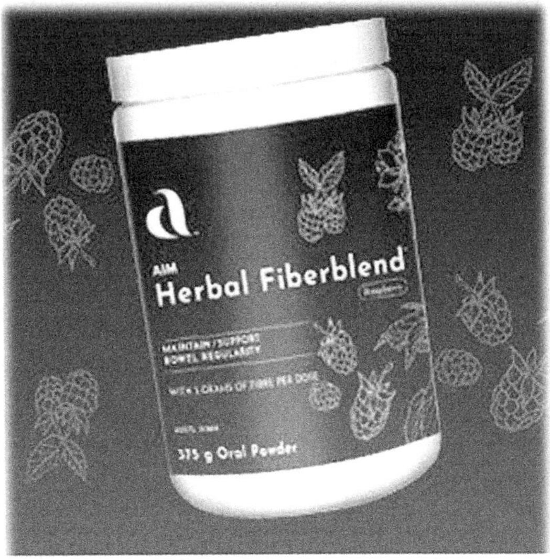

Digestive Detox

- **Herbal Release*** a combination of herbs that helps maintain a healthy **lymphatic** system. The lymphatic system is integral to maintaining our immune system.
- **Just Carrots** a carrot juice powder concentrate that contains important nutrients such as alpha and beta-carotene, calcium and iron.
- **LeafGreens** an all-natural powder concentrate that combines the nutrient-dense leaves of **barley, spinach, kale, arugula (rocket) and Swiss chard** along with **broccoli sprouts** for a wide spectrum of nutrients including vitamins, minerals, antioxidants, and a balanced plant-based protein, all for whole-body health.
- **Mag-nificence** complete cellular **Magnesium Chloride** supplements in **spray** and **lotion** for topical use on the skin, that provide a gentle way to raise your body's magnesium profile, which is critical to the utilisation and production of energy during cell metabolism.
- **ProPeas** a vegetable protein powder that provides 12 grams of protein, is low-carbohydrate, and low-fat. Ideal tool for **weight management** thanks to protein's ability to increase satiety, improve lean muscle, and increase metabolism.
- **ReAssure SP*** a unique and synergistic combination of saw palmetto berry oil extract, pumpkin seed oil, tomato lycopene, and zinc citrate for the maintenance of prostate health. Saw palmetto plant sterols have been shown to block the absorption of cholesterol through the intestine.
- **RediBeets** a concentrated beet juice powder with only the fibre removed, contains essential enzymes along with the natural form of betaine, which aids in cleansing the liver and reducing homocysteine levels.

Cerule

Information and Distributor Contact Details:

www.qk.cerule.com

Ph: 0427 443 302 (Australia)

quantumk88@gmail.com

Sponsor ID # **2477353**

Cerule products are also available in USA, UK, Europe, NZ, Taiwan and Canada

Cerule *Independent Business Owner*

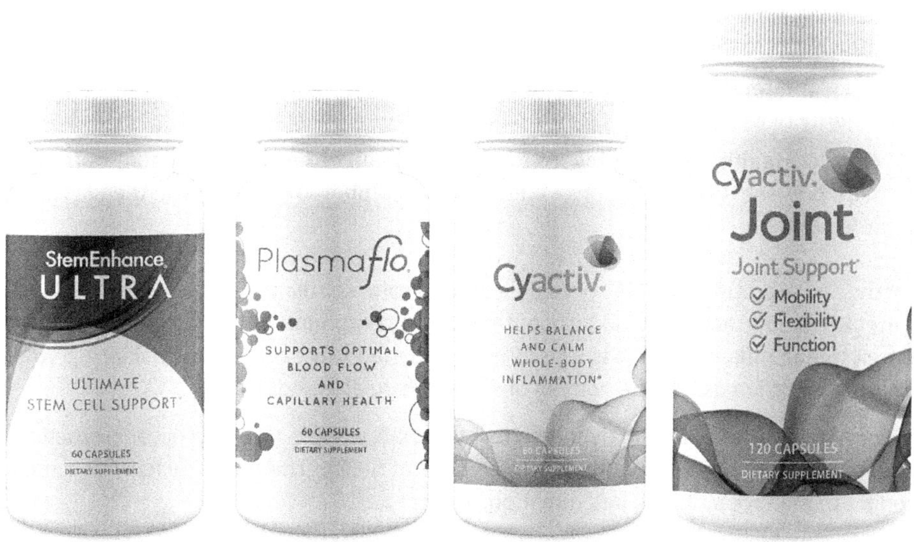

Stem Cell Release **Circulation** **Body Inflammation** **Joint Inflammation**

STEM CELL RELEASE – CIRCULATION – INFLAMMATION

Proven, One of a Kind Wellness Products

We Believe the Extraordinary is Possible!

StemEnhance® Ultra assists the body's inherent ability for long-term self-renewal by supporting the body's natural release of bone marrow adult stem cells. It concentrates and combines extracts from nature's most primitive superfoods, freshwater microalgae and marine macroalgae, providing the body with the ultimate in stem cell support.

1. StemEnhance® Ultra is the result of 16 years of research and constitutes the most efficacious and scientifically proven stem cell support product in the market.

2. Through multiple clinical trials StemEnhance® Ultra was documented to optimise stem cell function in the body by increasing the number of both CD34+ stem cells and Endothelial Progenitor Cells (EPCs) in the blood circulation, supporting optimum renewal and repair of tissues and organs.
3. StemEnhance® Ultra also contains Mesenkine™ (extract of spirulina) that was shown to increase the blood concentration of G-CSF that plays a key role in stem cell release.

PlasmaFloTM is a proprietary blend of proteolytic and fibrinolytic enzymes, concentrated plant extracts and potent antioxidants. Formulated to support the integrity of capillaries and improve the flowing properties of blood, PlasmaFlo™ helps the delivery of vital nutrients, oxygen and stem cells throughout the entire body for optimum health.

PlasmaFlo™ supports 3 vital vascular components:

1. Vascular **Flow** – PlasmaFlo™ provides enzyme nutrition to support the digestion of fibrin mesh in the bloodstream to improve circulation in capillaries.
2. Vascular **Integrity** – PlasmaFlo™ contains plant extracts that help support the structural integrity of capillaries.
3. Vascular **Health** – PlasmaFlo™ contains antioxidants to provide optimum nutrition to help prevent the formation of fibrin and combat oxidative stress and vascular inflammation.

Cyactiv® is a proprietary phycocyanin extract from spirulina. Phycocyanin is the blue pigment in blue-green algae and is a potent active compound proven to help balance and calm systemic inflammation associated with a myriad of health issues. Balancing whole-body inflammation assists the homing of stem cells to affected tissues.

Phycocyanin works as a selective inhibitor of COX-2 while a non-phycocyanin fraction of spirulina called LoxDown™, works as an inhibitor of 5-LOX. Therefore, Cyactiv® is a unique product to manage systemic inflammation.

Cyactiv® essentially helps modulate inflammation and provides antioxidant protection:

- Helps balance inflammation and maintain it within the normal range
- Supports the ability of stem cells to find and rejuvenate tissues in need of renewal
- Helps neutralize existing free radicals
- Provides cellular protection against the formation of new oxidative stress

----

Cyactiv® Joint is a natural and innovative solution composed of four extracts specifically formulated to support and nourish healthy joints:

1. **Eggshell Membrane** Supports cartilage strength and elasticity and provides structural support to bone, connective tissue and interstitial fluid. Eggshell membrane was clinically tested and shown to improve range of motion and joint function and increase levels of physical activity and overall joint comfort.
2. **Boswellia Serrata Extract** Improves comfort by reducing swelling and increasing blood supply to joint tissue. This extract also contains polysaccharides that increase absorption of active compounds. Boswellia serrata extract was clinically tested and

shown to reduce discomfort and swelling and increase levels of physical activity.

3. **Tart Cherry Extract** Rich in phenolic compounds, notably anthocyanins, flavonoids and natural melatonin, this powerful antioxidant speeds the recovery process by preventing the symptoms of exercise-induced muscle fatigue and damage. Tart Cherry extract was clinically tested to support physical performance in athletes by maintaining muscle strength, decreasing muscle soreness, recovery time and fatigue.
4. **Cyactiv – Spirulina Extract** Reduces existing and future production of free radicals by modulating the inflammatory enzyme COX-2. Contains bioactive compounds for cellular protection and anti-aging support. Cyactiv was clinically tested and showed a significant increase in joint comfort at rest and during physical activity and was associated with an increase in daily activity levels.

The above products are not intended to diagnose, treat, cure or prevent any disease.

Recommended Services

Andrena Forrest Soul Tone Voice Empowerment 0402550942
www.soultone.com.au

Paula Mack* Infinite Health & Harmony Body Code 0402556577
Infinitehealthandharmony@gmail.com

Stephanie Messenger* Vaccination Awareness 0412671922
www.naturematters.info

Joanne Luxton* The Emotion Code 0468990844
mindthebody3@gmail.com

Gerard Bini* Orgone Effects Australia 03 5977 7162
orgoneffectsaustralia.com.au

Shakti Selwood*
Iridology, Emotion Code, Body Code, Medical Intuitive 0427443302
shaktiselwood@gmail.com

**see promotion display below*

Some items are available from various outlets; however, Ramiah would sincerely appreciate your support for his introduction to these issues and products and the years of research and effort put into this book. Thank you☺

Contact Quantum Knowledge for assistance

Ph: 0427 443 302 (Australia) quantumk88@gmail.com

Shakti
Selwood

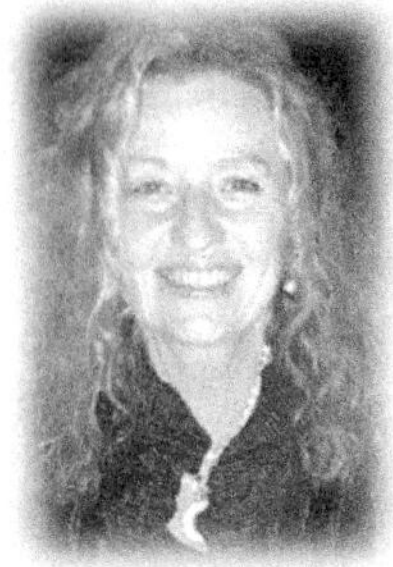

Iridology

Emotion Code & Body Code
0427 443 302
Find out what's making you sick!

Shakti

shaktiselwood@gmail.com

Iridology is extremely reliable in establishing function and many diseases of the body, including liver, intolerances and gut disorders and mental disorders like Alzheimer's and dementia. Iridologists may see the potential for poor function and disease before it fully takes hold, so the opportunity for repair may be available before it's too late.

Iridology, Emotion Code & Body Code sessions are available from Shakti's clinic on Tamborine Mtn, Gold Coast for private, Skype and phone sessions.

Shakti's abilities as a healing are truly extraordinary. Most people go through their whole lives without meeting someone like her. The fact that you are reading this means you are very fortunate as you are close to an experience that will change your life for the better in ways you could never have imagined.

The first time I saw Shakti, I will admit, I was extremely anxious about it as I felt instinctively that something significant would happen. It certainly did - she was able to heal a lifetime of suffering caused by destructive hidden emotional patterns and contracts, as well as lifting ingrained fears left behind from past traumatic events. The sense of freedom which has resulted has been amazing, and (to a tertiary educated professional) almost inexplicable.

No one else had ever been able to help with these issues - and some things you just can't fix alone! Sadly, when it comes to knowledge our society has such an overwhelming empirical bias that we tend to dismiss whatever we can't see under a microscope. That is like driving a car and looking for directions in the rear-view mirror! My wife and I have been so profoundly and positively affected by this work that we also brought our children to see Shakti for the age appropriate modalities she offers (e.g. self-sabotage healing and emotion code).

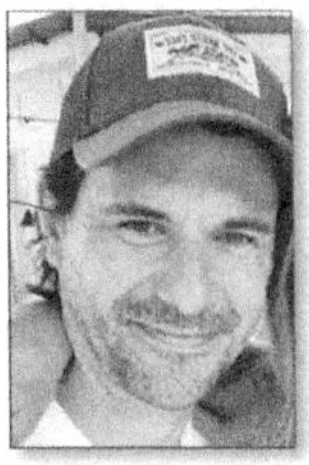

Since then, less than a year ago, everyone who knows them has commented on how much they have transformed, as a result of little signs like increased confidence and reduced anxiety, whingeing and sibling rivalry. It is clear to me that they have started to experience a new kind of sustained happiness that will benefit them for the rest of their lives. As a parent it has been so exciting to be able to help them in this way, before most of life's dramas can even affect them!

Thank you for everything you have done for us Shakti.

J Ford, Brisbane Qld Australia

Author's Contact Details

Ramiah J Selwood

Ph: **0428 667 234** Australia

www.cleanup-your-act.com *(book sales)*

www.quantumknowledge.com.au

www.abundanttimes.com

quantumk88@gmail.com

Ramiah regularly presents seminars, talks and international webinars. Ramiah is available to speak at conferences, conventions, meetings, gatherings and webinars. Search for Ramiah's YouTube channel.

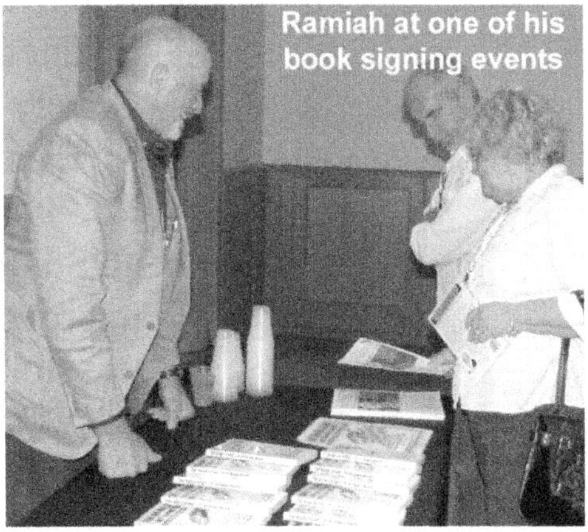

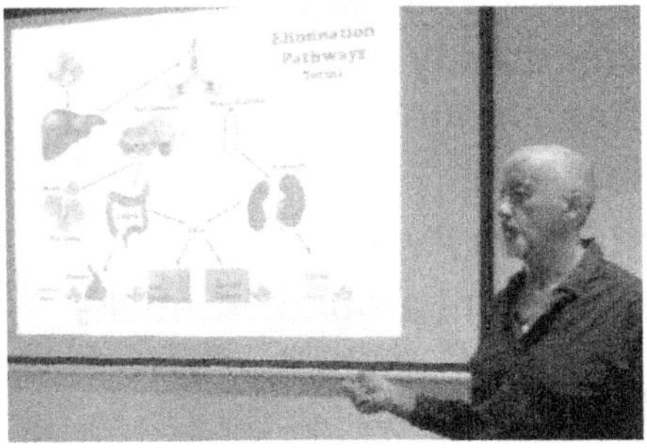

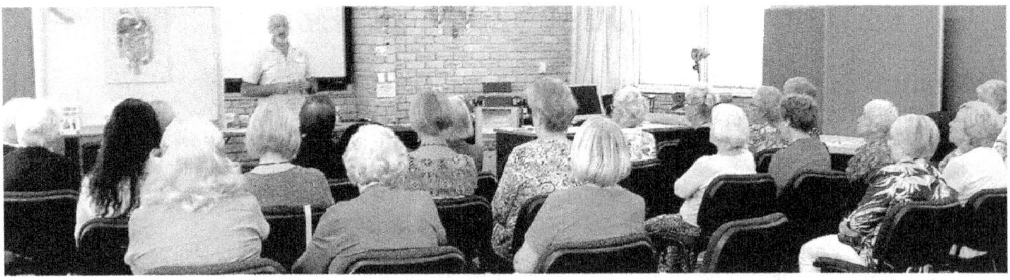

Testimonials

This is what readers have said...

"I have really enjoyed reading this book — it's definitely a life-changer – and most importantly, it REALLY stimulates the desire to improve my health, so effective is your book."

Isobel B, Melbourne, Australia

"Hi Ramiah, I bought your book "Clean up your act" through a friend a few years ago. Thank YOU for doing all your hard research & sharing it!

If only I had REALLY used it back then, I could've saved $$$$s spent on naturopaths. 1 very dodgy one who just wanted money."

Kelly B, Queensland, Australia

"Thank you so much Ramiah. That was amazing info and concisely helpful."
Brett J, Beechmont, Australia

"Your book was so instructive and interesting and your personal experience made it more credible."

Andre & Ramona, Vanuatu

"Shakti, I cannot stop thinking of you and your husband (Ramiah)... what a wonderful book. I can't put it down... I read it whenever I can and yesterday, I read so much, then again in bed and again this morning!

I am excited, happy, thrilled... call it what you want but I am feeling fabo and want to feel so much better in my health. I feel that for the first time I can truly get better from my restless arms and legs, and my IBS and every other health issue I have."

Colleen H, Tamborine, Australia

"I have been reading Ramiah's book. I have enjoyed it so much. It is so well written, so informative, it really is a great source of info, and through real experience!!! Inspirational, so much I can say. Thank you."

Ale, Upper Coomera, Australia

"Ramiah's book is GREAT! I've hardly been able to put it down!

It's so relatable, easy to read and great information. I am nodding the whole time agreeing as I believe exactly the same about my thinking, medication and good food."

Kim, Gold Coast, Australia

Hi Ramiah, "On a personal note, meeting you and Shakti at the markets that day has changed the way I look at life. It has led me to information, and then to self-development, and then to self-discovery, and hopefully to self-improvement.

Matthew is just getting better and better at everything all the time. We have enrolled him in regular school!!! (Matthew is autistic)

All this because one day we decided to drop into the markets and buy your book, and were lucky enough to have met Ramiah and Shakti."

Thank you ~ Love Nathan, Sammy, James and Matthew

It's Sylvia here. I came to visit you on Saturday at Markets. I purchased the Composure, Magnesium and Lavender oil from you. I applied the spray, took 4 capsules of the Composure and rubbed in lavender oil before bed - like you instructed on Saturday night. Can I say it was a 'Miracle' it worked for me. Slept like a baby, woke up refresh and alert, not drowsy and hard to wake up with the sleeping pill.

I'm so grateful and happy to meet and talk to you and to have come into your stall. Thank you so much. I can't thank you enough what you have done for me. I'll be taking the Composure from now on, not the chemical sleeping pill.

I have told my sister about my new transition to better health with natural herbs and organic ingredients. My sister will be coming in to see you soon to get her eyes checked and see what you can do for her. Till then. I'll see you again soon.

Warm regards, Sylvia ~ Sent from my iPhone

Sylvia also uses AIM Herbal FiberBlend and Probiotics too.

Clean Up Your Act – From Sickness to Vitality without Medication

Revised & Expanded

By Ramiah J Selwood

ISBN 978-0-646-91323-0

ISBN 978-0-646-91323-0

9 780646 913230 >

Made in the USA
Monee, IL
14 September 2026

63198319R00164